Civil Capacities in Clinical Neuropsychology

National Academy of Neuropsychology Series in Evidence-Based Practices

SERIES EDITOR

L. Stephen Miller

SERIES CONSULTING EDITORS

Glenn J. Larrabee

Martin L. Rohling

Civil Capacities in Clinical Neuropsychology: Research Findings and Practical Applications
Edited by George J. Demakis

Civil Capacities in Clinical Neuropsychology

Research Findings and Practical Applications

EDITED BY GEORGE J. DEMAKIS

OXFORD
UNIVERSITY PRESS

OXFORD
UNIVERSITY PRESS

Oxford University Press, Inc., publishes works that further
Oxford University's objective of excellence
in research, scholarship, and education.

Oxford New York
Auckland Cape Town Dar es Salaam Hong Kong Karachi
Kuala Lumpur Madrid Melbourne Mexico City Nairobi
New Delhi Shanghai Taipei Toronto

With offices in
Argentina Austria Brazil Chile Czech Republic France Greece
Guatemala Hungary Italy Japan Poland Portugal Singapore
South Korea Switzerland Thailand Turkey Ukraine Vietnam

Published by Oxford University Press, Inc.
198 Madison Avenue, New York, New York 10016
www.oup.com

ISBN 978-0-19-977406-7
A copy of this book's Cataloging-in-Publication Data is on file
with the Library of Congress.

To my parents,

Whose love of learning—including two dictionaries (one in English and one in Greek) within easy reach of the dinner table—inspired this book.

Contents

PART III: Applications

PART IV: Conclusions

Preface to the *National Academy of Neuropsychology Series on Evidence-Based Practices*

The field of Clinical Neuropsychology has advanced extensively and successfully in the worlds of psychology and neurology by following two major tenets. The first has been the constant focus on exploring and understanding the complex and intricate relationship between observed behavioral function and brain structure (and of course changes to that structure). From early observation of the relationship between injury and behavior to today's combination of psychometric testing, cognitive neuroscience, and functional neuroimaging techniques, this focus has served the field extremely well. The second has been the rigorous adherence to careful, replicable scientific principles of questioning and theorizing, data collection, and use of sophisticated statistical analysis in testing, evaluating, and interpreting information about brain/behavior relationships. It is in the spirit of this strong foundation of empirical evidence aimed at improving the quality of informed clinical decision making that the National Academy of Neuropsychology (NAN) Series on Evidenced-Based Practices developed and came to fruition.

For a long time, members of the neuropsychology community, and in particular the membership of the National Academy of Neuropsychology, have voiced a desire to have available to them thorough and accurate resources that are directly applicable to the everyday needs and demands of clinical neuropsychology, and that are presented in a meaningful and accessible way, offering the latest knowledge based on the most recent and rigorous scientific evidence within the field. The NAN Series on Evidence-Based Practices is meant to provide just such a series of resources.

At its formation, it was important to first identify an excellent publisher with a history of publishing significant psychological and scientific volumes who would share this vision and provide significant support for a quality product. After lengthy research and discussions with multiple publishers, the venerable Oxford University Press (OUP), one of the most renowned and respected publishing companies in existence, was selected by the NAN Board of Directors. For their part, OUP has committed to the long-term development and support of the NAN Series and, as can be seen in the pages herein, has spared no effort or expense to provide the finest quality venue for the success of the Series.

The Series is designed to be a dynamic and ever-growing set of resources for the science-based clinical neuropsychologist. As such, the volumes are intended to individually focus on specific significant areas of neuropsychological inquiry in depth, and together cover the majority of the broad clinical area of neuropsychology. This is a challenging endeavor, and one that relies on the foremost experts in the neuropsychological field to provide their insight, knowledge, and interpretation of the empirically supported evidence within each focused topic. It is our hope that the reader recognizes the many established scholars from our field who have taken on the task of volume editor or chapter author.

Although each volume is intended to provide an exhaustive review of its respective topic, there are a number of constants across the volumes. Importantly, each volume editor and the respective chapter authors have committed to constraining themselves to providing only evidence-based information that meets the definition of such. Second, each volume maintains a broad consistency in format, including an introductory chapter outlining the volume and a final discussion chapter summarizing the state of the art within the respective topic area. Each volume provides a comprehensive index, and each chapter provides relevant references for the reader. Third, each volume is designed to provide information that is directly and readily usable, in both content and format, to the clinical neuropsychologist in everyday practice. As such, each volume and each chapter within the volume are obliged to provide information in such a way as to make it accessible as a "pull off the shelf" resource. Finally, each volume is designed to work within a pedagogical strategy such that it educates and informs the knowledgeable neuropsychologist, providing a greater understanding of each volume's focus as well as meaningful (i.e., read "useful") information geared toward enhancing the practice of neuropsychology.

In keeping with the educational focus of the Series, an additional aspect is a collaboration of the Series contributors and the NAN Continuing Education Committee such that each Series Volume is available to be used as a formal continuing education text via the CEU system of NAN.

It is my hope, and the hope of the consulting editors who provide their time, expertise, and guidance in the development of the NAN Series, that this will become an oft used and ever expanding set of efficient and efficacious resources for the clinical neuropsychologist and others working with the plethora of persons with brain disorders and dysfunction.

L. Stephen Miller
Editor-in-Chief
National Academy of Neuropsychology
Book Series on Evidence-Based Practices

Preface to the First Volume in the *National Academy of Neuropsychology Series on Evidence-Based Practices Civil Capacities in Clinical Neuropsychology: Research Findings and Practical Applications*

The field of neuropsychology has taken on a greater and greater role in the evaluation of capacity and competency issues. Clinical neuropsychologists are, in ever increasing numbers, being asked to provide evaluation, interpretation, and subsequent recommendations for capacity and competency in individuals who have compromised brain function. Although information regarding many of these issues has been provided within the criminal domains, this has been relatively neglected in the civil domain. In response to this, the *National Academy of Neuropsychology Series on Evidenced-Based Practices*' inaugural volume has tackled this important area with *Civil Capacities in Clinical Neuropsychology: Research Findings and Practical Applications*. Under the guidance of the Volume Editor, George J. Demakis, *Civil Capacities in Clinical Neuropsychology: Research Findings and Practical Applications* provides a much needed, thorough examination of the state of the art of the field of civil capacity assessment. The definition of civil capacity, its changing scope, challenges, knowns and unknowns, and evaluation methods are thoroughly discussed. Information is presented on current research findings and empirically driven conceptualizations of, as well as limitations in, the effective assessment of capacity in this emerging area. Dr. Demakis is a clinical research neuropsychologist well published in the area of civil capacity. Additionally, he is an active practitioner whose primary work is in the evaluation of capacity-based issues from a neuropsychological perspective, making him an ideal editor for this much needed resource. He has gathered together an impressive group of chapter authors representing the breadth of the current knowledge base concerning civil capacity from an evidence-based perspective. The volume is aimed primarily at neuropsychologists, but should also find an audience among clinical psychologists, psychiatrists, and other mental health providers working with persons expressing brain dysfunction and facing issues of capacity or competency.

L. Stephen Miller
Editor-in-Chief
National Academy of Neuropsychology
Book Series on Evidence-Based Practices
June 2011

Acknowledgments

I am especially thankful to the series editor, Steve Miller, for providing me with the opportunity to edit the first book in this series and for his continued professional guidance and encouragement. His reviews of my work (and the work of other contributors) demonstrated a deep understanding of practice issues in clinical neuropsychology, and particularly how empirically supported approaches can be used to guide practice. Tracy O'Hara at Oxford University Press provided quick and timely feedback on the myriad issues that emerged during the creation of this book. I am particularly grateful for feedback provided by various professionals on my contributions including contributors Drs. Barton Palmer and Erik Everhart, as well as social worker Tienna Luong. Finally, my wife Maria's patience, support, and encouragement during this project matter more than I can express.

George J. Demakis
May 20, 2011
Charlotte, NC

Contributors

Frederick R. Benson, JD
Mecklenburg County Assistant Clerk of Superior Court
Legal Hearing Officer
Charlotte, NC

Jessica A. Clark, PhD
National Rehabilitation Hospital
Washington, DC

George J. Demakis, PhD
Department of Psychology
University of North Carolina Charlotte
Charlotte, NC

D. Erik Everhart, PhD
Department of Psychology
East Carolina University
Sleep Center
Pitt County Memorial Hospital
Greenville, NC

Alexandrea L. Harmell, BA
Department of Psychiatry
University of California, San Diego
La Jolla, CA

Jonathan M. Highsmith, MA
Department of Psychology
East Carolina University
Greenville, NC

Amy Knight, PhD
Department of Neurology
Alzheimer's Disease Center
University of Alabama at Birmingham
Birmingham, AL

Elissa A. Kolva, MA
Department of Psychology
Fordham University
Bronx, NY

Katie A. Lehockey, BS
Department of Psychology
East Carolina University
Greenville, NC

Daniel C. Marson, JD, PhD
Department of Neurology
Alzheimer's Disease Center
University of Alabama at Birmingham
Birmingham, AL

Paul J. Moberg, PhD
Brain-Behavior Laboratory
Neuropsychiatry Section
Department of Psychiatry
University of Pennsylvania School of Medicine
Philadelphia, PA

Alicia M. Moran, MA
Department of Psychology
East Carolina University
Sleep Center
Pitt County Memorial Hospital
Greenville, NC

Meryl O'Bryan, MA
Psychology Department
Claremont Graduate School
Claremont, CA

Barton W. Palmer, PhD
Department of Psychiatry
University of California, San Diego
La Jolla, CA

Carmelle Peisah, MD, FRANZCP
Academic Department for Old Age Psychiatry
University of New South Wales
Prince of Wales Hospital
Sydney, Australia

Gianni Pirelli, PhD
Greystone Park Psychiatric Hospital
Morris Plains, NJ

M. Joanne Romano, JD
Mecklenburg County Assistant Clerk of Superior Court
Legal Hearing Officer
Charlotte, NC

Barry Rosenfeld, PhD
Department of Psychology
Fordham University
Bronx, NY

Robert Ruchinskas, PsyD, ABPP
Department of Psychiatry
University of Medicine and Dentistry of New Jersey
Stratford, NJ

Gauri N. Savla, PhD
Department of Psychiatry
University of California, San Diego
La Jolla, CA

Sanjay Shah, JD, MS
Department of Psychology
Drexel University
Philadelphia, PA

Kenneth I. Shulman, MD, SM, FRCPsych, FRCPC
Department of Psychiatry
Sunnybrook Health Sciences Centre
University of Toronto
Toronto, ON, Canada

Karen A. Sullivan, PhD
School of Psychology and Counselling
Queensland University of Technology
Brisbane, Australia

Kristen Triebel, PsyD
Department of Neurology
Alzheimer's Disease Center
University of Alabama at Birmingham
Birmingham, Alabama

Penny L. Wolfe, PhD
Psychology Department
National Rehabilitation Hospital
Washington, DC

Stacey Wood, PhD
The Psychology Department
Scripps College
Claremont, CA

Patricia A. Zapf, PhD
John Jay College of Criminal Justice
The City University of New York
New York, NY

PART ONE

Background Issues

1

Introduction to Basic Issues in Civil Capacities

GEORGE J. DEMAKIS

INTRODUCTION

A number of years ago, after having completed a neuropsychological internship and postdoctoral fellowship, I was approached by a local mental health agency and asked to provide court-ordered capacity evaluations for (mostly) older adults. Although I was not formally trained in this area, I thought that my neuropsychology background and expertise would provide the necessary grounding for such work. I was right and I was wrong. Though I was knowledgeable about evaluating older adults with cognitive impairment, and felt confident in my abilities to do so, my knowledge and skills in forensic issues in this area were not as developed. Rather, my forensic training and background at that time were mostly in personal injury and disability work. Such began a steep learning curve into capacity and competency work: I sought supervision, consulted with colleagues and other professionals (mostly attorneys), attended workshops, read the professional literature on the topic, and, more recently, conducted research in this area. In hindsight, although I believe I have developed the essential skills necessary, I would not recommend my experiential process as the ideal learning method. This volume, then, is my attempt to provide others with the type of empirically grounded information I wish was available when I began doing civil capacity evaluations.

In many respects, clinical neuropsychologists are uniquely suited to evaluate civil capacities in light of their broad training in clinical psychology, psychological and cognitive assessment, and neurological disease and dysfunction. Such cases might include an older adult with dementia revising a will to favor one child in the context of family conflict, a young adult with chronic schizophrenia refusing to take medications because she believes that she is being poisoned, or a middle-aged man struggling to manage his finances after a severe traumatic brain injury. To render an opinion on capacity requires an understanding of the examinee's cognitive and psychological functioning, medical illnesses and treatment, current living situation, values and preferences, as well as social support and family dynamics. These complex cases (sometimes with multiple sources of conflicting data), as opposed to the obvious cases in examinees with severe mental retardation or end-stage dementia, are those most likely to be referred by judges and attorneys. Providing judicial decision makers assistance in such cases is challenging, but also plays to the strengths of clinical psychologists and, particularly, clinical neuropsychologists. This volume is about such work.

The current volume brings together several relatively recent professional and demographic developments. Demographically, we live in an aging society and the aging of the Baby Boom generation will increase the number of older adults (Vincent & Velkoff, 2010). By 2030, it is estimated that one in every five residents of the United States will be aged 65 or older and 7% will be aged 80 or older. Because dementia is highly correlated with age—dementia compromises cognitive functioning and eventually robs individuals of their ability to function independently—an increase in dementia will also likely increase capacity, competency, and guardianship issues. A second demographic trend is the increase in divorce—and subsequent remarriage for many—resulting in complex family structures involving both biological members and stepmembers (see Aulette, 2007, pp. 249–279). One family scholar described such blended families as follows: "Even when formed with the best of intentions, these families are delicate structures often riddled with mistrust, resentment, and conflicting loyalties that may challenge the marriages at their core" (Abbott, 2010, p. 303). Although there is little research on this topic, it would not be surprising if such families were at increased risk for disagreement and conflict surrounding estate planning, wills, and care placements for aged parents and relatives. These latter issues, particularly will disputes, may raise issues about testamentary capacity (see Chapter 5 by Peisah and Shulman).

Concurrent with these broad societal changes, neuropsychologists have become increasingly involved in forensic practice, the arena in which many civil capacity and competency evaluations occur. This has been documented through increases in the evaluation of forensic-related cases, as well as increases in the number of publications about forensic issues in professional journals and references to neuropsychology in federal and state legal cases (for a review, see Sweet and Giuffre Meyer, 2012). For instance, Sweet, King, Malina, Bergman, and Simmons (2002) found that the percentage of articles partially or substantially devoted to forensic issues in popular clinical neuropsychology journals (e.g., *The Clinical Neuropsychologist*) increased from 4% in 1990 to 14% in 2000. Although most of these articles dealt with malingering (86%), a small minority explicitly addressed capacity and related issues (14%). However, other articles focused on issues that may be relevant for the capacity evaluation such as confidentiality, the ecological validity of testing, and examiner qualifications. In terms of practice patterns, this forensic increase is clearest between surveys of clinical neuropsychologists conducted in 1994 and 1999 when the hours per week devoted to forensic activities jumped from an average of 3.5 hours to 5 hours (Sweet, Moberg, & Suchy, 2000). The most recent survey (Sweet, Giuffre Meyer, Nelson, & Moberg, 2011) presents the data in a different format that complicates direct comparisons of workload across time. Although this latter article also does not specify the types of cases evaluated, the fact that the "elderly dementias" are the most common referral source for adult neuropsychologists and that attorneys are among the top five referral sources for those in private practice and institution/private practice strongly suggests that these practitioners are addressing capacity issues. Given this, and the demographic changes described above that are likely to lead to more of these evaluations, it is concerning that there is no book that has brought together conceptual developments, empirically based findings, and practice recommendation in this area. This text is designed to fill this gap.

FORMAT AND EMPHASIS

This volume is divided into four sections. In the first, this Introduction and a broad overview of relevant legal issues and standards (Chapter 2 by Kolva and Rosenfeld) are presented to provide basic context and background information. Chapter 2, in particular, addresses the legal concept of informed consent, including its history, which provides an important backdrop for understanding capacity issues. In the second section (Chapters 3 to 8), a number of common civil capacities on which neuropsychologists commonly consult are detailed. These include financial decision making by Marson, Triebel, and Knight (Chapter 3), healthcare decision making by Palmer, Savla, and Harmell (Chapter 4), testamentary capacity by Peisah and Shulman (Chapter 5), driving by Wolfe and Clark (Chapter 6), and personal care and independence by Everhart, Lehockey, Moran, and Highsmith (Chapter 7). Chapter 8 by Demakis is the final chapter in this section and covers guardianship issues—a consideration (sometimes even more challenging than competency per se) the court may seek assistance with after an examinee is adjudicated incompetent. Each of these capacity chapters addresses relevant background issues, conceptual and/or theoretical advances, and empirical findings. An illustrative case study is also presented, as well as practical recommendations for clinicians completing these evaluations. This section of the book is designed to provide psychologists with the core knowledge and evidence-based recommendations (where possible) to best guide and support their opinion. Because the research literature on testamentary capacity is less developed than other areas of civil capacity, these recommendations are more conceptually based.

In the third section (Chapters 9 to 13), contributing experts provide a "nuts and bolts" perspective on the capacity evaluation and address common practical issues. These include the following: Chapter 9 by Wood and O'Bryan on an evaluative framework for the assessment of civil capacities; Chapter 10 by Sullivan on various psychometric and practical issues in the selection and use of civil capacity instruments; Chapter 11 by Ruchinskas on the use of data sources in addition to testing (e.g., collateral and clinical interview and review of medical records) that are key portions of capacity evaluations; Chapter 12 by Zapf and Pirelli on admissibility of expert testimony and best practices in report-writing and testifying; and

Chapter 13 by Moberg and Shah on common ethical issues facing the clinician performing these evaluations. Each chapter in this section provides practical and usable information.

The final section of the book is composed of two chapters. In Chapter 14, Benson and Romano, two clerks of the Superior Court (i.e., the legal officer and decision maker for competency cases in North Carolina), provide recommendations to improve the quality of psychological report-writing from their perspective as legal consumers. This unique chapter is a must read as it is from professionals who use and, in some cases, depend on psychological testimony to adjudicate competency. In the final chapter (Chapter 15), Demakis provides recommendations for future research to fill in gaps in the extant literature and to improve clinical decision making.

Although some of the information in this book may be relevant for neuropsychologists performing competency evaluations in criminal cases (e.g., to stand trial, to waive Miranda rights, to be sentenced), this volume is focused on the civil capacity evaluation. Readers interested in criminal capacity work from a neuropsychological perspective are referred to edited books such as *Clinical Neuropsychology in the Criminal Forensic Setting* (Denny & Sullivan, 2008) and *Forensic Neuropsychology Casebook* (Heilbronner, 2005). The former provides a broad overview of conceptual, ethical, psychological, and practical issues for practice in this area, and the latter presents (among various other case studies) four case studies of neuropsychological and competency issues of defendants undergoing various criminal proceedings.

INTRODUCTION TO BASIC ISSUES IN CIVIL CAPACITIES

In this Introduction, I set the stage for the remainder of the volume by introducing several key issues and concepts. Here I address basic terminology (i.e., the difference between capacity and competency), current practice patterns of psychologists in capacity evaluations, conceptual developments and related empirical findings, a framework for the evaluation process, and basic communication issues, particularly report-writing.

Definition and basic issues in capacity evaluations: Capacity and competency are sometimes used interchangeably for convenience (e.g., see Appelbaum, 2007), but they are typically considered to be different constructs. Capacity refers to a clinical decision made by a psychologist, physician, or other healthcare provider about an individual's ability to perform certain tasks or to make certain decisions. It may be viewed as a continuum, as individuals vary in the extent to which they possess a particular capacity. Capacity decisions are based on an assessment that may include, for instance, clinical interview, psychological testing, medical record review, and collateral interviews. As a result of the evaluation, the psychologist opines about the individual's capacity to, for instance, make healthcare decisions or to manage their finances independently. Such opinions may describe the nature and quality of decision making, including areas of persevered ability and areas of impairment. Capacity evaluations do not necessarily involve the court nor do all eventually lead to legal decisions about competency (see below); this is impractical and would likely overwhelm the courts. Many decisions about healthcare capacity such as the capacity to provide informed consent, to refuse treatment, or to leave the hospital against medical advice are typically handled clinically and may never go to court (e.g., see Farnsworth, 1990).

In contrast, competency refers to the ultimate judgment by a legal decision maker such as a judge or clerk concerning an individual's legal status (i.e., whether an individual is in fact competent or not). State statute defines competency; in North Carolina, an incompetent adult is an individual who "lacks sufficient capacity to manage the adult's own affairs or to make or communicate important decisions concerning the adult's person, family, or property" [North Carolina General Statutes 35A-1101 (7)]. Not surprisingly, these differ across jurisdiction (see Table 1.1 for three examples). These decisions have traditionally been of a dichotomous or "all-or-none" quality; in other words, an individual adjudicated incompetent is generally considered incompetent (however defined by the jurisdiction) in all areas of functioning. Such an individual is subsequently assigned a guardian who is responsible for all aspects of the individual's life—this is considered a general or plenary guardianship. More recently, however, there has been a move toward preserving retained capacities in individuals adjudicated incompetent to allow for individual autonomy and decision making (e.g., see Moye et al., 2007; Wingspan, 2002). In such partial or limited guardianships an individual may be adjudicated

Table 1.1 Examples of Competency Statutes in Three States

State	Statute
North Carolina	"Incompetent adult" means an adult or emancipated minor who lacks sufficient capacity to manage the adult's own affairs or to make or communicate important decisions concerning the adult's person, family, or property whether the lack of capacity is due to mental illness, mental retardation, epilepsy, cerebral palsy, autism, inebriety, senility, disease, injury, or any similar cause or condition. [North Carolina General Statutes 35A-1101 (7)]
Nevada	"Incompetent" means an adult person who by reason of mental illness, mental deficiency, disease, weakness of mind. or any other cause is unable to, without assistance, properly manage and take care of his or her property, or both. The term includes a person who is mentally incapacitated. (Nevada Revised Statutes 159.019)
Ohio	"Incompetent" means any person who is so mentally impaired as a result of a mental or physical illness or disability, or mental retardation, or as a result of chronic substance abuse, that the person is incapable of taking proper care of the person's self or property or fails to provide for the person's family or other persons for whom the person is charged by law to provide, or any person confined to a correctional institution within this state. [Ohio Revised Code 2111.01(D)]

incompetent, but may retain certain rights (assuming that they have the requisite capacity), such as the ability to manage a small amount of money or to make decisions about where to live. The incompetency adjudication process and subsequent guardianship determination are detailed in Chapters 8 and 14. Importantly, the legal decision maker may use the psychologist's capacity evaluation to assist in his or her competency determination. In fact, they may actually order an evaluation to assist their decision making in complex or difficult cases.

How psychologists actually evaluate civil competencies: Unfortunately, relatively little research has been done in this area and it does not provide much specific guidance for clinicians conducting these evaluations. One study by Moberg and Kniele (2006)—described as an "informal online survey of psychologists" (p. 102)—found that only 30% indicated that they regularly perform civil or criminal capacity evaluations from the court or attorneys. However, capacity questions and issues were reported to occur regularly in the course of standard clinical examinations. Not surprisingly, dementia, traumatic brain injury (TBI), and stroke/cerebrovascular disease were the conditions in which these issues were most likely to arise. Of the various domains of neuropsychological functioning, executive functioning was considered the most important, followed by various others (in order): intelligence, memory, language, and personality. Unfortunately, this study did not separate findings for civil versus criminal evaluations. In a study of how Australian neuropsychologists evaluate decision-making, Mullaly et al. (2007) found that the majority use a "history taking" interview, standardized tests, information from files, and a semi-structured interview. Fewer psychologists use functional assessments. In terms of tests, the Wechsler Adult Intelligence Scale, Wechsler Memory Scale, Trail-Making Tests, and Controlled Oral Word Association Test are the most frequently used. Thirty-nine percent (the highest) take 6–8 hours to complete a capacity evaluation. A final study by Christie, Savill, Buttress, Newby, and Tyerman (2001) surveyed 92 clinical neuropsychologists (an approximate 30% response rate) in the United Kingdom on how they assess driving capacity after TBI. Most (70%) reported that they based their capacity decision on routine neuropsychological evaluation and, of these respondents, 58% thought that measures of attention and visuospatial measures were most useful. Interestingly, over half of all respondents did not feel confident about their ability to evaluate driving capacity, although those who saw more cases were more likely to be confident than those who saw fewer cases. Overall, although these studies provide some information about what some psychologist are doing "on the ground," they are limited because of relatively low (if not unknown) response rates and lack of knowledge about the representativeness of these respondents. Moreover, because the data are self-report, the content and quality of their reports are not known nor is how judicial decision makers use these findings and opinions known.

Conceptual models of capacity and cognitive underpinnings: Given the diversity and complexity of civil capacities, model-building and other conceptual work in this area is difficult and there is no "one-size-fits-all" approach. This is not surprising given that each capacity addressed in this volume has multiple components;

for instance, testamentary capacity requires memory to recall the content of one's estate and perhaps prior wills, language to express one's desires, and, if complex, higher-order reasoning to make decisions about its disposition. In contrast, driving capacity relies heavily on sensory abilities, particularly vision, basic motor coordination and functioning, as well as attention and visuospatial processing. Even within the same capacity, there is likely to be variability in the requisite capacities. For instance, the cognitive skills and financial sophistication required to manage, for instance, a single disability check without other assets are considerably less than what is required to manage multiple investments, landholdings, and multiple sources of income. Increased capacity is also probably necessary in cases in which there are other multiple and competing demands on the individual, such as often occurs in the context of family conflict.

Despite this diversity in type and degree of capacity, good examples of work in this area include the early MacArthur Treatment studies for capacity to make medical treatment decisions (Appelbaum & Grisso, 1995; Grisso, Appelbaum, Mulvey, & Fletcher, 1995; Grisso & Appelbaum, 1995) and Marson and colleagues' work on financial capacity (Marson et al., 2000; Marson & Herbert, 2005). For the latter, financial capacity is conceptualized as consisting of three levels: specific financial abilities, general domains of financial activities, and overall or global financial capacity. Based on this model, an instrument, the Financial Capacity instrument, was developed that includes a variety of specific tasks of financial ability within various domains. For instance, the Basic Monetary Skills domain includes specific tasks that require naming coins/currency and counting coins/currency, whereas the Bill Payment domain includes tasks that require understanding bills and preparing bills for mailing. Through use of psychometrically based cutoffs on this measure, participants can be classified as capable, marginally capable, or incapable. It is important to note that these distinctions are not equivalent to the ultimate legal determination of competency, but provide a useful tool toward understanding performance on these measures. The validity of the prototype instrument (and its revision) has been demonstrated as those diagnosed with moderately severe Alzheimer's disease perform worse than those with mildly severe Alzheimer's disease who in turn do worse than older control participants (Marson et al., 2000). Over the course of a year in a longitudinal study, individuals with mild Alzheimer's disease were also increasingly likely to be considered incapable in most of the specific financial domains (Martin et al., 2008).

Grisso and Appelbaum's (1998) work has also been important in developing conceptual models of capacity and their work was initially on capacity to consent to treatment in psychiatrically ill patients. Based on their review of the relevant literature and case law, they focused on the following four functional abilities (p. 31): the ability to express a choice; the ability to understand information relevant to the treatment decision; the ability to appreciate the significance of the information for one's own situation, including possible consequences of various treatment options; and the ability to reason with the relevant information to weigh treatment options logically. Grisso and Appelbaum (1998) carefully note that there is no simple relationship between these abilities and examinees' capacity to consent to treatment for two reasons. First, examinees do not possess these in an "all-or-none fashion" and they usually manifest all of them, but in varying degrees. Moreover, varying levels of these abilities are needed based on their situation and the complexity of the required medical decision, particularly for risky treatments. Second, courts vary in the degree to which they require these abilities; legal and ethical standards are applied differently across various jurisdictions, making a broad summary in this area difficult. In any case, these four abilities provide a fair sampling of the abilities necessary to decide about medical decision making. It is important to note that these authors (and others) typically do not specify what the outcome of the medical decision making should be (i.e., the correct or wise choice). In other words, examinees are free to make decisions that most others would not make or that some might consider "poor" as long as they demonstrate adequate reasoning, understanding, and appreciation to make such decisions.

Palmer and Savla (2007) examined the literature that correlated neuropsychological performance with the above model of healthcare decision making. They concluded that there were fairly consistent correlations between neuropsychological measures and key aspects of decision making (e.g., understanding, appreciation, and reasoning), but that these were nonspecific. For instance, executive processing was not specifically related to appreciation, a higher-order type of reasoning. It was interesting, however, that in schizophrenia, cognitive functioning was more highly correlated with decisional ability than psychiatric functioning. However, this finding should be interpreted cautiously, as patients with severe psychiatric illness probably were not enrolled in the various studies and thus the samples of individuals were likely biased toward psychiatric stability. Grisso and Appelbaum (1995) found this same pattern in hospitalized patients with depression (i.e., the capacity to consent to treatment was related to cognitive, but not psychiatric symptom), but not in schizophrenia. In this latter disorder, self-reported symptom severity was negatively correlated with treatment consent capacity. This finding is at odds with the conclusions of Palmer and Savla (2007), but this study did not use particularly robust measures of cognitive functioning as they conceptualized "verbal cognitive functioning" as a composite measure of three Wechsler Adult Intelligence Scale subtests. See Chapter 4 for an additional discussion of these issues.

Research has also examined how well neuropsychological measures are related to financial capacity. Mackin and Arean (2009) examined financial capacity in older adults with late life major depression. These individuals performed more poorly on a financial capacity instrument, the Money Management scale of the Independent Living Scales, than age-matched controls, but no differently on a variety of standard neuropsychological tests. Attention and executive processing measures also predicted scores on this measure in a regression analysis even after sociodemographics, arithmetic achievement performance, and depression severity were accounted for. Using patients with Mild Cognitive Impairment, Okonkwo, Wadley, Griffith, Ball, and Marson (2006) also found that tests of attention and executive processing predicted select aspects of financial capacity performance, but on a different measure of financial capacity, the Financial Capacity Instrument.

The predicted domains were financial conceptual knowledge, bank statement management, and bill payment. See Chapter 3 for a detailed discussion of these issues.

Although there is clearly still work to do in this area (see Chapter 15), the above research on medical and financial decision making is promising for neuropsychologists as it suggests the importance of cognitive functioning for these capacities. Some research, in fact, demonstrates that cognitive functioning may be more important than psychiatric functioning. The relationship between cognitive functioning and the other capacities is addressed in the various chapters in the second part of this volume.

Specific tools for assessing capacity: Several different types of measures have been developed to evaluate capacity. The first type requires that the examinee, or an informant, rate the ability to perform some task or tasks. An early example of this is the Blessed Dementia Scale (Blessed, Tomlinson, & Roth, 1968), which has an informant rate changes in everyday activities (e.g., household tasks and managing small sums of money) and habits (e.g., eating and dressing). Although this and similar measures have some psychometric support and are easy to administer and score, they are subject to rater biases and inaccuracies. Certainly, relying solely on such a measure would not be sufficient for a capacity evaluation. A more frequently used measure is a structured or semi-structured interview that requires the examinee to respond to either the situation facing the examinee or a hypothetical vignette. An example of the former is the MacArthur Competence Assessment Tool for Treatment (Grisso & Appelbaum, 1998) in which the examinee is first informed about their condition and is then asked a variety of questions about it to gauge his or her ability to make a choice, as well as his or her understanding, appreciation, and reasoning. The Hopemont Capacity Assessment Interview (Edelstein, 1999) is an example of the latter and uses a semi-structured interview. The examinee is asked to respond to questions in hypothetical vignettes about either medical decision making or financial issues. As examples, in the medical vignette, the examinee is asked to reason about cardiopulmonary resuscitation, whereas in the financial vignette he or she is asked to reason about lending a substantial sum of money to a family member. Taken together, these types of measures are attractive as they flow from a conceptual understanding of the capacity and, in some cases, directly evaluate the capacity in question. Chapters 3, 4, and 7 detail some of these measures and issues associated with their use.

A final type of commonly used measure is one that is performance based, or at least has performance-based elements. The Independent Living Scales (Loeb, 1996), for example, requires (among other things) the examinee to perform a variety of financial, health and safety, and "everyday" tasks. These include writing out a check, computing financial balances, demonstrating how to call 911, and addressing an envelope. Other items on this measure are more knowledge based and require the examinee to, for instance, specify what he or she would do in various health and household emergencies. Other performance-based tasks are more targeted and specifically assess one type of capacity. For instance, the Financial Capacity Instrument designed by Marson (Marson et al., 2000;

Triebel et al., 2009) in its most recent form includes 20 tasks ranging from simple to complex, such as counting money, checkbook management, and bill payment. A performance-based task of activities of daily living is the Direct Assessment of Functional Status (Loewenstein et al., 1989), which requires the examinee to perform a variety of tasks such as dressing, grooming, and feeding. An advantage of such measures is that they directly assess the capacity in question, though sometimes they may not be practical to administer and issues of ecological validity are sometime still raised. For instance, does the capacity to write checks accurately in a controlled setting necessarily correlate with the ability to perform such a task in daily life? Chapters 3 and 7 provide additional detail about the strengths and weaknesses of performance-based measures. The interested reader is also referred to the Grisso's (2003) book *Evaluating Competencies: Forensic Assessment and Instruments* for a comprehensive discussion of psychometric and conceptual issues in capacity test development (see also Chapters 3 and 10).

Whatever types of psychological measure are used to assess capacity, it is important to view them as one component of the evaluation. Performance on such measures must be integrated with other sources of data such as medical records, collateral interviews, and behavioral observations. Moreover, performance on such tests, no matter how strong the supporting reliability and validity, does not translate to legal competency. Kapp and Mossman (1996) caution that the use of such measures—"capacimeters" in their terminology—may lead to their automatic and reflexive use by legal and clinical consumers without broader consideration of the examinee and his or her situation. In other words, there is a danger that an inordinate amount of weight will be placed on the tests results alone. We agree that test results should always be viewed in a broad context, but also do not want to diminish the unique contributions that clinical neuropsychologists can make in capacity cases. More than any other mental health professional, we are in the unique position to not only use tests to measure constructs such as capacity, but also to realize the limitations of such testing. Clearly, the framework for such evaluations includes more than only psychological or functional testing (see below and Chapter 9).

A framework for evaluating civil capacities: Again, because of the diversity of civil capacities, as well as the diversity of issues within each capacity (e.g., the capacity to make a decision about receiving a prescribed antibiotic versus undergoing major surgery that has a variety of risks and benefits), there is no "one-size-fits-all" evaluative framework. Moreover, some evaluations, particularly regarding healthcare decision making, may need to be completed rapidly without benefit of formal psychological or functional testing. At a minimum though, for most evaluations (except driving), it would seem that a thorough clinical interview and/or behavioral observation of an individual who is unable to communicate would appear essential. This would allow at least some determination about whether an examinee is able to express a choice, as well as understand, reason, and appreciate the issue at hand. Ideally, however, the evaluation process should be more detailed. An excellent resource for such a detailed framework is the joint effort by the American Psychological Association and the American Bar Association.

This group published handbooks for psychologists, lawyers, and judges that provide considerable information, guidance, and recommendations for these professionals conducting competency evaluations with older adults (American Bar Association Commission on Law and Aging—American Psychological Association, 2008). In the handbook for judges, the group identified the six pillars of a capacity assessment: medical condition, cognition, everyday functioning, values and preferences, risk and level of supervision, and means to enhance capacity. Clinical psychologists, and neuropsychologists in cases in which cognitive issues are more relevant, can play an important role in assisting the judge or other judicial decision maker with these so-called pillars. However, more than a clinical interview is typically necessary to assist with these; psychological, functional, and/or neuropsychological evaluations, medical record reviews, and collateral interviews are typically indicated. See Chapter 9 for a full discussion of a broad evaluative framework for capacity evaluations, as well as Chapter 11 for challenges in obtaining information in the above framework including limitations on the use of medical records, sometimes questionable accuracy of collateral-report and self-report, and the reliability of clinical diagnoses.

Reporting writing and communication: Communicating one's finding after the evaluation is a key part of the capacity evaluation and is usually in the form of a written report, but may also include in-person testimony. Because such testimony is not typical in capacity cases, the report should stand alone and be well written and organized, clearly address the relevant issue(s), and be jargon free. Chapter 14 is written from the perspective of two judicial decision makers and consumers of psychological reports—a perspective that, in my view, is sometimes missing in psychology circles. In addition to the above recommendations about the report, it stresses the importance of describing the tests administered and what they assess in plain English and addressing factors that may contribute to poor performance, such as sensory or physical impairments. Other potential limitations that should be addressed (if present) include psychological factors such as anxiety or paranoia, fatigue, and the effects of medications. These consumers are clearly not solely looking for a test score on a so-called "capacimeter."

A key issue in report writing is addressing the so-called ultimate issue or, in these types of reports, if the examinee is competent or incompetent. There are conflicting opinions about whether psychologists (or any other type of expert) should offer such opinions as some argue that they are moral and legal issues under the sole purview of the courts (see Slobogin, 1989). Chapter 12 addresses this issue from a psychological perspective and Chapter 14 does so from a legal consumer perspective. The latter authors do not oppose such opinions; they acknowledge that such opinions are helpful, but that they ultimately make their own decision based on all the provided evidence and the relevant statue. Chapter 12 details some of the arguments in favor of and against psychologists offering opinions on the ultimate issue. Briefly, one argument against offering such opinions is that they are legal and moral decisions outside the expertise of psychologists. An argument for offering such opinions is that they are the inevitable result of conducting evaluations and that in seeking to avoid ultimate issue testimony, oblique or "couched" opinions might replace clear and explicit opinions. Although a full discussion of this issue is beyond the scope of this Introduction, psychologists working in forensic settings conducting capacity evaluations certainly need to be familiar with this issue. Understanding relevant state statutes and local practices on experts offering opinions about the ultimate issue provide a good source of information to guide one's practice.

CONCLUSIONS

The purpose of this volume is to bring together neuropsychological research, conceptual and empirical developments on a variety of different capacities, and information on legal statutes to aid clinical neuropsychologists in performing capacity evaluations. Although similar work has been done for neuropsychologists in the criminal arena, this has yet to be done for civil capacities. With the graying of our population and the increase in forensic work among neuropsychologists, capacity evaluations and issues are probably already a part of many practitioners' work and this will likely increase in the future. In sum, it is hoped the current volume will foster improved evidence-based practice in this area for both the beginning and more seasoned clinician.

References

Abbott, E. (2010). *A history of marriage*. Toronto, Ontario: Penguin.

American Bar Association/American Psychological Association Assessment of Capacity in Older Adults Project Working Group. (2008). Assessment of older adults with diminished capacity: A handbook for psychologists. *American Bar Association Commission on Law and Aging—American Psychological Association.*

Appelbaum, P. (2007). Assessment of patients' competency to consent to treatment. *The New England Journal of Medicine, 357*, 1834–1840.

Appelbaum, P. S., & Grisso, T. (1995). The MacArthur Treatment Competence Study. I. Mental illness and competence to consent to treatment. *Law and Human Behavior, 19*, 105–126.

Aulette, J. R. (2007). *Changing American families* (2nd ed.). Boston: Pearson.

Blessed, G., Tomlinson, E., & Roth, M. (1968). The association between quantitative measures of dementia and of senile change in the cerebral grey matter of elderly subjects. *British Journal of Psychiatry, 114*, 797–811.

Christie, N., Savill, T., Buttress, S., Newby, G., & Tyerman, A. (2001). Assessing fitness to drive after head injury: A survey of clinical psychologists. *Neuropsychological Rehabilitation, 11*, 45–55.

Denney, R. L., & Sullivan, J. P. (2008). *Clinical neuropsychology in the criminal forensic setting*. New York: Guilford.

Edelstein, B. (1999). *Hopemont Capacity Assessment Interview manual and scoring guide*. Morgantown, WV: West Virginia University.

Farnsworth, M. G. (1990). Competency evaluations in a general hospital. *Psychosomatics, 31*, 60–66.

Grisso, T. (2003). *Evaluating competencies: Forensic assessments and instruments.* New York: Kluwer Academic/Plenum.

Grisso, T., & Appelbaum, P. (1995). The MacArthur Treatment Competence Study. III. Abilities of patients to consent to psychiatric and medical treatments. *Law and Human Behavior, 19,* 149–174.

Grisso, T., & Appelbaum, P. S. (1998). *Assessing competency to consent to treatment: A guide for physicians and other health professionals.* New York: Oxford.

Grisso, T., Appelbaum, P. S., Mulvey, E. P., & Fletcher, T. (1995). The MacArthur Treatment Competence Study. II. Measures of abilities related to competence to consent to treatment. *Law and Human Behavior, 19,* 127–148.

Heilbronner, R. L. (2005). *Forensic neuropsychology casebook.* New York: Guilford.

Kapp, M. B., & Mossman, D. (1996). Measuring decisional capacity: Cautions of the construction of a "capacimeter." *Psychology, Public Policy, and Law, 2,* 73–95.

Loeb, P. A. (1996). *Independent Living Scales manual.* San Antonio, TX: Psychological Corporation.

Loewenstein, D. A., Amigo, E., Duara, R., Guterman, A., Hurwitz, D., Berkowitz, N., Wilkie, F., et al. (1989). A new scale for the assessment of functional status in Alzheimer's disease and related disorders. *Journal of Gerontology: Psychological Sciences, 44,* 114–121.

Mackin, R. S., & Arean, P. A. (2009). Impaired financial capacity in late life depression is associated with cognitive performance on measures of executive functioning and attention. *Journal of the International Neuropsychological Society, 15,* 793–798.

Marson, D. C., & Herbert, K. (2005). Assessing civil competencies in older adults with dementia: Consent capacity, financial capacity, and testamentary capacity. In G. J. Larrabee (Ed.), *Forensic neuropsychology: A scientific approach* (pp. 334–377). New York: Oxford University Press.

Marson, D. C., Sawrie, S. M., Snyder, S., McIntruff, B., Stalvey, T., Boothe, A., Aldridge, T., Chatterjee, A., & Harrell, L. E. (2000). Assessing financial capacity in patients with Alzheimer's disease: A conceptual model and prototype instrument. *Archives of Neurology, 57,* 877–884.

Martin, R., Griffith, R., Belue, K., Harrelle, L., Zamrini, E., Anderson, B., Bartolucci, A., & Marson, D. (2008). Declining financial capacity in patients with mild Alzheimer's disease: A one-year longitudinal study. *American Journal of Geriatric Psychiatry, 16,* 209–219.

Moberg, P. J., & Kniele, K. (2006). Evaluation of competency: Ethical considerations for neuropsychologists. *Applied Neuropsychology, 13,* 101–114.

Moye, J., Wood, E., Edelstein, B., Wood, S., Bower, E. H., Harrison, J. A., & Armesto, J. C. (2007). Statutory reform is associated with improved court practice: Results of a tri-state comparison. *Behavioral Sciences and the Law, 25,* 425–426.

Mullaly, E., Kinsell, G., Berberovic, N., Cohen, Y., Dedda, K., Froud, B., Leach, K., & Neath, J. (2007). Assessment of decision-making capacity: Exploration of common practices among neuropsychologists. *Australian Psychologist, 42,* 178–186.

Nevada Revised Statutes 159.019.

North Carolina General Statutes 35A-1101(7).

Ohio Revised Code 2111.01(D).

Okonkwo, O. C., Wadley, V. G., Griffith, H. R., Ball, K., & Marson, D. C. (2006). Cognitive correlates of financial abilities in mild cognitive impairment. *Journal of the American Geriatrics Society, 54*, 1745–1750.

Palmer, B. W., & Savla, G. (2007). The association of specific neuropsychological deficits with capacity to consent to research or treatment. *Journal of the International Neuropsychological Society, 13*, 1047–1059.

Slobogin, C. (1989). The "Ultimate Issue" issue. *Behavioral Sciences and the Law, 7*, 259–266.

Sweet, J. J., & Giuffre Meyer, D. (2012). Trends in forensic practice and research. In G. J. Larrabee (Ed.), *Neuropsychology: A scientific approach.* (2nd ed.) (pp. 501–516). New York: Oxford University Press.

Sweet, J. J., Giuffre Meyer, D., Nelson, N. W., & Moberg, P. J. (2011). The TCN/AACN 2010 "Salary Survey": Professional practices, beliefs, and incomes of U. S. neuropsychologists. *The Clinical Neuropsychologist, 25*, 12–61.

Sweet, J. J., King, J. H., Malina, A. C., Bergman, M. A., & Simmons, A. (2002). Documenting the prominence of forensic neuropsychology at national meetings and in relevant professional meetings from 1990 to 2000. *The Clinical Neuropsychologist, 16*, 481–494.

Sweet, J. J., Moberg, P. J., & Suchy, Y. (2000). Ten-year follow-up survey of clinical neuropsychologists: Part II. Private practice and economics. *The Clinical Neuropsychologist, 14*, 479–495.

Triebel, K. L., Martin, R., Griffith, H. R., Marceaux, J., Okonkwo, O. C., Harrell, L., et al. (2009). Declining financial capacity in mild cognitive impairment: A 1-year longitudinal study. *Neurology, 73*, 928–934.

Vincent, G. K., & Velkoff, V. A. (May, 2010). The older population in the United States: 2010 to 2050. Population estimates and projections. *Current Population Reports.* Washington, D.C.: Bureau of the Census.

Wingspan—The Second National Guardianship Conference. (2002). Wingspan—The second national guardianship conference recommendations. *Stetson Law Review, 31*, 595–609.

2

Legal Perspectives on Civil Capacity and Competence

ELISSA A. KOLVA AND BARRY ROSENFELD

In 1981, Darrell Burch was found wandering along a Florida highway, injured and disoriented. He was brought to a local mental health center where he was "hallucinating, confused, psychotic, and believed he was in 'heaven'" (*Zinermon v. Burch*, 1990, p. 118), and later signed voluntary admission and consent-to-treatment forms at Florida State Hospital (Isaac & Brakel, 1992). Following his release from the hospital 5 months later, Burch sued the hospital physicians and administration, alleging that they knew or should have known that he was incompetent to provide informed consent to his admission as was required by Florida state law. His argument rested on the presumption that had he been treated as an incompetent patient (rather than a voluntary one) he would have been afforded the various procedural safeguards that accompany involuntary hospitalization. Burch's civil lawsuit claimed that he had been deprived of his liberty without due process, and sought redress through the federal courts. The U.S. Supreme Court upheld Burch's claim that the deprivation of liberty without due process (i.e., valid consent or an involuntary placement hearing) constituted a legitimate basis for his federal lawsuit. The Court's subsequent ruling in *Zinermon v. Burch* (1990) highlights the legal and ethical consequences of the failure to assess decision-making capacity. This ruling necessitates the assessment of functional capacities relevant to the patient's ability to perform a task or make a decision, as the mere presence of a mental disability does not indicate incompetence (Melton, Petrila, Poythress, & Slobogin, 2007, pp. 336–337).

Clinicians working in healthcare settings are charged with assessing whether a patient is capable of making critical decisions about his or her life. This can include determining whether a patient can make medical decisions or refuse needed care, whether a doctor should rely more heavily on a family member's judgment in a medical setting, or testifying in court that a person's decision-making capacity is so impaired that he or she loses the ability to make autonomous decisions and that role should be assumed by a guardian. In other contexts, clinicians may be asked to determine whether an adult is capable of making important financial or personal decisions, such as issuing or changing a will or deciding whether to engage in sexual activity. This chapter introduces the core legal issues surrounding capacity and competence, primarily as they pertain to medical, financial, and other types of legally relevant decision making. We review the development of the legal theories of competence and capacity as they relate to individuals' ability to make decisions. This includes the origins of the doctrine of informed consent, the legal standards and procedures used to assess and determine competence, and the legal implications of a finding of incompetence. Additionally, the admissibility of psychological evidence will be addressed, as will the roles and responsibilities of the attorney and guardian *ad litem*. It should be noted that although this chapter addresses decision-making competence in a wide range of areas, the majority of clinical literature and case law has focused on competence to consent to medical treatments and financial decision making.

COMPETENCE VS. CAPACITY

The terms *capacity* and *competence* are often used interchangeably when applied to decision making, but the distinctions between these terms have important legal implications (Appelbaum, 2007). In the medical decision-making literature, capacity is a clinical term that generally refers to the patient's cognitive abilities, or in the medical treatment setting, the ability to make a given treatment decision (Rosenfeld, 2004, p. 112). In contrast, competence is a legal term that refers to a patients' inability to make decisions for himself or herself. Competency is typically determined by a judge (Rosenfeld, 2004, p. 112).

ORIGINS OF MEDICAL DECISION-MAKING COMPETENCE

The doctrine of informed consent imposes tort liability on a physician for battery or negligence if the physician treats a patient who has not validly given consent. The doctrine of informed consent rests on three core elements: first, consent must be voluntarily provided; second, the patient must be provided with sufficient knowledge to make a decision as discussed above; and third, the patient must have sufficient decisional capacity to make a competent decision (Melton, 2007, p. 377). Accordingly, it is critical for healthcare professionals to assess whether a patient has sufficient decision-making capacity to give a valid consent. The case law in which the doctrine of informed consent arose correspondingly developed legal standards for decision-making capacity in medical settings.

Informed consent is rooted in the English common law and stems from the writ of trespass for assault and battery. In the first case to apply this principle to healthcare, *Slater v. Baker & Stapleton* (1767), two physicians were accused of breaking a patient's healing fracture without his consent. Rather than applying the rule of nonconsensual touching as the basis for an assault and battery charge, the judge in *Slater* cited the physicians' failure to obtain the patient's consent

(Appelbaum, Lidz, & Meisel, 1987, pp. 36–37). In their discussion of *Slater*, Appelbaum et al. (1987, pp. 36–37) noted that the judge's language in his decision laid the foundation for the doctrine of informed consent, which would not be crystallized for another 150 years. In describing his decision, the judge stated "indeed it is reasonable that a patient should be told what is about to be done to him that he may take courage and put himself in such a situation as to enable him to undergo the operation" (Appelbaum et al., 1987, p. 37).

Although the foundation for informed consent was laid in *Slater*, and arose in two early U.S. cases (*Mohr v. Williams*, 1905; *Pratt v. Davis*, 1906), the origins of this doctrine in U.S. law is usually attributed to the seminal opinion delivered by Judge (later U.S. Supreme Court Justice) Benjamin Cardozo in the New York State Court of Appeals case, *Schloendorff v. Society of N.Y. Hospital* (1914). In *Schloendorff*, the plaintiff was informed by her physicians that an ether examination was needed in order to determine the nature of a lump in her stomach. The patient reportedly agreed to the examination, but not to surgery to remove the lump. During the examination the physicians identified the lump as a fibroid tumor and removed it. Unfortunately, the plaintiff subsequently developed gangrene in her arm that necessitated the amputation of several fingers and resulted in intense pain and suffering. In the patient's lawsuit against the hospital, the court ruled that the physicians' actions went beyond mere negligence and constituted an act of trespass. Judge Cardozo's now-famous ruling stated "every human being of adult years and sound mind has a right to determine what shall be done with his own body; and a surgeon who performs an operation without his patient's consent, commits an assault, for which he is liable in damages" (p. 93).

Concern regarding the application of informed consent later turned to research participation following recognition of the atrocities and human rights abuses carried out by Nazi Germany during World War II (Appelbaum et al., 1987, pp. 212–213). The actions conducted by Nazi doctors were exposed during one of the Nuremberg Trials, in which 23 German physicians were tried for crimes against humanity (Slovenko, 2005). In *United States v. Karl Brandt* (1947), the prosecution aimed to determine a universal standard for justifying human experimentation by citing evidence that the defendants subjected concentration camp prisoners to inhumane, often fatal experiments without their consent. Following these trials, which resulted in guilty verdicts for 15 of the 23 doctors (including seven death sentences), two American physicians (and prosecution witnesses) authored the Nuremberg Code, detailing guidelines for ethical human experimentation (Slovenko, 2005). These guidelines, which established the precedence of the rights of the subject over the interests of science, also emphasized the importance of informed consent as a requirement for ethical research conduct (Appelbaum et al., 1987, pp. 212–213). The code states that research participants should be informed of the "nature, duration and purpose of the experiment; the method and means by which it is to be conducted; all inconveniences and hazards reasonably to be expected; and the effects upon his person which may possibly come from his participation in the experiment" (Reiser, Dyck, & Curran, 1977, pp. 272–273). These criteria, as well as the voluntary nature of research participation, although not immediately adopted as standard practice in the United States, influenced the development of the doctrine of informed consent with regard to patient care.

In the decade following the Nuremburg trials, a series of legal cases outlined the contours of how and what information physicians are expected to communicate to their patients. In one of these cases, *Salgo v. Leland Stanford Jr. University Board of Trustees* (1957), the California Court of Appeals stipulated that the consent obtained by physicians must be "informed" (Appelbaum et al., 1987, pp. 38–39), which they defined as providing the patient with "any facts which are necessary to form the basis of an intelligent consent by the patient to the proposed treatment" (p. 578). This standard was further clarified in *Canterbury v. Spence* (1972), a case in which a patient suffered complications following back surgery. In *Canterbury*, the United States Court of Appeals for the District of Columbia concluded that physicians should inform the patient of all potential risks of a procedure that a reasonable person would likely find significant when making a medical decision. The court stated "true consent to what happens to one's self is the informed exercise of a choice, and that entails an opportunity to evaluate knowledgably the options available and the risks attendant upon each. The average patient has little or no understanding of the medical arts, and ordinarily only his physician to whom he can look for enlightenment with which to reach an intelligent decision" (p. 780). This "reasonable person" standard for the disclosure of information has become a central element of modern tort law, as the standard against which to judge allegations of inadequate physician disclosure regarding the risks of a medical procedure (Mazur, 2003).

More recently, case law surrounding informed consent has continued to define the contours of what must and what need not be disclosed. Although the duty of a physician to disclose information about the relevant risks and benefits of a proposed treatment prior to obtaining a patient's consent is well established (Twerski & Cohen, 1999), case law has gradually expanded the range of information that might be considered relevant. For example, recent cases have highlighted the need to disclose information regarding the physician's experience (or lack thereof), his or her success using a proposed intervention, and the economic interests of the institution in which treatment might occur (Petrila, 2003). Twerski and Cohen (1999) have labeled this wave of case law the second revolution in informed consent. Although such expansions of the legal doctrine are clearly occurring, there now exist wide variations across jurisdictions in terms of precisely what information might be considered relevant in any given treatment decision. But regardless of how such cases affect institutional policies or patient–physician communication, they are merely the backdrop for a clinical evaluation of decision-making capacity.

DECISION-MAKING CAPACITY

The numerous cases that gave rise to the legal doctrine of informed consent have pointed the way for the types of assessments that mental health clinicians conduct when assessing decision-making capacity. Assessment of decision-making capacity is required when a patient's ability to make an important decision (e.g., about medical treatment, living independently, or financial matters) is questioned. The case law on medical decision making and informed consent indicates that the critical question for the clinician is determining whether the patient has sufficient decisional capacity to make a competent decision (Petrila, 2003). When patients lack sufficient capacity to make a competent decision, alternative provisions must be implemented. The assessment of capacity to make treatment decisions and the provisions for dealing with incompetent patients are the focus of the remainder of this chapter.

Clinician Assessment of Capacity

The term capacity has been applied to a wide range of settings and situations, most of which pertain, in one way or another, to the ability of an individual to carry out a task. In the context of decisional capacity, this involves making nontrivial decisions, whether regarding healthcare, finances, or other legally relevant matters. Of course, the specific skills or abilities required for a determination of capacity will typically differ depending on the nature of the decision. In the context of medical treatment decision making, capacity refers to the patient's ability to provide meaningful and, hence, legally valid informed consent. The underlying abilities that make up this construct have been the subject of considerable scrutiny by both healthcare providers and legal decision makers.

Capacity generally refers to the patient's cognitive abilities, or in the treatment setting, the ability to make a given treatment decision (Rosenfeld, 2004, p. 112). A patient's capacity to make treatment decisions is often assessed by treating or evaluating clinicians, such as in cases in which the patient consents to or refuses a recommended treatment (Grisso & Appelbaum, 1995). There is often considerable variability in the assessment of decision-making capacity, due in part to the paucity of well-accepted assessment methods. Ideally, clinicians assess their own patients' decision-making capacity, allowing a more thorough understanding of the patient's goals and values, as well as the current decision in the context of past decisions. This context allows clinicians to consider the continuity of their patient's decisions, and identify when a decision seems to diverge from goals and values that the patient has expressed in the past. However, in some instances patients are forced to make important treatment decisions in an emergent situation, often with a doctor they have only recently been introduced to, effectively removing the patient's life-context from the assessment process. Moreover, when a long-standing physician–patient relationship does exist, treating clinicians are vulnerable to the temptation of projecting their own feelings or expectations onto their patients, or misinterpreting psychological changes that influence decision making (Rosenfeld, 2004, pp. 114–115). For example, treating physicians may interpret their patient's onset of depressive symptoms as a natural reaction to declining health rather than identifying depression as a potentially treatable disorder that has clouded the patient's judgment.

These inherent limitations in the effectiveness of treating physician assessments of capacity, coupled with a lack of familiarity as to how decision-making capacity should be assessed (which is a common complaint of healthcare providers), have led many institutions to utilize specialized professionals for the assessment of decision-making capacity—at least for instances in which capacity is unclear or a patient's refusal of recommended treatment raises concern. Such institutional services are typically the domain of Consultation-Liaison (C-L) services, and are typically staffed by psychiatrists or psychologists who have learned, among other specialized evaluation skills, techniques for assessing decision-making capacity. Although C-L services often provide little of the context for understanding a patient's decision, the increased sophistication and expertise brought to bear on the assessment process typically outweigh the potential for diminished contextual information.

Legal Determination of Competence

Whereas capacity refers to a clinical decision based on the treating or evaluating clinician's judgment, the term *competence* refers to a legal determination made by a judge or other legal decision maker (Rosenfeld, 2004, p. 112). Most patients do not require a formal clinical evaluation of decision-making capacity when making healthcare or financial decisions. The capacity of an adult with no obvious cognitive, psychiatric, or physical limitations, who is accepting the treatment recommendation of a physician, is rarely questioned. Conversely, the incompetence of a nonresponsive patient is indisputable. However, when there is a legitimate question as to a patient's competence that cannot be resolved by a clinical evaluation of capacity, or where there are strongly conflicting opinions as to what treatment should be pursued on behalf of an incompetent patient, judicial guidance may be sought.

In reality, the courts are invoked to settle disputes about decisional competence relatively infrequently, particularly when there is general agreement between the healthcare providers, the patient (if he or she is able to express an opinion), and the family members involved in the patient's care. However, when disputes occur, such as a patient's refusal to accept a potentially beneficial treatment that their family members also favor (as is common among psychiatric patients, for example), or a division exists among family members as to whether their relative's expressed wishes should be respected, the legal system is forced to adjudicate the patient's decision-making competence (as often happens among patients with a life-threatening medical illness). The court's decision will typically include both a determination of competence or incompetence and, in the case of incompetence, the appointment of a surrogate decision maker or guardian. This legal declaration of incompetency requires a formal judicial hearing, as the denial of an individual's rights without due process of law violates the Fourteenth Amendment of the U.S. Constitution.

Legal Standards of Competence

Legal standards defining competence differ between jurisdictions; there are no universally accepted standards for incompetency (Appelbaum et al., 1987, pp. 83–84). However, the different standards that have been applied in court cases are generally grouped into five broad categories (Appelbaum & Grisso, 1988; Appelbaum et al., 1987, pp. 84–86; Roth, Meisel, & Lidz, 1977): ability to express a choice, ability to understand and recall information disclosed, ability to provide rational reasons for one's choice, ability to appreciate the significance of the decision, and ability to rationally manipulate information into a decision that is consistent with one's values and preferences. These standards, which are typically thought of as representing a hierarchy of "tests" of competence (with the rigor of the test applied corresponding to the importance of the decision), are each described below.

Expressing a choice. The simplest test of competency, often considered appropriate only for decisions in which the risks and benefits are modest, is the ability to articulate a choice. This standard offers the most respect for the patient's autonomy of decision making by requiring only minimal cognitive abilities without regard for the quality of a decision or the reasoning behind it. Applying this standard, incompetence would occur only in cases in which the individual was incapable of articulating a choice (either verbally or behaviorally) or adhering to a decision long enough for the choice to be implemented. Roth et al. (1977) cited the case of *Wyatt v. Aderholt* (1974) as an example of this standard, as the court prohibited the sterilization of legally incompetent or noncomprehending individuals unless they expressed a genuine desire to undergo the procedure. Under this standard, a patient may be deemed incompetent due to impairments of consciousness, severe thought disorder, a disruption of short-term memory, or extreme ambivalence (Appelbaum & Grisso, 1988).

Understanding information. Perhaps the most widely used standard for assessing decision-making competence is the ability to understand information relevant to the decision. According to this standard, to accept or reject a proposed treatment the patient must understand the information that has been disclosed. This test of competence typically requires the individual to simply repeat or paraphrase information, and hence relies heavily on memory, attention, and overall intelligence (Appelbaum & Grisso, 1988). Indeed, many healthcare providers utilize this standard, whether purposefully or intuitively, in their own assessments of decision-making capacity by asking their patients to repeat information that has just been disclosed as a means of testing their understanding of the information. What is less clear, however, is how to determine the minimally adequate threshold for differentiating competence from incompetence (i.e., is the proportion or number of correct responses sufficient?).

Ability to provide rational reasons. Roth and colleagues (1977) describe the ability to provide rational reasons for one's decision as a standard that has been commonly accepted by the courts, but one that has also frequently been maligned by theorists (e.g., Appelbaum & Grisso, 1988). Although this standard is relatively easily ascertained, and has an obvious intuitive appeal (e.g., asking "why" as a natural extension of asking patients what decision they intend to choose), the requirement that patients provide a rational explanation may contradict the emphasis on autonomy that underlies the doctrine of informed consent. Patients who are confused or have distorted thinking (e.g., psychosis or severe depression) may be unable to meet the demands of this standard. This standard involves the process of weighing information to reach a decision. Thus, competence should be determined by an evaluation of the logical consistency of the process by which a decision was made, rather than an evaluation of the outcome of the process (i.e., the decision). As a result of the common failure to distinguish between outcome and process, theorists have increasingly dismissed the ability to provide rational reasons as a valid test of competence, despite the acceptance of this standard in many jurisdictions.

Appreciating the situation. A somewhat more abstract test of competence rests on the patient's ability to assign personal meaning to the information that has been presented. "Appreciation" refers to the ability of patients to understand the implications of their treatment decisions, which includes both acknowledging the underlying illness and the possible effects each alternative has for their own lives (often including the effects that a decision might have on others). Patients who lack abstract reasoning abilities due to a cognitive or psychiatric disorder, or have a delusional perception of their health state, may fail to meet this standard of competence even when they can accurately paraphrase the risks and benefits that have been disclosed. In *United States v. George* (1965), a U.S. District Court in Connecticut applied an early example of this standard, finding that the patient was competent to refuse life-saving treatments because his refusal rested on his religious beliefs. His refusal of a life-saving blood transfusion on religious grounds was described as an idiosyncratic decision that would not be widely accepted by others, yet he demonstrated an appreciation of the nature of his circumstances and the implications of his choice.

Rational manipulation of information. The most rigorous standard for assessing decisional competence requires an ability to rationally manipulate the information that has been presented. Under this standard, patients are required to demonstrate not only an understanding and appreciation of the information disclosed, but are able to balance the pros and cons of treatment alternatives in the context of their own personal goals and values. This standard differs from the ability to provide rational reasons in that patients need not offer a rationale that would be accepted by others, but rather can provide a rationale that is consistent with their own values, even if others might not accept their logic. For example, in cases similar to *United States v. George* (1965) described previously, medically ill patients are routinely given the option to refuse even seemingly benign life-sustaining interventions provided they can demonstrate that their refusal of treatment is in keeping with their long-standing religious values and personal beliefs. On the other hand, patients who have never held such beliefs, yet offer such a rationale as the basis for their request to refuse treatment, might be seen as making a decision that deviates from their personal goals and core values and thus may fail to meet standards for competence. Furthermore, because of the emphasis on rational thinking, patients with thought disorder, confusion, delirium, dementia, or even significant mood or anxiety symptoms may fail to meet this standard.

Application of Legal Standards of Competence

The application of these legal standards by the courts is often vague and inconsistent as a result of the absence of any landmark jurisprudence concerning *how* a patient's competence should be judged (Grisso & Appelbaum, 1995; Lo, 1990). The majority of landmark cases regarding end-of-life decision making have concerned patients who were clearly incompetent due to unconsciousness or focused on the necessity of treatment rather than the patient's capacity to make decisions. When issues of competence have been raised, the courts have focused largely on the particular facts of the case (e.g., the setting, patient characteristics, and the decision to be made) rather than the standard by which competence should be judged.

Although the courts have given little guidance for choosing one test of competence over another, many experts agree that more stringent requirements for competence should be applied to more important decisions (Grisso & Appelbaum, 1998, p. 137; Rosenfeld, 2004, p. 113). Yet increasing the cognitive demands upon a patient for a determination of competence may have the unintended effect of diminishing self-determination and autonomy. In fact, Saks (1991) has argued that a *lower* standard for competency should be applied to important decisions because individuals have the greatest investment in these decisions and restricting decision-making autonomy in important decisions may have a negative impact on the patient's self-esteem. On the other hand, Roth et al. (1977) recommended the use of differing competency standards based on the risk/benefit ratio of the proposed treatment and whether the patient accepts or rejects the treatment. They suggested that a lower standard should be applied to a decision to accept treatment and a more stringent standard should be applied to reject recommended treatment. Although debates continue to exist as to how a "sliding scale" of competence should be operationalized, the idea of matching the legal test or standard with the seriousness of the consequences that hinge on a patient's decision was endorsed by the Presidential Commission for the Study of Ethical Problems in Medicine and Biomedical and Behavioral Research (1982) and has often been applied by the courts.

Despite the intuitive appeal of a sliding scale of competence, the hierarchical nature of these tests of competence may be clearer in theory than in practice. Grisso and Appelbaum (1995) compared the different legal standards for competence in their study of an instrument designed to assess four of these standards (expression of a choice, understanding, appreciation, and rational manipulation of information). They found that the different tests of competence do not necessarily form a coherent hierarchy, as patients who appeared to be impaired according to a "lower" test were not necessarily impaired on a more stringent test. On the other hand, the use of compound tests (i.e., requiring that patients meet more than one test of competence) inevitably increases the number of patients classified as impaired.

INCOMPETENCE AND THE LOSS OF DECISION-MAKING AUTHORITY

De Facto vs. De Jure Incompetence in Medical Settings

As discussed previously, the right to self-determination is highly valued in American society and the presence of a mental disability does not automatically nullify that right. Even in the context of a mental disorder, adults are presumed to be competent until proven otherwise. Although assessments of decisional capacity are often initiated by treating clinicians (often in response to a refusal of recommended treatment), only a judge or other legal decision maker can adjudicate a person incompetent. Yet in most instances, questions of competence are not decided by the legal system. In medical settings, where decision making is typically a process in which family members actively participate and heated disagreements about what course of treatment is best are uncommon occurrences, clinicians frequently rely on family members whenever the patient is unable to participate fully (Appelbaum, 2007; Lo, 1990). Indeed, if physicians sought a judicial review every time there was a question of incompetence, both the legal and medical systems would be overwhelmed. The utilization of a substitute decision maker without a formal judicial finding of incompetence is referred to as *de facto* incompetence, and is distinguished from *de jure* incompetence, which occurs when individuals are deprived of their decision-making capacity as a matter of law.

In the event that an individual is declared legally incompetent, a substitute (surrogate) decision maker is required. When an advanced directive (AD) or living will is in place, the provisions of the AD are generally activated upon a finding of incompetence, often including the designation of a guardian (described in more detail in the next section). In the absence of an advanced directive, family members are usually appointed as surrogate decision makers, with the hierarchy of family surrogate decision makers dictated by state law. In most states, the order of surrogacy for an adult is as follows: spouse, adult children, parents, siblings, and then other relatives (Appelbaum, 2007). However, in several leading court cases, courts have ignored the preferences of the relatives of incompetent patients. Despite evidence that the decisions rendered by the relatives might reflect the patients' preferences, the courts have occasionally rejected decisions to forgo life-sustaining treatments (e.g., *Cruzan v. Harmon,* 1988; *In re O'Connor,* 1988). When caregivers have diverging opinions about what treatments should be sought, legal intervention is typically necessary.

Legal Removal of Decision-Making Authority

The doctrine of informed consent arises from tort law in which a private individual is acting on another. However, medical decision making is also relevant in the context of constitutional law when the state is exercising its power to remove an individual's ability to make his or her own decisions. The American legal system places a premium on respecting an individual's autonomy and freedom of choice. The Fifth and Fourteenth Amendments to the U.S. Constitution assert that federal and state and local governments (respectively) cannot deprive persons of life, liberty, or property without due process of law. Because a declaration of incompetence essentially strips an individual of certain liberties (e.g., the ability to make medical or financial decisions), this cannot occur in the absence of the legal procedures put into place to protect an individual's liberty and autonomy. Thus the constitutional requirement of due process embodied in the Fifth and Fourteenth Amendments is responsible for the need for competency and guardianship hearings and corresponding evaluations by medical and mental health professionals.

Guardianship

Once an individual has been adjudicated incompetent, the court restricts rights through the denial of decision-making autonomy (Appelbaum & Grisso, 1988). A surrogate decision maker (or guardian) is required whenever patients are deemed incompetent to make some types of decisions (Appelbaum, 2007). Because guardianship entails a loss of autonomy, the courts have typically required a high standard of proof—clear and convincing evidence—before such decisions can be made (Tor & Sales, 1994).

Most jurisdictions distinguish between "plenary" or general guardianship and limited guardianship (Melton et al., 2007, p. 370). Plenary guardianship allows the guardian comprehensive control over the incapacitated person (usually termed the "ward") and is the more widely used approach, despite also being more restrictive. Limited guardianship, on the other hand, is restricted to a particular type of decision (e.g., medical treatment decisions). In a limited guardianship, a guardian can be appointed to make any type of personal decision for the incompetent person, but is most often appointed for financial or medical decision making. In principal, an individual could be found incompetent to make financial decisions but competent to make treatment decisions (or the reverse). Rather than tailored to the individual needs of the patient, most guardianships are plenary rather than limited or restricted (Moye et al., 2007). Tor and Sales (1994) outlined several reasons for the widespread use of plenary guardianship. These include the vague standards for both guardianship and decisional capacity, a presumed bias toward a finding of incompetence among judges, a lack of resources to implement specific guardianship, and a failure of respondents (i.e., the proposed ward) and their experts to detail the specific needs and limitations of the respondent (e.g., providing only broad statements about the individual's functioning).

Because guardianship proceedings are relatively informal, they can be initiated by any interested party, not just family members or healthcare professionals (Melton et al., 2007, pp. 371–375). There are no consistent, well-established standards as to how and when respondents will be informed of guardianship proceedings or informed of their right to counsel or trial by jury. Court-appointed guardians may be family members, members of government agencies, social workers, lawyers, or in rare cases sheriffs. Each of these parties may have different advantages and disadvantages, depending on the circumstances of the individual case. For example, a family member may have more information about the patient's treatment decision-making preferences, but because of the personal connection to the patient, the family member may have personal motives and attachments that color the decisions rendered. Conversely, an independent guardian may increase objectivity, but often at the expense of familiarity with the patient's history and values.

The court also has the power to limit the ability of the guardian to make treatment decisions on behalf of the patient. In the case of Richard Roe (*In the Matter of Guardianship of Richard Roe III*, 1981), a young man suffering from schizophrenia and declared legally incompetent, his father was appointed as his guardian but was not allowed to make decisions regarding his son's medication. Although the father was able to make decisions regarding his son's finances, he was unable to consent to the administration of antipsychotic medication over his son's objections. The court retained the ability to make Roe's treatment decisions, and stated "a guardian of a mentally ill person does not have inherent authority to consent to the forcible administration of antipsychotic medication to his noninstitutionalized ward in the absence of an emergency" (p. 417).

The guardianship process underwent significant revisions following a 1987 report by the Associated Press exposing numerous abuses in the guardianship process, including findings that half of all persons under guardianship were not represented by an attorney, 25% had never had a hearing, and 13% had received no notice of the proceedings (Bayles & McCartney, 1987). Many states subsequently adopted reforms including appropriate notification, including standardized notice forms and petition requirements, as well as the right of the respondent to be present at the hearing, to present evidence, and to cross-examine witnesses (York, 2006).

TYPES OF CAPACITY

Capacity to Accept and Refuse Treatment

Prior to the 1970s, psychiatric hospitals were occasionally penalized for failing to involuntarily medicate patients that had been committed to their care (see Isaac & Brakel, 1992). It was assumed that once a patient was involuntarily committed to the hospital, psychoactive medication could be administered freely without consulting the patient or his or her family. This practice changed following the U.S. Supreme Court's decision in *Rennie v. Klein* (1978), after the Court ruled that involuntarily committed psychiatric patients retained the right to refuse medication provided they did not pose a risk of harm to themselves or others. The court stated that involuntary medication in situations in which the government has *not* shown the patient to be incompetent violated the patient's constitutional rights. Before employing the coercive power of the state to force a patient to take medication, the government must clear the procedural hurdle of proving that the patient lacks competence to make his or her own decisions.

The guardians of legally incompetent patients also have the ability to refuse treatment, provided their refusal is consistent with the presumed wishes of the incompetent patient (Wortzel, 2006). In *Superintendent of Belchertown State School v. Saikewicz* (1977) the guardian of a legally incompetent man with profound mental retardation was able to refuse life-prolonging treatment for his ward's incurable acute myeloblastic leukemia. In their decision, the court recognized that the guardian has the right to make decisions in accordance with what the patient would want if he or she were competent. Guardians may make medical decisions for incompetent patients except in the case of deprivation of life-saving treatment (*Charles S. Soper, as Director of Newark Developmental Center* et al. *v. Dorothy Storar*, 1981).

The adoption of a patient's wishes by a guardian or surrogate decision maker is termed substituted judgment. In some jurisdictions, surrogate decision makers are specifically instructed to attempt to make the decision that the patient, if competent, would make whereas other jurisdictions rely on a "best interest" standard, asking the surrogate to make decisions that are in the patient's best interest. Of course, substitute judgment is far simpler when an advance directive is in place to specify treatment preferences, but even the existence of such documents does not eliminate questions about what and how a surrogate should decide on behalf of the incompetent patient. Although advance directives provide broad directions about treatment preferences, they rarely provide specific guidance that is pertinent to a particular decision in a specific set of circumstances.

Testamentary Capacity

Testamentary capacity is the term used to describe an individual's legal and mental capacity to make or alter a will. The general standard for testamentary capacity is that the testator or testatrix understands (or understood, if the individual is deceased when the question of capacity is raised) the nature and consequences of executing a will, knows the nature and extent of the property that he or she was disposing of, and knows those who would be considered the natural objects of his or her bounty and his or her relations with them (*Matter of Slade*, 1984). In contrast to the wide range of standards for assessing the capacity to make treatment decisions, this standard is generally thought to be "indisputable" in evaluating testamentary capacity (*In re Estate of Kumstar*, 1985). Standards for testamentary capacity are also considered to be less restrictive than those required for treatment decision making. In the case of *In re Estate of Colby* (1997), the decedent was determined to lack decisional competency and was assigned a guardian; however, she still retained testamentary capacity. The court stated that the presence of a guardian "does not collaterally stop her from arguing that the decedent possessed testamentary capacity at the time of the executed codicils, since a finding of incapacity . . . is based upon different factors from those involved in a finding of testamentary capacity" (*In re Estate of Colby*, 1997, p. 2).

Financial Capacity

When a person is unable to manage his or her own business or financial affairs, he or she is considered to lack financial capacity. In these cases guardianship of the estate or a conservatorship (the terminology used differs by state) is necessary. Conservatorship statutes date back to ancient Greece, and the government's interest in the control of an incapacitated person's money and property is well established (York, 2006). A conservatorship is a legal arrangement in which a manager or conservator handles the personal and/or business affairs of the ward or beneficiary (Friedman & Savage, 1988). In some states (e.g., California, Tennessee) conservatorship refers to the establishment of a surrogate decision maker with regard to matters of the disabled adult's person, property, or both; most laws are similar to those established for guardianship (Friedman & Savage, 1988; York, 2006). However, some states refer to conservatorship primarily in the discussion of financial capacity. According to the Uniform Probate Code (2006), a guardian is defined as a person who is qualified, pursuant to appointment by a court, to make all decisions on behalf of the incompetent person whereas a conservator is a person appointed by the court solely to manage the estate of a protected (i.e., incompetent) person.

The court may appoint a conservator in either a limited or unlimited role, if the individual meets either of the following conditions:

A) By clear and convincing evidence, the individual is unable to manage property and business affairs because of an impairment in the ability to receive and evaluate information or make decisions, even with the use of appropriate technological assistance, or because the individual is missing, detained, or unable to return to the United States; and
B) By a preponderance of evidence, the individual has property that will be wasted or dissipated unless management is provided or money is needed for the support, care, education, health, and welfare of the individual or of individuals who are entitled to the individual's support and that protection is necessary or desirable to obtain or provide money (Uniform Probate Code, 2006, Section 5-401).

Petitions for conservatorship can be brought by any person who believes that an allegedly incompetent person is in need of assistance. In recent years, clinicians have begun to devote more attention to the assessment of financial capacity and have developed validated interviews to assess the functional abilities related to financial capacity (Marson et al., 2009). Despite these improvements in the legal system, little attention has been paid to how clinicians or evaluators assess financial capacity or to how to measure the functional abilities required for competent financial decision making.

LEGAL ISSUES IN CAPACITY EVALUATIONS

Standards for the Admissibility of Scientific Testimony

The admissibility of psychological testimony in a court of law, whether related to decision-making capacity or any other topic, is typically governed by the Federal Rules of Evidence (1992); although variations exist across states, most states use an approximation of the Federal Rules of Evidence. These broad standards have been further clarified by relevant case law, primarily *Daubert v. Merrell Dow Pharmaceuticals* (1993). Under Rule 401 of the Federal Rules of Evidence, evidence is admissible if it is "relevant." Rule 702 defines relevancy as it pertains to the role of expert testimony regarding scientific evidence (Federal Rules of Evidence, 1992). According to Rule 702, "[i]f scientific, technical, or other specialized knowledge will assist the trier of fact to understand the evidence or to determine a fact in issue" an expert "may testify thereto." Rule 702 also requires that expert testimony "assist the trier of fact to understand the evidence or to determine a fact in issue." Thus, under rules 401 and 702, expert testimony must be relevant and tied to the facts of the case, and must aid the judge or jury in resolving a factual dispute. In essence, the evidence to be presented must be helpful in deciding the case (McCann, 1998). However, the appropriateness of the content of the proffered testimony, and in particular whether it is sufficiently reliable and relevant, is determined by the trial judge. Indeed, the judge is charged with determining both the adequacy of the expert as well as the reliability of the evidence to be presented.

The scientific basis for expert evidence was first addressed by the U.S. Supreme Court in *Frye v. U.S.* (1923). In *Frye* the Court ruled that the polygraph test, which had been developed only a few years earlier, was not admissible as scientific evidence and could not be relied upon by an expert because the test was not "generally accepted" by the profession. The Court stated: "just when a scientific principle or discovery crosses the line between the experimental and demonstrable stages is difficult to define. Somewhere in this twilight zone the evidential force of the principle must be recognized, and while the courts will go a long way in admitting experimental testimony deduced from a well-recognized scientific principle or discovery, the thing from which the deduction is made must be sufficiently established to have gained general acceptance in the particular field in which it belongs" (p. 1014). This broad legal standard has provided judges with considerable flexibility with regard to the admissibility of expert testimony, but has also led to difficulty determining when "general acceptance" had been achieved. Although the *Frye* standard was the result of a Federal court decision, it has been adopted as the appropriate standard for the admissibility of expert testimony in many states including Florida, California, Arizona, New York, and Nebraska (McCann, 1998).

Discrepancies between the *Frye* standard and the Federal Rules of Evidence were resolved by the Supreme Court in *Daubert v. Merrell Dow Pharmaceuticals* (1993). According to *Daubert*, the testimony proffered by an expert witness must meet a two-pronged test of admissibility that finds the testimony both reliable and relevant. The first prong of the *Daubert* test, the relevancy of the evidence, deals with whether an expert's evidence "fits" the facts of the case. Relevant evidence was defined as "that which has any tendency to make the existence of fact that is of consequence to the determination of the action more probable or less probable than it would be without the evidence" (p. 2795). The second prong pertains to the reliability (a legal term more akin to the psychological concept of validity) of the evidence, and states that in order for expert testimony to be reliable, the expert must have derived his or her conclusions from the scientific method.

The *Daubert* decision described four factors that could be used by judges to determine whether the expert's conclusions were based on scientific knowledge: (1) whether the evidence or technique has been the subject of empirical testing; (2) whether the theory or technique has been subjected to peer review and publication; (3) whether there is available information about the known or potential error rate and whether appropriate norms and standards are available; and (4) whether the theory is generally accepted by the relevant scientific community (*Daubert v. Merrell Dow Pharmaceuticals*, 1993). The Court cautioned that this list was not "a definitive checklist or test," and many factors could bear on the inquiry. In their decision, the Court acknowledged that the *Daubert* test was imperfect because "there are important differences between the quest for truth in the courtroom and the quest for truth in the laboratory. Scientific conclusions are subject to perpetual revision. Law, on the other hand, must resolve disputes finally and quickly. . . . We recognize that, in practice, a gate keeping role for the judge, no matter how flexible, inevitably on occasion will prevent the jury from learning of authentic insights and innovations" (*Daubert v. Merrell Dow Pharmaceuticals*, 1993, pp. 2798–2799). This decision has engendered considerable controversy regarding the admissibility of certain types of scientific evidence.

Under *Daubert* and its progeny, the role of judges was not only to permit reliable testimony, but to exclude unreliable testimony. The Court has also extended the principles of *Daubert* to expert testimony of nonscientists (e.g., *Kumho Tire Co. v. Carmichael,* 1999). The goal of these opinions was to protect the integrity of the legal process and eliminate the admission of unreliable expert testimony that is often contrary to public policy (Grove & Barden, 1999). Although the *Daubert* standard has rarely been applied to cases involving civil competency, the recent proliferation of standardized measures and techniques described elsewhere in this volume may give rise to a growing number of legal challenges.

Guidelines for the Use of Psychological Testing in Forensic Assessment

The American Psychology-Law Society and Division 41 of the American Psychological Association (APA) developed and recently revised the *Specialty Guidelines for Forensic Psychology*, a set of guidelines designed to be consistent with the *Ethical Principles of Psychologists* but more specific to monitoring the professional conduct of forensic psychologists when in court, when party to legal proceedings, and when working in correctional and forensic mental health facilities (American Psychological Association, in press). The guidelines in legal settings provide an aspirational model for psychological practice.

A more concrete set of recommendations for determining the admissibility of the results of psychological testing was developed by Heilbrun (1992). First, assessments should be commercially available and documented in at least two sources. Such a test should also have a manual describing its development, psychometric properties, and method of administration. It should also be listed in a reliable source such as the *Mental Measurements Yearbook* (Conoley, Kramer, & Mitchell, 1989). Second, the reliability of the test should be strongly considered. Tests with a reliability coefficient less than 0.80 should not be considered reliable. If less reliable tests are used, there should be a strong justification provided. Third, the test should be relevant to the legal issue or a construct underlying the legal issue. Fourth, test administration and interpretation should be standardized. Fifth, objective tests and actuarial data, when appropriate, are preferable to more subjective tests and interpretation. Finally, response style should always be assessed to identify cases of distortion, and should influence interpretation of test results (Heilbrun, 1992).

Role of the Attorney

The conventional attorney–client relationship is based on the premise that the client is capable of understanding advice from counsel and of making important decisions. In the event that this relationship is threatened due to diminished capacity (of the client), the role of the attorney is generally governed by the American Bar Association's (ABA) Model Rules of Professional Conduct, Rule 1.14 (Client with Diminished Capacity; American Bar Association, 2010). The rules of professional conduct may vary by state, and thus an attorney should monitor the Rules of Professional Conduct for the state in which he or she is practicing. The ABA's model rule has three central guidelines for attorneys working with clients with diminished capacity. First, when a client's decisional capacity is impaired, the attorney should attempt to maintain a conventional relationship with the client. This includes treating the client attentively and with respect. Second, the lawyer should take reasonable protective action if the client's diminished capacity places him or her at risk of substantial physical, financial, or other harm. This may include consulting with other individuals who may be in a position to protect the client and, when appropriate, seeking the appointment of a guardian or conservator. If a legal representative has been appointed, the attorney should consult with that individual in matters related to the client. Third, despite the client's diminished capacity, information relating to the attorney's representation of the client is protected by rules governing the confidentiality of attorney–client information. Any information revealed by the attorney must be done only to the extent necessary to protect the client's interests. Confidentiality must be observed even in cases in which the client elects to involve family members or other persons to participate in the discussions with the attorney.

If the court determines that the legal representation of an incompetent person is insufficient, it may appoint a guardian *ad litem* to represent the interests of the person (Uniform Probate Code, 2006). The role of the guardian *ad litem* is generally governed by one of two models, the "zealous advocate" or the "best interest" model (Saxon, 2008). Under the "best interest" model the guardian *ad litem* functions as an investigator or officer of the court. He or she investigates facts impartially and reports back to the court. His or her duty lies with the court, not as an advocate for the potentially incompetent person. However, the guardian *ad litem* is still responsible for informing the person about the nature of the proceedings as well as his or her rights, and may submit a written report of his or her findings to the court. This process enables the court to make objective decisions in the best interest of the incompetent person. In contrast, the "zealous advocate" model requires the guardian *ad litem* to represent his or her client in the same manner as any other client in a pending legal proceeding. There are no guidelines outlining the selection of the model, thus this is a recent topic of debate. In many cases, due to this ambiguity, attorneys choose which model to use (Saxon, 2008).

SUMMARY

Over the past few decades, researchers, clinicians, and legal scholars have become increasingly focused on issues related to decisional capacity and competency in civil settings. Although this focus has been predominantly on conceptualizing, measuring, and assessing competence in the context of healthcare decision making and informed consent, there is growing interest in financial decision making. Without an awareness of the legal parameters of competency determinations, clinicians are ill equipped to assist the courts. This chapter provides only broad guidance regarding the legal parameters of civil competence and considerable variations exist across jurisdictions. Clinicians must familiarize themselves with these variations in order to adequately research, assess, and make decisions about the complex issues involved in civil competence determinations.

References

American Bar Association. (2010). Model rules of professional conduct. *Center for Professional Responsibility*. Retrieved from http://www/abanet.org/cpr/mrpc/rule_1_14.html.

American Psychological Association. (in press). Specialty guidelines for forensic psychology. *American Psychologist.*

Appelbaum, P. S. (2007). Clinical practice: Assessment of patients' competence to consent to treatment. *New England Journal of Medicine, 357,* 1834–1840.

Appelbaum, P. S., & Grisso, T. (1988). Assessing patients' capacities to consent to treatment. *The New England Journal of Medicine, 319,* 1635–1638.

Appelbaum, P. S., Lidz, C. W., & Meisel, A. (1987). *Informed consent: Legal theory and clinical practice.* New York: Oxford University Press.

Bayles, F., & McCartney, S. (1987, September). Guardians of the elderly: An ailing system. *Associated Press,* pp. 1–26.

Canterbury v. Spence. 464 F.2d 772 (D.C. Cir. 1972).

Charles S. Soper, as Director of Newark Developmental Center et al. *v. Dorothy Storar,* N.Y., 420 N.E.2d 64, 1981.

Conoley, J. C., Kramer, J. J., & Mitchell, J. V. (Eds.) (1989). *The tenth mental measurements yearbook.* Lincoln, NE: University of Nebraska Press.

Cruzan v. Harmon, 760 S.W. 2d 408, 416417 (Mo. 1988).

Daubert v. Merrell Dow Pharmaceuticals, 113 U.S. 2786 (1993).

Federal Rules of Evidence. (1992). Boston: Little Brown.

Friedman, L., & Savage, M. (1988). Taking care: The law of conservatorship in California. *Southern California Law Review, 61*, 273–290.

Frye v. United States, 293F 1013 (D.C. Cir. 1923).

Grisso, T., & Appelbaum, P. S. (1995). Comparison of standards for assessing patients' capacities to make treatment decisions. *American Journal of Psychiatry, 152,* 1033–1037.

Grisso, T., & Appelbaum, P. S. (1998). *Assessing competence to consent to treatment: A guide for physicians and other health professionals.* New York: Oxford University Press.

Grove, W. M., & Barden, R. C. (1999). Protecting the integrity of the legal system: The admissibility of testimony from mental health experts under Daubert/Kumho analyses. *Psychology, Public Policy, and Law, 5*, 224–242.

Heilbrun, K. (1992). The role of psychological testing in forensic assessment. *Law and Human Behavior, 16,* 257–270.

In re Estate of Colby, 240 A.D.2d 338, 660 2d 3 (N.Y. Sup.1997).

In re Estate of Kumstar, 66.2d 691, 487 N.E.2d 271 (N.Y. 1985).

In re O'Connor, 531 NE2d 607 (N.Y. 1988).

In the Matter of Guardianship of Richard Roe III, 421 N.E.2d 40 (Mass. 1981).

Issac, R. J., & Brakel, S. J. (1992). Subverting good intentions: A brief history of mental health law "reform." *Cornell Journal of Law and Public Policy, 2,* 89–119.

Kumho Tire Co. v. Carmichael, 526 U.S. 137 (1999).

Lo, B. (1990). Assessing decision-making capacity. *Law, Medicine & Health Care, 18,* 193–201.

Marson, D. C., Martin, R. C., Wadley, V., Griffith, H. R., Snyder, S., et al. (2009). Clinical interview assessment of financial capacity in older adults with mild cognitive impairment and Alzheimer's disease. *Journal of the American Geriatric Society, 57*, 806–814.

Matter of Slade, 483 2d 4th Dept. 513 (N.Y. Sup. 1984).

Mazur, D. J. (2003). Influence of the law on risk and informed consent. *British Medical Journal, 327,* 731–734.

McCann, J. T. (1998). Defending the Rorschach in court: An analysis of admissibility using legal and professional standards. *Journal of Personality Assessment, 70,* 125–144.

Melton, G. B., Petrila, J., Poythress, N. G., & Slobogin, C. (2007). *Psychological evaluations for the courts.* New York: The Guilford Press.

Mohr v. Williams, 104 N.W. 12 (Minn. 1905).

Moye, J., Wood, E., Edelstein, B., Wood, S., Bower, E. H., et al. (2007). Statutory reform is associated with improved court practice: Results of a tri-state comparison. *Behavioral Sciences and the Law, 25,* 425–436.

Petrila, J. (2003). The emerging debate over the shape of informed consent: Can the doctrine bear the weight? *Behavioral Sciences and the Law*, 21, 121–133.

Pratt v. Davis, 118 161, 79 N.E. 562 (Ill. App. 1906).

President's Commission for the Study of Ethical Problems in Medicine and Biomedical and Behavioral Research (1982). United States Code Annotated. U S. 1982; Title 42 Sect. 300v.

Reiser, S. J., Dyck, A. J., & Curran, W. J. (1977). *Ethics in medicine: Historical perspectives and contemporary concerns.* Cambridge, MA: The MIT Press.

Rennie v. Klein, 462 F Supp 1131(D NJ, 1978), 476 F Supp 1294 (D NJ, 1979), affirmed in part, 653 F 2d 836 (3rd Cir, 1981), vacated and remanded, 102 S Ct 3506 (1982), 700 F 2d 266 (3rd Cir, 1983).

Rosenfeld, B. (2004). *Assisted suicide and the right to die: The interface of social science, public policy, and medical ethics.* Washington, D.C.: American Psychological Association.

Roth, L. H., Meisel, A., & Lidz, C. W. (1977). Tests of competency to consent to treatment. *American Journal of Psychiatry, 134,* 279–284.

Saks, E. R. (1991). Competency to refuse treatment. *North Carolina Law Review, 69,* 945–999.

Salgo v. Leland Stanford Jr. University Board of Trustees, 154 2d 560 (Cal. App. 1957).

Saxon, J. (2008). *North Carolina Guardianship Manual.* UNC-Chapel Hill, Chapel Hill, NC.

Schloendorff v. Society of New York Hospital, 211 125, 105 NE 92 (NY 1914).

Slater v. Baker & Stapleton, 95 860 (Eng. 1767).

Slovenko, R. (2005). The evolution of standards for experimental treatment or research. *The Journal of Psychiatry & Law, 33,* 129–174.

Superintendent of Belchertown State School et al. v. Joseph Saikewicz, 370 N.E.2d 417, (Mass. 1977).

Tor, P. B., & Sales, B. D. (1994). A social science perspective on the law of guardianship: Directions for improving the process and practice. *Law and Psychology Review, 18,* 1–41.

Twerski, A. D., & Cohen, N. B. (1999). The second revolution in informed consent: Comparing physicians to each other. *Northwestern University Law Review,* 94, 1–54.

Uniform Probate Code. (2006). National Conference of Commissioners on Uniform State Laws, Chicago, IL.

United States v. George, 239 F.Supp. 752 (D. Conn.1965).

United States v. Karl Brandt et al., in U.S. Adjutant General's Department, Trials of War Criminals before the Nuremberg Military Tribunals under Control Council Law No. 10 (October 1946–April 1949). Vol. 2, *The Medical Case.* Washington, D.C.: U.S. Government Printing Office, 1947.

Wortzel, H. (2006). The right to refuse treatment. *Psychiatric Times, 23,* 30–32.

Wyatt v. Aderholt, 503 F.2d 1305, 1308 (5th Cir. 1974).

York, T. M. (2006). Conservatorship proceedings and due process: Protecting the elderly in Tennessee. *University of Memphis Law Review, 36,* 491–542.

Zinermon v. Burch, 494 U.S. 113 (1990).

PART TWO

Civil Capacities and Guardianship

3

Financial Capacity

DANIEL C. MARSON, KRISTEN TRIEBEL, AND AMY KNIGHT

INTRODUCTION

Financial capacity is a medical–legal construct that represents the ability to independently manage one's financial affairs in a manner consistent with personal self-interest and values (Marson & Hebert, 2008). Financial capacity thus involves not only performance skills (e.g., counting coins/currency accurately, completing a check register accurately, paying bills) but also judgment skills that optimize financial self-interest, and values that guide personal financial choices. Financial experience and skills can vary widely among cognitively normal individuals and are associated with factors of education and socioeconomic status (American Bar Association/American Psychological Association Assessment of Capacity in Older Adults Project Working Group, 2008). From a legal standpoint, financial capacity represents the financial skills sufficient for handling one's estate and financial affairs, and is the basis for determinations of conservatorship of the estate (or guardianship of the estate, depending on the state legal jurisdiction). Broadly construed, financial capacity also conceptually encompasses more specific legal capacities such as contractual capacity, donative capacity, and testamentary capacity. Thus, financial capacity is an important area of assessment in the civil legal system (American Bar Association/American Psychological Association Assessment of Capacity in Older Adults Project Working Group, 2008; Marson & Hebert, 2008), and one that neuropsychologists are increasingly called upon to evaluate (Marson, 2002).

From a clinical standpoint, financial capacity is a highly cognitively mediated capacity that is vulnerable to neurological, psychiatric, and medical conditions that affect cognition such as dementia, stroke, traumatic brain injury, and schizophrenia. In particular, financial capacity issues arise frequently in the context of older adults with cognitive loss and dementia. Family members of such older adults often raise concerns about an elderly person's new problems managing household finances, making poor financial decisions, or being exploited. Clinicians are increasingly asked by families, other clinicians, attorneys, and judges to evaluate and offer clinical opinions regarding financial capacity (American Bar Association/American Psychological Association Assessment of Capacity in Older Adults Project Working Group, 2008; Marson & Hebert, 2008; Widera, Steenpass, Marson, & Sudore, 2011).

In this chapter, we examine the clinical assessment of financial capacity from a neuropsychological perspective. Specifically, we discuss the conceptual bases of financial capacity and a clinical conceptual model of financial capacity, briefly describe financial capacity assessment approaches and instruments available for use by neuropsychologists, review existing financial capacity research with particular attention to recent neuropsychological and neuroimaging findings, offer guidelines and recommendations for assessment of financial capacity in the neuropsychological setting, and conclude with an illustrative neuropsychological and capacity case report. Given the focus of the limited financial capacity literature on older adult patients with dementia, and the authors' own clinical and research focus in this area, the chapter concentrates on financial capacity issues in the elderly. However, most of the principles and findings articulated in the chapter are applicable to other younger clinical populations, such as traumatic brain injury.

CONCEPTUAL BACKGROUND

The capacity to manage financial affairs comprises a broad range of conceptual, pragmatic, and judgment abilities, used across a range of everyday settings, that are critical to the independent functioning of adults in our society (Marson, 2001; Marson, Hebert, & Solomon, 2011; Marson et al., 2000). A range of studies have suggested that financial capacity is an "advanced" or instrumental activity of daily living (IADL) (Marson et al., 2000; Wolinsky & Johnson, 1991). Advanced ADLs are mediated by higher cognitive functions and can be distinguished from "household" ADLs (e.g., meal preparation, shopping, housekeeping) and "basic" ADLs (e.g., bathing, dressing, walking) (Wolinsky & Johnson, 1991). Financial capacity entails a broad set of abilities ranging from basic skills of identifying and counting coins/currency, to conducting cash transactions, to higher level abilities of managing a checkbook and bank statement, to very complex activities of making investment decisions. As might be expected, such abilities can vary enormously across individuals, depending on a person's socioeconomic status, occupational attainment, and overall financial experience (Marson, 2001; Marson et al., 2000). Along with medical decision making, driving, and mobility, financial capacity is a core aspect of individual autonomy in our society (Marson, 2001; Marson et al., 2011; Marson et al., 2000).

Definitions of Financial Capacity

From a legal standpoint, financial capacity represents the financial skills sufficient for handling one's estate and financial affairs, and is the basis for determinations of conservatorship (or guardianship, depending on the legal jurisdiction) (American Bar Association/American Psychological Association Assessment of Capacity in Older Adults Project Working Group, 2008). Broadly construed, financial capacity also conceptually encompasses other more specific legal capacities such as contractual capacity, donative capacity, and testamentary capacity. Thus, financial capacity is an important area of assessment in the civil legal system (Marson, 2001; Marson & Hebert, 2008, Marson et al., 2011; Marson et al., 2000).

Historically, the legal standard for financial capacity in conservatorship statutes was generally (and vaguely) cast as the capacity to manage "in a reasonable manner all of one's financial affairs" (American Bar Association/American Psychological Association Assessment of Capacity in Older Adults Project Working Group, 2008). A more modern and specific standard is set forth in Section 410(2) of the Uniform Guardianship and Protective Proceedings Act (UGPPA), which states that a court may appoint a conservator if the court determines that "the individual is unable to manage property and business affairs because of an impairment in the ability to receive and evaluate information or make decisions, even with the use of appropriate technological assistance"; and the individual has property that will be wasted or dissipated unless management is provided, or funds are needed for the support of the individual or of others entitled to the individual's support (Uniform Guardianship and Protective Proceedings Act, 1997; American Bar Association/ American Psychological Association Assessment of Capacity in Older Adults Project Working Group, 2008; Marson, 2001; Marson et al., 2011; Marson et al., 2000).

From a clinical standpoint, there is currently no widely accepted clinical definition for financial capacity. Since Lawton's seminal 1969 paper on definitions of IADLs (Lawton & Brody, 1969), it is striking how little conceptual and definitional work has been conducted in the area of financial capacity. Marson and his group have recently proposed the following definition: "the capacity to manage money and financial assets in ways that meet a person's needs and which are consistent with his or her values and self-interest" (Marson, 2001; Marson et al., 2011; Marson et al., 2000; Widera et al., 2011). This working definition incorporates performance and judgment aspects characteristic of financial capacity (see below), as well as consideration of a person's longstanding values.

Performance and Judgment Aspects of Financial Capacity

Financial capacity can be understood to have both a performance aspect and a judgment aspect. To possess financial capacity, a person must be able to *perform* a variety of tasks and skills in order to meet his or her needs. Such tasks and skills include understanding basic financial concepts, possessing basic monetary skills, carrying out cash transactions , and paying bills. However, in addition to such performance skills, an individual must also be able to exercise *judgment* and decision making to promote his or her own financial well-being. Thus, in addition to performance skills, the individual must be able to carry out financial activities in ways that promote and protect his or her self-interest (Marson, 2001; Marson et al., 2011; Marson et al., 2000).

These performance and judgment dimensions of financial capacity are distinct. By way of example, a patient with schizophrenia may have a number of intact financial performance skills (count coins/currency, carry out cash transactions, use a money order or checkbook), but due to mental illness and substance abuse problems, may also be unable to exercise good judgment and utilize the skills in ways that meet basic needs and protect his or her self-interest. Such a patient may impulsively spend his or her disability entitlement check within a few days of receipt, resulting in a disruption of his or her medication regimen and nutrition, causing in turn psychiatric decompensation, and threatening the continuity of housing such that he or she may become homeless (Marson, 2001; Marson et al., 2011; Marson et al., 2000).

Conceptual Model of Financial Capacity

As noted, despite its salient relationship to everyday living and independence, there has been a surprising lack of conceptual and empirical study of financial capacity. Early work in the area of IADLs offered elementary and unsatisfactory schema such as "financial management skills," without providing needed conceptual structure or detail. We present below a clinically based conceptual model of financial capacity in older adults (Marson, 2001; Marson et al., 2000; Martin et al., 2008). This model has been the basis for instrument development and for ongoing studies of financial capacity in mild cognitive impairment (MCI), Alzheimer's disease (AD), and other clinical populations (Dreer, DeVivo, Novack, & Marson, in press; Marson, 2001; Marson et al., 2011; Marson et al., 2000).

Because financial capacity represents a broad continuum of activities and specific skills, it may be best conceptualized as a series of domains of activity, with each having specific clinical relevance (Griffith et al., 2003; Marson, 2001; Marson et al., 2000). Examples of these domains include basic monetary skills, carrying out cash transactions, managing a checkbook, managing a bank statement, and exercising financial judgment. This domain-based approach is clinically oriented and is consistent with the presumed multidimensionality of financial capacity and its variability across individuals. It is also consistent with the legal principle of limited financial competency adopted within most state legal jurisdictions, which recognizes that an individual may be competent to carry out some financial activities and not others (Grisso, 1986; Marson, 2001; Marson et al., 2011; Marson et al., 2000).

In addition to domains of activity, our model identifies specific financial abilities, or tasks (Marson, 2001; Marson et al., 2000). Tasks reflect more basic financial skills that compromise domain-level capacities. For example, the domain of "financial conceptual knowledge" draws upon specific abilities, such as understanding simple concepts (e.g., a loan or savings) and pragmatically applying such concepts in everyday life (e.g., selecting interest rates, identifying a medical deductible, and making simple tax computations). The domain of financial judgment consists of tasks related to detection/awareness of financial fraud, or of making informed investment choices. Therefore, tasks represent abilities that taken together constitute broader, clinically relevant domains of financial activity. We have defined tasks as being simple or complex, depending on the level of cognitive resources they appear to require (Marson, 2001; Marson et al., 2011; Marson et al., 2000).

Our model also considers financial capacity at the global level (Griffith et al., 2003; Marson, 2001). Competency is ultimately an overall categorical judgment or classification made by a clinician or legal professional. Thus, the conceptual model of financial capacity currently has three levels (Griffith et al., 2003): (1) specific financial abilities or tasks, each of which is relevant to a particular domain of financial activity; (2) general domains of financial activity, which are clinically relevant to the independent functioning of community-dwelling older adults; and (3) overall financial capacity, which reflects a global measure of capacity based on the summation of domain- and task-level performance. Our conceptual model of financial capacity, presented in Table 3.1, is composed of nine domains, 18 tasks, and two global levels (Griffith et al., 2003; Marson, 2001; Marson et al., 2011; Marson et al., 2000; Martin et al., 2008). This model has been the basis for financial capacity instrument development, including the Financial Capacity Instrument (FCI-9), which is discussed later in this chapter.

ASSESSMENT APPROACHES AND INSTRUMENTS

Assessment Approaches

At least three different measurement approaches exist for clinically assessing financial capacity. These approaches are (1) patient and informant-based ratings and reports of financial skills, (2) direct assessment of financial skills using performance-based instruments, and (3) clinical interview approaches that involve clinician interviewing to obtain information about a patient's financial skills and functioning. A patient and informant-based report of everyday financial functioning in community settings can be gathered through written questionnaire or rating forms. Performance-based instruments provide a direct and quantitative assessment of specific financial skills that are norm-referenced and usually more finely grained than rating forms. Clinical interviews combine the strengths of both informant rating/report and direct performance approaches, by drawing upon the interviewing skills of a clinician who can also choose to use various direct assessment techniques to examine financial skills. In the sections below, we provide an overview of the three assessment approaches and highlight examples of instruments developed for each approach. However, before doing so, we first address the key conceptual issue of assessing premorbid financial capacity.

Importance of Assessing Premorbid Financial Capacity

Regardless of the assessment approach, the goal of a financial capacity assessment is to evaluate a patient's current financial functioning in reference both to the patient's current environmental demands and to the patient's premorbid financial

Table 3.1 Conceptual Model of Financial Capacity: Eighteen Tasks, Nine Domains, Two Global Scores

	Task Description	Task Difficulty
Domain 1 Basic Monetary Skills		
Task 1a Naming coins/currency	Identify specific coins and currency	Simple
Task 1b Coin/currency relationships	Indicate relative monetary values of coins/currency	Simple
Task 1c Counting coins/currency	Accurately count groups of coins and currency	Simple
Domain 2 Financial Conceptual Knowledge		
Task 2a Define financial concepts	Define a variety of simple financial concepts	Complex
Task 2b Apply financial concepts	Practical application/computation using concepts	Complex
Domain 3 Cash Transactions		
Task 3a One-item grocery purchase	Enter into simulated 1 item transaction; verify change	Simple
Task 3b Three-item grocery purchase	Enter into simulated 3 item transaction; verify change	Complex
Task 3c Change/vending machine	Obtain change for vending machine use; verify change	Complex
Task 3d Tipping	Understand tipping convention; calculate/identify tips	Complex
Domain 4 Checkbook Management		
Task 4a Understand checkbook	Identify and explain parts of check and check register	Simple
Task 4b Use checkbook/register	Enter into simulated transaction; pay by check	Complex
Domain 5 Bank Statement Management		
Task 5a Understand bank statement	Identify and explain parts of a bank statement	Complex
Task 5b Use bank statement	Identify specific transactions on a bank statement	Complex
Domain 6 Financial Judgment		
Task 6a Detect mail fraud risk	Detect and explain risks in mail fraud solicitation	Simple
Task 6b Detect telephone fraud risk	Detect and explain risks in telephone fraud solicitation	Simple

Table 3.1 Conceptual Model of Financial Capacity: Eighteen Tasks, Nine Domains, Two Global Scores (Cont'd)

	Task Description	**Task Difficulty**
Domain 7 Bill Payment		
Task 7a Understand bills	Explain meaning and purpose of bills	Simple
Task 7b Prioritize bills	Identify overdue utility bill	Simple
Task 7c Prepare bills for mailing	Prepare simulated bills, checks, envelopes for mailing	Complex
Domain 8 Knowledge of Assets/Estate	Indicate/verify asset ownership, estate arrangements	Simple
Domain 9 Investment Decision Making	Understand options; determine returns; make decision	Complex
Global 1 Sum of Domains 1–7	Overall functioning across tasks and domains	Complex
Global 2 Sum of Domains 1–7 + 9	Overall functioning across tasks and domains	Complex

Reprinted with permission from Griffith et al. (2003), the American Academy of Neurology.

experience and abilities. As noted above, the financial experience of individuals can vary widely, based on educational, occupational, socioeconomic status, and other factors. Thus, in conducting an evaluation, one of the clinician's first objectives is to establish a patient's premorbid financial experience and ability levels. Using this information, the clinician can form an impression of premorbid function against which current financial activities and performance levels can be measured and compared. In addition, information on premorbid financial function can inform the areas of evaluation and test measures used. For example, if a patient has never used a checkbook/register to pay bills, or has traditionally delegated this task to a spouse, it would be inappropriate to assess this ability and conclude that impaired performance is the product of a mental disorder or illness. Instead, the examiner should inquire as to whether the individual has used other forms of bill payment, such as money orders or debit cards, and tailor the evaluation accordingly. The ultimate goal for the clinician is to form a clear picture of the patient's premorbid level of financial functioning in order to select appropriate assessment measures and to draw meaningful conclusions regarding the patient's overall current financial capacity and possible deficits or declines in financial skills.

Informant-Based Assessment

The informant report approach to financial assessment involves gathering data about a person's real-life financial functioning through self-report, collateral report, or both. Ideally, the informant provides information about prior optimal levels of financial skill, how financial functioning has changed over time, as well as current activities and skills. The primary advantages of patient and informant report are the potential ecological validity of the information received and the relative ease of administration and minimal cost to obtain such valuable functional information. In current clinical practice, most information regarding financial functioning is derived from patient and collateral report, whether obtained during a standard clinical interview or through a questionnaire/report form.

Detailed questionnaires of financial functioning are not widely available. Most functional inventories that assess a broad spectrum of basic and advanced activities of daily living include only a very limited review of financial abilities. One of the earliest functional report forms was the Lawton & Brody Instrumental Activities of Daily Living Scale (Lawton & Brody, 1969), which included one finance item asking about the respondent's independence in financial matters such as paying bills, making purchases, or handling money. The Blessed Dementia Scale, another early survey of functional and behavior change, included just one question related to finance, "Inability to cope with small sums of money" (Blessed, Tomlinson, & Roth, 1968). Although surveys of instrumental activities of daily living frequently reference overall financial functioning, rarely do they include more than one or two items. A self-report or informant questionnaire is usually not standardized or norm-referenced, and thus results cannot be generalized across patients and settings. Finally, the questionnaire approach is further limited by anosognosia and reporter bias affecting the accuracy of financial information received (Wadley, Harrell, & Marson, 2003). For example, our group found that both patients with AD and their family members had difficulty making reliable estimations of patients' financial abilities. Patients with AD overestimated their financial abilities due to their increasing anosognosia (a neurologically based deficit in a patient's awareness of illness or disability), while family member estimates were more accurate but demonstrated problems with judgment reliability over time, possibly due to the stresses of caregiving (Wadley et al., 2003).

Example of Informant Rating/Report Instrument

The Disability Assessment for Dementia (DAD) (Gelinas, Gauthier, McIntyre, & Gauthier, 1999). The DAD is an interview-based questionnaire (40 items) that evaluates functional disability through a proxy-respondent. A recent critical review of IADL questionnaires rated the DAD as best overall for its psychometric properties (Sikkes, de Lange-de Klerk, Pijnenburg, Scheltens, & Uitdehaag, 2009). The DAD questionnaire was developed as a disease-specific scale aimed at community-dwelling dementia patients in the early stages of AD. This measure of functional disability is based on the model of health proposed by the World Health

Organization (WHO). Basic and instrumental activities of daily living are examined in relation to executive skills (initiation, planning and organization, effective performance) to permit identification of problematic areas. The DAD includes four items related to finance. Administration of the DAD takes approximately 15 minutes. Only actual performance over the past 2 weeks is reported and activities are evaluated as performed without any assistance or reminder being provided from caregivers.

Performance-Based Assessment

Performance-based instruments directly assess functional abilities in a clinical or laboratory setting. These instruments ask individuals to perform a series of conceptual and pragmatic tasks equivalent to those performed in the home and community setting. Performance-based measures are standardized, quantifiable, repeatable, and norm-referenced, and thus results can be generalized across patients and settings. Performance-based assessment of financial abilities may be included as part of a global functional status assessment, or financial skills may be explored alone or in greater detail with specific financial capacity instruments.

An advantage of an objective performance measure is the freedom from subjective reporter bias. Performance-based instruments can provide information that is more objective and frequently more reliable than third-party observations or examinees' self-reports. Thus, a person's performance on specific financial tasks can illuminate possible concerns with patient and informant reports, and be highly relevant to diagnostic formulations, recommendations, and treatment strategies. In addition, the findings from these measures are much more precise and finely grained than patient and collateral reports. For example, change over time can be evaluated with much more precision using performance-based measures.

There are also weaknesses to performance-based measurement. One issue is the requirement for a specialized measure and materials, and a trained administrator, which together make performance instruments more challenging, expensive, and time consuming to administer. A second and key issue is ecological validity, as tasks are completed in clinical or laboratory settings versus real world home and community settings (American Bar Association/American Psychological Association Assessment of Capacity in Older Adults Project Working Group, 2008). In general, performance-based instruments provide evidence of adequate reliability, but there is less empirical evidence regarding the predictive validity of each scale in terms of real world functioning (Moore, Palmer, Patterson, & Jeste, 2007). Measures conducted in a laboratory or clinical office setting cannot take into account either the contextual cues or distractions within the home environment that may assist or interfere with a person's abilities to perform everyday financial tasks. Successful performance on a functional measure may demonstrate ability under controlled and potentially optimal conditions, but may not always accurately predict actual daily functioning. Ultimately, it is the ability of patients to engage in self-initiated instrumental activity in community environments that is critical for independence.

General Performance Instruments with Financial Items

Direct Assessment of Functional Status-Revised (DAFS-R) (Loewenstein et al., 1989; McDougall, Becker, Vaughan, Acee, & Delville, 2010). The DAFS is a performance measure of higher level daily living skills in older adults with dementia. The original DAFS (Loewenstein et al., 1989) measured instrumental activities for individuals with AD and related disorders, but showed a ceiling effect for older adults living independently in the community. The 85-item DAFS was subsequently revised to be more challenging and to place greater emphasis on medical management skills. The resulting instrument, the DAFS-R, comprises 55 items in total, with 13 items related to financial abilities such as money handling, writing a check, and balancing a checkbook. The DAFS-R requires that the patient attempt each financial item (e.g., the patient is given a blank check to fill out). The entire assessment is estimated to require 30–35 minutes to complete. A psychometrically trained administrator administers the test. The DAFS-R shows a more normal distribution than the original DAFS and no ceiling effect with community-living older adults.

Independent Living Scales (ILS) (Loeb, 1996). The ILS is a performance-based instrument designed to assess the degree to which adults are capable of caring for themselves and their property (Loeb, 1996). The ILS consists of 68 items, including 17 items comprising the subscale for Managing Money. There are also subscales for Memory/Orientation, Managing Home and Transportation, Health and Safety, and Social Adjustment. Summation of the five subscales reflects the individual's overall capacity to function independently in the community. The items were constructed specifically to be consistent with legal standards to enhance its value for expert testimony about capacities of the elderly in legal guardianship cases. The estimated assessment time is 45 minutes. Different aspects of competence can be identified and compared, using normative data and cut scores for the different subscales. Normative data are provided for adults 17 years of age and older without clinical diagnosis, as well as for those who have a psychiatric diagnosis, dementia, mental retardation, or traumatic brain injury.

Specific Performance-Based Measures of Financial Capacity

Financial Capacity Instrument (FCI) (Marson et al., 2000). The FCI is a standardized psychometric measure designed specifically to assess everyday financial activities and abilities in older adults with mild cognitive impairment and dementia. The FCI is based on a conceptual model that views financial capacity at three levels (see Table 3.1): specific financial abilities (tasks), broader financial activities (domains) important to independent functioning, and overall financial capacity (global score) (Marson, 2001; Marson et al., 2000). The current version of the FCI (FCI-9) directly assesses financial abilities across 20 tasks, nine domains, and two global scores. The FCI items range from testing more basic skills such as naming and counting coins/currency, and making one-item grocery purchases, to more complex skills such as managing a checkbook and register, managing a bank statement, and preparing bills for mailing. The primary global score measures overall performance across the first seven domains: basic monetary skills, financial conceptual knowledge, cash transactions, checkbook management, bank statement management, financial judgment, and bill payment. Two optional domains of the FCI are knowledge of personal assets and estate arrangements and investment decision making. Trained technicians administer and score the FCI. Administration time for the full FCI is 50 minutes for normal elderly patients and 60+ minutes for patients with dementia. Scoring of task, domain, and global performance is manualized and norm referenced. The FCI has demonstrated good internal, test–retest, and interrater reliabilities, as well as good content and construct validity (Marson, 2001; Marson et al., 2000). The FCI has been used in a range of research studies involving older adults with dementia (Griffith et al., 2003; Marson, 2001; Marson et al., 2000; Martin et al., 2008; Sherod et al., 2009; Triebel et al., 2009), and more recently patients with traumatic brain injury (TBI) (Dreer et al., in press).

Financial Competence Assessment Inventory (FCAI) (Kershaw & Webber, 2008). The FCAI is an individually administered performance instrument developed by investigators in Australia to assess different dimensions of financial abilities. The FCAI consists of 38 financial items in six domains: everyday financial abilities, financial judgment, estate management, debt management, cognitive functioning related to finances, and support resources. The FCAI can be used to determine strengths and weaknesses within six different components of financial competence, and also to assess support needs. Although the FCAI is suitable for individuals with and without cognitive impairment, it has been validated as a means of distinguishing individuals who are financially competent from those who are incompetent (i.e., individuals with a legally appointed guardian or conservator). The FCAI evaluates various aspects of financial competence linked to legal criteria for decisional competence, including "understanding," "appreciation," "reasoning," and "expressing a choice." The FCAI also measures other functional abilities that influence financial competence, such as support from others and functional cognitive abilities (i.e., basic reading and writing and numeracy).

Hopemont Capacity Assessment Interview (HCAI) (Edelstein, 1999). The HCAI is a semi-structured measure that uses vignettes to evaluate medical and financial decision-making capacity. The financial decision-making component is presented as three scenarios with related questions. The questions are modeled after four legal standards related to understanding relevant information, appreciation of consequences of alternatives, reasoning or weighing of costs and benefits, and the ability to make a choice. For each scenario the individual is asked basic questions about what he or she has heard, and is then asked to explain costs and benefits, make a choice from options presented in the scenario, and explain the reasoning behind that choice. The HCAI uses a semi-structured format for presenting general instructions, the scenarios, and follow-up questions on the rating form. Norms were intentionally not developed by Edelstein and his colleagues because of concerns about potential misuse.

Recent Review of Existing Performance Instruments Assessing Financial Capacity

A literature review conducted by Moore et al. (2007) recently identified and evaluated standardized performance-based instruments to assess functional living skills across a range of adult populations. The authors reviewed a total of 31 functional instruments (20 multi-domain batteries and 11 domain-specific instruments) and made specific recommendations regarding the use of currently available instruments. Although basic financial ability was assessed in a majority of batteries, the authors recommended the DAFS (Loewenstein et al., 1989), Everyday Functioning Battery (Heaton et al., 2004), and ILS (Loeb, 1996) as offering the most comprehensive financial assessment within the multidomain batteries. The FCI (Marson et al., 2000) was recommended as a domain-specific instrument for a thorough evaluation of financial capacity.

Clinical Interview Assessment of Financial Capacity

As noted above, financial capacity may also be directly assessed by a clinician via a specialized clinical interview. In addition to structured questions, such an interview can also include the semi-structured examination of specific performance skills. However, it remains distinct from formal performance assessment instruments that require standardized administration, a trained psychometrician, and more intensive material requirements. Clinical interview approaches also differ in that they do not yield quantitative scores, but rather categorical impairment ratings reflecting the clinician's judgments regarding a patient's various skills (e.g., capable/intact, marginally capable/marginal, incapable/impaired). Such categorical outcomes have clinical utility as they logically connect to issues of capacity, and can be more readily understood and applied by other clinicians and professionals than can informant ratings or quantitative performance scores.

Clinical Interview Measure for Assessing Financial Capacity

Semi-structured Clinical Interview for Financial Capacity (SCIFC) (Marson et al., 2009). The SCIFC was designed by Marson and colleagues as a clinician based, semi-structured interview and is based on the same conceptual model of financial capacity as the FCI. A semi-structured interview format provides the structure necessary for obtaining reliable and valid assessments, but also permits the clinical flexibility needed for individualized assessments of patients in the clinical setting. The SCIFC assesses eight financial domains, overall financial capacity, and also the patient's need for a formal financial conservatorship/guardianship. The eight domains assessed are basic monetary skills, financial conceptual knowledge, cash transactions, checkbook management, bank statement management, financial judgment, bill payment, and knowledge of personal assets and estate arrangements. The SCIFC takes approximately 25 minutes to administer by a clinician. The domain-based approach allows the clinician to preselect areas of assessment as needed, and to differentiate areas of independence and preserved autonomy from areas of deficit. The SCIFC combines verbally administered items (e.g., "What is money?") with performance items using simple props and testing materials (e.g., "Please identify these coins and currency."). Clinicians follow general scoring criteria for individual items but retain substantial autonomy regarding their clinical judgments of performance at the domain and overall capacity level. Clinical judgments for domain and global performance variables are categorical (capable, marginally capable, or incapable). The SCIFC has demonstrated good reliability as well as content and construct validity (Marson et al., 2009).

EMPIRICAL RESEARCH ON FINANCIAL CAPACITY

In this section, we discuss the existing empirical research on financial capacity. As noted above, until recently there have been relatively few studies in this area. As reflected below, most of the small body of work has been conducted in older adult and dementia populations (Griffith et al., 2003; Marson, 2001; Marson et al., 2000; Martin et al., 2008; Sherod et al., 2009; Triebel et al., 2009), with a few additional studies conducted in populations with severe mental illness (Barrett et al., 2009; Patterson, Goldman, McKibbon, Hughes, & Jeste, 2001).

Financial Capacity in Alzheimer's Disease and Mild Cognitive Impairment

Financial capacity in mild and moderate AD. Over the past 10 years, several studies using the FCI have investigated financial capacity in patients with AD (Marson, 2001; Marson et al., 2000). The original FCI (FCI-6) assessed six domains and 14 tasks (Marson et al., 2000) (the global level was introduced in later versions of the FCI). In an initial study, a sample of 23 older controls and 53 AD patients (30 with mild dementia and 23 with moderate dementia) was administered the FCI-6 (Marson et al., 2000). Mild AD patients performed equivalently to control subjects on the basic monetary skills domain, but significantly below controls on the other five domains. Moderate AD patients performed significantly below controls and mild AD patients on all domains. On the FCI tasks, mild AD patients performed equivalently to controls on simple tasks such as naming coins/currency, counting coins/currency, understanding parts of a checkbook, and detecting the risk of mail fraud. Mild AD patients performed significantly below controls on more complex tasks such as defining and applying financial concepts, obtaining change for vending machine use, using a checkbook, understanding and using a bank statement, and making an investment decision. Moderate AD patients performed significantly below controls and mild AD patients on all tasks (Marson, 2001; Marson et al., 2011; Marson et al., 2000).

Using a cut-score method derived from control group performance (Marson, 2001; Marson et al., 2000), the quantitative performance of the AD patients was translated into categorical outcomes (capable, marginally capable, incapable) on each domain. In the context of a prototype instrument and small control sample, the authors advised that these outcomes should be interpreted cautiously. However, mild AD patients demonstrated an interesting pattern of categorical impairment across the domains. Less than 30% of mild AD patients were found capable on complex domains of checkbook management and bank statement management, and less than 15% were found capable on financial judgment. Moderate AD patients, in turn, demonstrated very high rates of incapable outcomes on all FCI domains (range 90–100%). The relationship of the AD patients' dementia level to their capacity outcomes was statistically robust for all domains (Marson et al., 2011; Marson et al., 2000).

To our knowledge, this was the first empirical study of financial capacity in patients with AD, and very possibly the first empirical study of financial skills in any clinical population (Marson, 2001). The findings suggest that significant impairment of financial capacity occurs in AD, even in the early stages of the disease. Mild AD patients appear to experience deficits in complex financial abilities (tasks) and some level of impairment in almost all financial activities (domains). Moderate AD patients appear to experience loss of both simple and complex financial abilities and severe impairment across all financial activities. Based on these initial findings, Marson proposed two preliminary clinical guidelines for the assessment of financial capacity in patients with mild and moderate AD (Marson et al., 2000):

> (1) Mild AD patients are at significant risk for impairment in most financial activities, in particular complex activities like checkbook and bank statement management. Areas of preserved autonomous financial activity should be carefully evaluated and monitored.
> (2) Moderate AD patients are at great risk for loss of all financial activities. Although each AD patient must be considered individually, it is likely that most moderate AD patients will be unable to manage their financial affairs. (p. 883)

Declining financial capacity in patients with mild AD. A recent longitudinal study by Martin et al. (2008) using the FCI demonstrated that financial capacity declines rapidly in patients with mild AD over a one year period. Financial capacity was assessed at baseline and 1-year follow-up in a sample of 55 individuals with mild AD and 63 healthy older adults. Baseline results from this study replicated our prior findings and indicated that patients with mild AD exhibit near global financial capacity deficits relative to same-aged cognitively intact peers. At one year follow-up, participants in the mild AD group exhibited marked declines in overall financial capacity and on the majority of financial capacity domains. In contrast, the healthy older adults exhibited intact and stable financial performance over the course of the study. Overall, the mild AD group exhibited relatively rapid decline over one year, with an overall 10% decline from their original baseline performance relative to controls (Marson et al., 2011; Martin et al., 2008).

Financial capacity in patients with mild cognitive impairment. Financial capacity has also been investigated in patients with MCI. As noted above, MCI represents an intermediate and often transitional phase between normal cognitive aging and dementia (Petersen et al., 2001). Patients with MCI show less functional impairment than is characteristic of dementia but nevertheless show clear declines in instrumental activities of daily living over time (Daly et al., 2000; Griffith et al., 2003; Marson et al., 2011; Petersen et al., 2001; Ritchie, Artero, & Touchon, 2001).

In an initial study, financial capacity was assessed using the FCI-9 in a cross-sectional sample of 21 older controls, 21 patients with amnestic MCI (aMCI), and 22 patients with mild AD (Griffith et al., 2003; Marson et al., 2011). We found that at the task level, controls performed significantly better than the mild AD group on most abilities, with the exception of simple tasks of basic monetary skills, cash transactions, and telephone fraud (Griffith et al., 2003; Marson et al., 2011). Controls performed significantly better than the MCI group on tasks of applying financial concepts, understanding and using a bank statement, understanding bills, and preparing bills for mailing. The MCI group, in turn, demonstrated significantly higher scores than the AD group on tasks of understanding and applying financial concepts, using a vending machine, understanding and using a checkbook, understanding and using a bank statement, prioritizing bills, and preparing bills for mailing. There were no tasks on which the MCI group performed better than controls. At the broader domain level, controls performed significantly better than mild AD subjects on all domains except knowledge of assets and estate. Controls performed significantly better than the MCI group on the domains of financial concepts, checkbook management, bank statement management, financial judgment, and bill payment. There were no domains on which the MCI group performed better than controls. In turn, the MCI group performed significantly better than mild AD patients on all domains except financial judgment and knowledge of assets and estate. For overall financial capacity (domains 1–7), control participants performed significantly better than MCI and AD participants, and MCI participants performed significantly better than AD participants.

This study represents one of the first published reports of performance-based evidence for higher order functional decline and capacity loss in MCI. Using a direct assessment approach, patients with aMCI demonstrated significant, albeit mild, deficits on some (but not all) financial abilities compared to age, education, gender, and racially matched healthy controls. MCI patients showed a decline in overall financial capacity of 1.74 SD units compared to control subjects. These results suggest that initial declines in financial capacity begin in MCI prior to the development of a frank dementia (Griffith et al., 2003; Marson et al., 2011).

Declining financial capacity in aMCI. Financial capacity has also been shown to decline in a subset of aMCI patients who converted to AD over a one year period (Triebel et al., 2009). Using the FCI, this longitudinal study investigated change in financial capacity in relation to conversion from MCI to dementia. Performance on the FCI domain and global scores was compared within and between groups of cognitively healthy controls, MCI patients who converted to Alzheimer-type dementia (MCI converters), and MCI patients who did not convert to dementia (MCI nonconverters) using multivariate repeated measures analyses (age as a covariate). These analyses revealed significant group differences on FCI variables and also group-by-time interactions.

As shown in Table 3.2, controls at baseline performed better than MCI converters and nonconverters on almost all FCI domains and on both FCI total scores, replicating prior cross-sectional findings in patients with MCI (Griffith et al., 2003), and indicating that impairment of financial capacity in MCI had already occurred prior to baseline assessment. At one year follow-up, MCI converters demonstrated decline relative to controls and MCI nonconverters for checkbook management and for both FCI total scores. A strong trend emerged for bank statement management. MCI converters showed declines in procedural skills associated with checkbook management and bank statement management, such as calculating the correct balance in a checkbook register. Declines did not occur in the conceptual understanding of a checkbook or a bank statement. This study indicated that declines in financial capacity are detectable in patients with aMCI in the year prior to conversion to AD.

Neuropsychological Predictors of Financial Capacity

Given the limited research on financial capacity as a construct, and the limited number of available instruments, there have been correspondingly few neuropsychological studies of this capacity (Marson et al., 2011). However, a relatively recent study by the Marson group using the FCI examined cognitive predictors of financial capacity in a sample of healthy older controls (n = 85), aMCI patients (n = 113), and mild AD patients (n = 43) (Sherod et al., 2009). The goal of this study was to develop and compare multivariate cognitive models of financial capacity across the continuum from normal aging to dementia. Robust cognitive models of financial capacity emerged for each group. Written arithmetic skill (WRAT-3 Arithmetic) was the primary predictor of financial capacity across all three models, accounting for 27% of variance (control model), 46% (mild AD model), and 55% (aMCI model). Visuomotor tracking/executive function (Trails A/B) was a secondary cognitive predictor of financial capacity across the two patient models. Short-term verbal memory and visuomotor tracking/executive function were secondary predictors for the normal aging group. This study demonstrated that similar neurocognitive predictor models of financial capacity emerge across the dementia spectrum of normal cognitive aging, MCI, and mild AD. In particular, the findings strongly implicated written arithmetic skills as a critical cognitive function subserving financial capacity performance in both normal cognitive aging and neurodegenerative disease.

Neuroimaging and Financial Capacity

Some exciting initial neuroimaging research has recently been conducted examining the relationships between brain structure and financial capacity (Griffith et al., 2010). In this study, magnetic resonance imaging (MRI) structural volumetrics were examined in relation to FCI performance in patients with aMCI. Using 3.0-Tesla MRI, T1 images were acquired in 38 patients with aMCI and 28 older controls matched for age, sex, and race. This study examined volumes of cortical

Table 3.2. One-Year Change in FCI Variables across Groups

		Controls		MCI Nonconverters		MCI Converters			
		Time 1	Time 2	Time 1	Time 2	Time 1	Time 2		
	Range	*n* = 76	*n* = 76	*n* = 62	*n* = 62	*n* = 25	*n* = 25	Baseline*	Interaction†
D1. Basic Monetary Skills	0–34	32.1 (2.7)	32.7 (2.3)	30.6 (3.8)	30.3 (3.9)	29.2 (4.7)	28.4 (5.6)	<0.001[a]	0.064
D2. Financial Concepts	0–2	29.3 (2.5)	29.9 (2.1)	27.9 (4.0)	27.5 (4.5)	24.9 (5.7)	24.7 (5.6)	<0.001[b]	0.174
D3. Cash Transactions	0–24	21.7 (2.0)	21.7 (2.2)	20.5 (3.0)	19.9 (3.3)	18.7 (4.7)	17.6 (4.7)	<0.001[b]	0.134
D4. Checkbook Management	0–50	48.2 (2.7)	48.2 (2.6)	46.9 (3.6)	47.0 (3.8)	44.6 (6.1)	40.8 (7.9)	<0.001[a]	0.001 [c]
D5. Bank Statement Management	0–39	35.4 (3.1)	34.7 (3.3)	31.9 (5.4)	31.6 (6.0)	28.0 (6.8)	24.9 (9.5)	<0.001[b]	0.021
D6. Financial Management	0–16	13.9 (2.4)	14.7 (1.6)	13.9 (2.9)	14.1 (2.9)	12.5 (2.8)	12.4 (3.6)	0.002 [a]	0.190
D7. Bill Payment	0–46	44.4 (2.4)	43.9 (4.0)	40.2 (6.2)	41.3 (6.1)	35.8 (9.0)	33.5 (10.6)	<0.001[b]	0.124
D9. Investment Decisions	0–17	14.3 (2.4)	14.5 (2.4)	12.9 (3.1)	12.2 (3.3)	11.6 (4.4)	10.5 (4.4)	<0.001[a]	0.056
FCI Total Score (Domains 1–7)	0–241	225.0 (9.9)	225.9 (11.9)	212.0 (20.9)	211.5 (22.2)	193.7 (29.6)	182.3 (39.0)	<0.001[b]	0.002 [c]
FCI Total Score (Domains 1–7, 9)	0–258	239.3 (10.9)	240.4 (13.0)	224.9 (22.8)	223.7 (24.2)	205.3 (32.4)	192.8 (42.3)	<0.001[b]	0.001[c]

*Baseline group comparison on FCI variables between controls, MCI nonconverters, and MCI converters.
†Time × diagnostic group interaction over one year on FCI variables between control, MCI nonconverter, and MCI converter groups.
MANCOVA (age entered as covariate) was the statistic employed.
[a]Controls > MCI nonconverters, MCI converters.
[b]Controls > MCI nonconverters > MCI converters.
[c]MCI converters showed greater decline compared to controls and MCI nonconverters.
Reprinted with permission from Triebel et al. (2009), the American Academy of Neurology.

regions identified in fMRI activation studies (Greicius, Supekar, Menon, & Dougherty, 2009; Rombouts, Barkhof, Goekoop, Stam, & Scheltens, 2005) and structural imaging studies (Greicius et al., 2009; Seeley, Crawford, Zhou, Miller, & Greicius, 2009) as components of the default mode network (DMN) that shows early change in AD. Specific neuroanatomical areas examined were the hippocampi, posterior cingulate/precuneus, medial frontal lobes, and angular gyri. MRI images were obtained the same day or within 2 months of participants' FCI assessment.

Images were processed using structural volumetrics and voxel-based morphometry (VBM). With respect to volumetrics, angular gyrus volumes in the parietal lobe correlated most strongly with the FCI score (posterior cingulate/precuneus correlated at 0.32 and medial frontal lobe region at 0.31). Using stepwise regression, angular gyrus volume was the sole predictor of FCI score in the aMCI group, accounting for 19% of variance. Regarding VBM, a positive association with FCI score was detected for a cluster at Montreal Neurological Institute (MNI) coordinates corresponding to the angular gyrus in the parietal cortex. The findings were both intriguing and neuropsychologically plausible: volume of the angular gyrus, a neuroanatomical region that subserves numeracy and higher order arithmetic functions in the brain, is linked to financial capacity performance in patients with prodromal AD.

The study also sought to identify specific cognitive mediators of the brain volume–financial capacity relationships. Both Spatial Span (Wechsler, 1997) and WRAT-3 Arithmetic (Wilkinson, 1993) met assumptions for possible mediation, correlating significantly both with angular gyri volume as well as with FCI score. The Sobel test (Sobel, 1982) was used to determine whether these variables mediated the angular gyrus–FCI relationship. WRAT-3 Arithmetic was statistically significant, whereas Spatial Span showed a trend ($p = 0.07$). Thus, the Arithmetic score was a partial mediator and Spatial Span a possible partial mediator of the angular gyrus–FCI score relationship in patients with MCI.

To our knowledge, this is the first imaging study that has sought to identify relationships between brain volume, cognitive impairment, and financial capacity. In addition to its significance to the study of financial capacity, the study augurs the potential contribution of advanced techniques in neuroscience to our understanding of capacity issues more generally.

Studies of Financial Capacity in Other Clinical Populations

There has been empirical research in the area of financial capacity of patients with severe mental illness. Barrett et al. (2009) examined financial abilities using the Direct Assessment of Functional Status (DAFS) scale in patients with schizophrenia or schizoaffective disorder (Barrett et al., 2009). The purpose of the study was to investigate the criterion validity of the financial skills subscale of the DAFS in differentiating 25 outpatients with severe mental illness who managed their finances independently from 24 outpatients who needed assistance managing finances and had a court-appointed guardian or representative payee. In addition, 25 participants without mental illness were used as a control group. Logistic regression analyses, Bayesian statistics, and Receiver Operating Characteristic analyses revealed moderate classification accuracy with the DAFS financial skills subscale in a sample with mild cognitive impairment. The Mini-Mental State Examination (MMSE) was less accurate than the DAFS financial skills subscale at predicting group status. The authors concluded that the DAFS financial skills subscale could be used by clinicians to assess financial capacity of individuals with severe mental illness.

Patterson and his group at the University of California San Diego have also examined financial capacity in psychiatric populations, but as part of a broader assessment of functional abilities [UCSD Performance-Based Skills Assessment (UPSA)] (Patterson et al., 2001). In the initial validation study, the UPSA was administered to 50 middle-aged and older outpatients with schizophrenia or schizoaffective disorder and 20 normal controls. Patients with schizophrenia or schizoaffective disorder performed significantly below controls on all five domains of the UPSA, including the financial domain. This battery is now an established part of many clinical trials in schizophrenia and related mental disorders.

GENERAL RECOMMENDATIONS FOR NEUROPSYCHOLOGICAL ASSESSMENT OF FINANCIAL CAPACITY

1. At the outset, identify and clarify the specific referral question(s) relevant to financial capacity.

Clinicians should identify and clarify financial capacity issues at the outset of the evaluation. In some cases, multiple "financial" issues may be intertwined, and sorting them out ahead of time will be essential to conducting an effective evaluation. For example, seek to identify how general or narrow the issue may be. For example, is this a matter related to overall financial capacity and need for a conservatorship, or a more narrow issue of contractual capacity for a specific transaction, or both? Is the referral seeking a prospective evaluation of an individual's financial capacity, or a retrospective judgment of his or her financial capacity at some earlier point of time?

2. At the outset, identify the patient's premorbid level of financial capacity.

It is important for the clinician to form a clear picture of the patient's premorbid level of financial functioning as part of conducting the evaluation. Knowledge ahead of time of a patient's premorbid financial skills will inform the kinds of questions and testing that should be pursued in answering the referral questions. For example, if a patient has never managed a checkbook during his or her life, it does not make sense to test the patient's ability to complete a checkbook register, and we cannot attribute deficits on such a checkbook task to the effects of a neurocognitive disorder. Thus knowledge of premorbid financial functioning is essential for the clinician to draw meaningful conclusions regarding the patient's current financial capacity and possible deficits or declines in financial skills.

3. In prospectively assessing financial capacity, focus on functional information from capacity-specific measures as the core evidence.

In assessing financial capacity, the core evidence will be functional data regarding the patient's specific financial skills and abilities, viewed in relation to the current demands of his or her economic and psychosocial context (Grisso, 2003). Accordingly, it is important to ask financial capacity questions, and administer financial capacity measures, that will provide this capacity-specific evidence. Thus, in addition to general clinical interview questions, the use of informant questionnaires/rating forms and direct performance measures related to financial capacity is essential. A number of these measures are discussed above.

Neuropsychologists must be wary of relying on capacity-remote cognitive measures, such as the much vaunted Trails B, as an acceptable proxy for capacity-specific financial information. Trails B does not convey any capacity-specific information regarding an individual's financial functioning. It is not itself a replacement for collateral report or direct performance evidence of financial functioning. Similarly, diagnosis by itself, such as TBI or schizophrenia, cannot be dispositive of a question of financial capacity. The specific functional abilities constituent to financial capacity in the individual's personal context must be evaluated (Grisso, 2003), and this requires capacity-level information. Put differently, diagnosis and neuropsychological test findings are secondary levels of evidence in a financial capacity assessment.

4. In retrospective evaluations of financial capacity, obtain capacity, neuropsychological, mental status, and other evidence contemporaneous with the financial transaction at issue in the case.

In retrospective evaluations, the clinician is asked to evaluate whether a patient had financial capacity at an earlier point in time. Such retrospective assessments most frequently arise in forensic cases in which a legal issue of capacity has been raised. Such evaluations can be challenging, depending on the nature and extent of the available evidence of capacity relevant to the past transaction. The clinician in such cases should seek to obtain all of the capacity, neuropsychological, mental status, medical, and lay testimony evidence that exists that is relevant to and contemporaneous with the legal transaction at issue. An informative discussion of retrospective evaluation of capacity can be found in the American Bar Association/American Psychological Association Capacity Assessment Handbook for Psychologists (American Bar Association/American Psychological Association Assessment of Capacity in Older Adults Project Working Group, 2008).

5. Neuropsychological testing can inform all financial capacity evaluations by providing explanatory links between the diagnostic condition and specific impairments in financial capacity.

Although neuropsychological test results by themselves do not represent or implicate capacity findings, they play a very valuable role in capacity evaluations and should be incorporated into such assessments wherever possible. Neurocognitive findings can provide the explanatory links that tie a condition such as acute traumatic brain injury to specific impairments in financial skills. Thus, an acutely injured patient with moderate or severe TBI, involving intraparenchymal hemorrhage and frontal contusions, may demonstrate a neurocognitive profile reflecting characteristic impairments in attention, short-term memory, and executive function. These cognitive deficits can then be meaningfully related to corresponding deficits in the TBI patient's financial knowledge, performance, and judgment skills, as elicited by financial capacity questions and measures. In conjunction with other evidence, specific neurocognitive deficits can also raise persuasive inferences that certain financial skills, such as awareness of fraud risk or complex financial decision making, were probably impaired at critical points in a patient's disease process.

SUMMARY

Financial capacity is a medical–legal construct that represents the ability to independently manage one's financial affairs in a manner consistent with one's self-interest and values (Marson & Hebert, 2008). In this chapter, we have examined conceptual, clinical assessment, and research aspects of financial capacity from a neuropsychological perspective, using dementias of aging as our primary clinical focus. Conceptually, we have emphasized the importance of financial capacity as an IADL critical to both independent functioning and personal autonomy, and noted that it comprises important performance and judgment dimensions. We have articulated a working conceptual model of financial capacity that can inform clinical practice and that has been the basis of a growing body of empirical research.

From a clinical standpoint, we underscored the importance of evaluating or estimating premorbid financial capacity prior to conducting a financial capacity evaluation. We then presented three assessment approaches of informant report, direct performance, and clinical interview, along with brief descriptions of actual instruments representative of each approach. The neuropsychological case study appended at the end of the chapter demonstrates the use of performance-based assessment of financial capacity, as well as an approach to report organization and writing in this area.

In terms of research, we focused on empirical studies of financial capacity in older adults with MCI and dementia, as the majority of extant studies of financial capacity are found in this population. A study of neurocognitive predictors of financial capacity found that a common predictor model based on written arithmetic and executive function measures was predictive of performance across the dementia spectrum of normal cognitive aging, aMCI, and AD. Finally, an exciting research development is the emerging use of neuroimaging techniques as a means to better understand the specific changes in the brain that ultimately lead to "downstream" impairment of financial skills and capacity in patients with neurodegenerative disease. Using these techniques, investigators are positioned to develop a true "neuroscience" of financial capacity that will advance both clinical practice and research.

EXAMPLE OF A NEUROPSYCHOLOGICAL REPORT THAT INCLUDES A FINANCIAL CAPACITY ASSESSMENT

The following is an edited and anonymized neuropsychological report concerning an older adult with dementia that includes a prospective assessment of his financial capacity.

Background Information

Mr. Patient, a 75-year-old widowed white male and construction business owner with a sixth-grade education, was referred as an outpatient to the Neuropsychology Clinic by his daughter, Ms. Daughter, and her attorney, Mr. Legal, Esq., for evaluation of the patient's cognitive and emotional status and capacity to manage his business and financial affairs.

Mr. Patient reportedly has a 3- to 5-year history of memory problems, which reportedly developed insidiously and have become progressively worse. He reportedly has not been previously evaluated for these problems.

In interview, Mr. Patient stated that he does not have any problems with his memory. He also generally denied any other cognitive or functional problems. He stated that he does not have any help at home, but that his daughter comes by sometimes to help him pay bills or to bring him groceries. He denied problems with his driving. Regarding mood or personality changes, he reported that he is "doing fine" and denied any symptoms of depression or anxiety.

Mr. Patient's daughter, Ms. Daughter, described a much more serious situation. Ms. Daughter said that her father has had memory problems for at least 5 years, and that his memory has become noticeably worse over the past 3 years. She said that she first noticed something was different when she left her accounting job in the family business in 1998 over some disagreements with her uncle James, who co-owns the business with her father. She said that her father did not seem to be supporting her, which was uncharacteristic of him. She said that she later realized that her father was forgetting about these disagreements and his role in resolving them. Ms. Daughter reported that he currently asks the same question repeatedly, forgets conversations, and constantly misplaces items. She said that he has more trouble remembering people's names. She said that he has comprehension problems, but pretends to understand people when they talk to him. She reported that when they go to restaurants, he gets lost on his way back from the restroom. She reported that he has not driven since July 2000 when he had lung surgery. She said that just prior to that, he complained to her about getting lost while driving in a familiar area.

Regarding functional changes, Ms. Daughter reported that her father has no meaningful activities around the home. He has had full-time caregivers since July 2000. She noted that he still cannot remember their names. She reported that prior to these home healthcare arrangements, her father was not bathing and was wearing the same clothes every day. She reported that she has handled all of her father's bills since October 2000. She said that she also tries to supervise his business transactions. Ms. Daughter reported that her father co-owns an excavation business, Happy Valley Construction, with his brother James. The business is located in Columbus, Georgia. Mr. Patient reportedly has a separate business where he also buys, develops, and sells real estate. She stated that her father has agreed on several occasions to consult her before signing any business documents, but then forgets to do so.

Ms. Daughter reported several poor business decisions her father has made recently. She said that in the past year he sold a piece of real estate for $10,000 that was worth $250,000. She also reported that he has made almost $500,000 in loans to the family business over the past 2 years, and that these loans have not been repaid. She reported that her father initially loaned $200,000 to Happy Valley in 1998, $90,000 of which went to his nephew, who also works for the company. She stated that there does not appear to be a note for the loan to his nephew. She reported that the remaining $300,000 was loaned out in October 2000. Ms. Daughter said that she has also recently discovered a buy/sell agreement, signed by her father while she was out of town, that states that if her father dies, the company will go to her uncle James and the money owed by the company to her father will be forgiven. She noted that in this buy/sell agreement, some property that belongs to her father is listed instead as company property.

Regarding mood or personality changes, Ms. Daughter reported that her father is more laid back and even indifferent. She said that he used to be very focused on and concerned about his business affairs, but now does not seem concerned about them. She denied symptoms of anxiety or depression, but noted that he naps a lot during the day. She also stated that he always wants to eat because he forgets that he has already eaten.

Social/Academic/Occupational History: *Mr. Patient reportedly was born and raised in Columbus, Georgia. He reported that he had four brothers and sisters. The patient's father was a farmer and iron smith. The patient was reportedly married for 40 years when his wife died in 1990. He reported that he has two daughters and one son with a disability. He currently lives alone.*

Mr. Patient reportedly completed 6 years of education. He reportedly buys and sells real estate and co-owns an excavation business called Happy Valley Construction Company.

Prior Medical History: *Mr. Patient's medical history reportedly is significant for diabetes and a history of blood clots. His surgical history reportedly includes four-way coronary artery bypass graft (1989) and partial lung resection (2000).*

The patient reportedly does not drink alcohol and does not smoke. There is reportedly no history of alcohol or other substance abuse.

Family medical history is reportedly positive for myocardial infarction in his brother, stomach cancer in his sister, skin cancer in his sister, and possible AD in his mother.

Psychiatric History: *Mr. Patient reportedly has no history of mental health treatment. As noted above, he reportedly has had no prior evaluations for his memory problems.*

Medications: *Mr. Patient takes coumadin, Exelon, Tenormin, ginkgo biloba, Ambien, Detrol, and Claritin.*

Behavioral Observations

Mr. Patient presented as a well-groomed, nicely dressed 75-year-old white man. He was accompanied to the evaluation by his daughter.

In the interview, the patient's speech was fluent and reasonably goal-directed but lacked spontaneity. Responses were impoverished. Comprehension appeared generally intact. Affect was mildly constricted, and mood was cordial but with occasional irritability. Insight was judged to be very poor. There was no indication or report of formal hallucinations or delusions, or of a thought or perceptual disorder. There was no indication or report of suicidal ideation, plan, or intent.

During testing, Mr. Patient was alert and pleasant but would quickly become irritable and uncooperative. He exhibited mild performance anxiety. He displayed task frustration by abandoning or avoiding tasks. He showed no response to encouragement from the psychometric technician. He displayed an inability to complete some tasks due to comprehension problems. He made a few perseverative and intrusion errors. He required constant redirection to the task. He showed a complete lack of test-taking strategies.

Mr. Patient was irritable and at times uncooperative during the testing. At one point, he refused to continue testing and started to leave, but was persuaded by his daughter to continue. Because of his reluctance to participate, and the examiner's concern that he would prematurely terminate the testing, only an abbreviated test battery could be administered. Nevertheless, sufficient information was obtained to respond fully to the referral questions. Overall, the patient appeared to put forth a variable but acceptable effort during the testing. Much of his reluctance to participate related to tasks that he appeared unable to perform. Overall, the current test results are an accurate representation of Mr. Patient's current levels of cognitive and emotional functioning and of his current financial abilities.

Tests Administered

California Verbal Learning Test–II (CVLT-II)
Clinical Interview
Cognitive Competency
Executive Clock Drawing Task (CLOX)

Financial Capacity Instrument
Geriatric Depression Scale (GDS)
Mattis Dementia Rating Scale (DRS)
Token Test
Trails A and B
WAB Auditory Comprehension
Wide Range Achievement Test-3 (Reading subtest)

IMPRESSIONS AND SUMMARY

Neuropsychological Findings

1. Probable Dementia, Currently Moderate (DRS = 89/144, CDR = 2.0)

The neuropsychological test results were consistent with probable moderate dementia. Evidence for this impression included severe impairment on a dementia screening instrument and impairments in high-load verbal learning, recall, and recognition memory (severe to profound), simple short-term verbal recall (severe), orientation to time (severe), orientation to place (severe), simple auditory comprehension (severe), reading abilities (moderate), visuospatial construction of a clock drawing (mild), simple visuomotor tracking (mild), propositional auditory comprehension (moderate), and spontaneous construction of a clock drawing (severe). The patient was unable to complete a measure of visuomotor tracking/set flexibility. In addition, the patient's daughter reported that he has had progressive memory and other cognitive problems for as long as 5 years.

Functional testing and interview data were also consistent with moderate dementia. Mr. Patient was severely impaired on a cognitive measure of everyday problem-solving abilities. On a functional measure of financial capacity, the patient showed intact performance only on simple tasks of naming coins/currency, coin/currency relationships, and single and multiitem grocery purchases. He demonstrated significant impairment on tests of counting coins/currency, understanding financial concepts, making change for a vending machine, tipping, conceptual understanding of a checkbook/register, pragmatic use of a checkbook/register, conceptual understanding of a bank statement, use of a bank statement, detection of telephone fraud, conceptual understanding of bills, identifying and prioritizing bills, and knowledge of his personal financial assets and activities.

In addition, Mr. Patient's daughter indicated that he currently has no meaningful activities around the home and requires home healthcare aides around the clock. She reported that prior to these arrangements, the patient was not bathing and wore the same clothes every day.

2. Possible AD

Mr. Patient's neurocognitive profile was consistent with possible AD. High-load verbal learning, recall, and recognition memory were moderately to severely impaired and he was unable to benefit from semantic or recognition cueing. He showed 0% recall after a short delay, which is consistent with the rapid decay of information over delay seen in AD. In addition, he had 0% short-term recall of verbal items from the memory subtest of the DRS. Characteristic impairments were found on measures of executive function (simple visuomotor tracking, propositional auditory comprehension, spontaneous clock drawing, and visuomotor tracking/set flexibility). Due to the patient's reluctance to cooperate with testing, a more comprehensive evaluation of memory, attention, expressive language, and verbal intellectual abilities was not possible.

The clinical course was consistent with AD. Mr. Patient's cognitive difficulties reportedly have progressed slowly and insidiously over the past 5 years. He also has a family history of possible AD.

In the examiner's judgment, it is likely that Mr. Patient has AD. However, he needs a neurological work-up for dementia before the clinical diagnosis can be established more conclusively.

Capacity Findings

3. Probable Current Incapacity to Manage Financial Affairs

History, interview information, and test data indicated that Mr. Patient is currently incapable of managing his financial affairs and making business-related decisions. In the interview, Mr. Patient demonstrated inaccurate knowledge of his financial and business affairs. For example, the patient indicated that he goes into work at his excavation business every day, even occasionally running construction equipment, whereas the patient's daughter reported that he is retired and that his brother operates and manages the business on his own. She reported that her father continues to manage his own finances, but makes poor business decisions (e.g., he recently sold some property for 10% of its value). She reported that her father has agreed several times not to sign anything without letting her review it first, but then forgets to consult her. She said that he has also made several large loans to his business recently, but seems generally unaware of these loans and the fact that they are not being repaid.

Direct performance testing revealed an overall severe impairment in financial capacity. Mr. Patient was impaired on tests of counting coins/currency, understanding financial concepts, making change for a vending machine, tipping, conceptual understanding of a checkbook, use of a checkbook, conceptual understanding of a bank statement, use of a bank statement, detection of telephone fraud, conceptual understanding of bills, identifying and prioritizing bills, and knowledge of personal financial activities. He demonstrated intact performance only on relatively simple tasks of naming coins/currency, coin/currency relationships, and single and multiitem cash purchases.

Taken together, these findings indicate that Mr. Patient is no longer capable of managing his business and financial affairs, and are consistent with his moderate dementia and near global cognitive deficits. Given Mr. Patient's progressive dementia, this finding of financial incapacity is unlikely to change.

Recommendations

1. *We recommend that Mr. Patient be referred to the Memory Disorders Clinic for a full neurological and dementia evaluation.*
2. *Continued pharmacotherapy with cholinesterase inhibitors appears to be appropriate.*
3. *Mr. Patient and his family should consider legally securing his business, financial, and personal affairs as soon as possible. Mr. Patient could potentially benefit from both a guardianship and a conservatorship.*
4. *Mr. Patient's cognitive and emotional status should continue to be closely monitored. This evaluation would provide a useful baseline if follow-up testing were indicated.*

The above case study/report was adapted from the handbook Assessment of Older Adults with Diminished Capacity: A Handbook for Psychologists, American Bar Association/American Psychological Association Assessment of Capacity in Older Adults Project Working Group. (2008). Washington, D.C.: American Bar Association and American Psychological Association. It is reprinted here with the permission of the copyright holders.

ACKNOWLEDGMENTS

This study was supported by the National Institute on Aging [2 RO1 AG021927 (Marson, PI), and P50 AG16582 (Marson, PI)] and the National Institute on Child Health and Human Development (R01HD053074) (Marson, PI). The authors express gratitude to the hundreds of participants and families who contributed to the financial capacity research studies discussed above.

References

American Bar Association/American Psychological Association Assessment of Capacity in Older Adults Project Working Group. (2008). *Assessment of older adults with diminished capacity: A handbook for psychologists.* Washington, D.C.: American Bar Association and American Psychological Association.

Barrett, J. J., Hart, K. J., Schmerler, J. T., Willmarth, K., Carey, J. A., & Mohammed, S. (2009). Criterion validity of the financial skills subscale of the direct assessment of functional status scale. *Psychiatry Research, 166*, 148–157.

Blessed, G., Tomlinson, B. E., & Roth, M. (1968). The association between quantitative measures of dementia and of senile change in the cerebral grey matter of elderly subjects. *British Journal of Psychiatry, 114*, 797–811.

Daly, E., Zaitchik, D., Copeland, M., Schmahmann, J., Gunther, J., & Albert, M. (2000). Predicting conversion to Alzheimer disease using standardized clinical information. *Archives of Neurology, 57*, 675–680.

Dreer, L. E., DeVivo, M. J., Novack, T. A., & Marson, D. (in press). Assessment of financial capacity in patients with TBI: A six-month longitudinal study. *Rehabilitation Psychology.*

Edelstein, B. (1999). *Hopemont Capacity Assessment Interview manual and scoring guide.* West Virginia University: Author.

Gelinas, I., Gauthier, L., McIntyre, M., & Gauthier, S. (1999). Development of a functional measure for persons with Alzheimer's disease: The disability assessment for dementia. *American Journal of Occupational Therapy, 53*, 471–481.

Greicius, M. D., Supekar, K., Menon, V., & Dougherty, R. F. (2009). Resting-state functional connectivity reflects structural connectivity in the default mode network. *Cerebral Cortex, 19*, 72–80.

Griffith, H. R., Belue, K., Sicola, A., Krzywanski, S., Zamrini, E., Harrell, L., et al. (2003). Impaired financial abilities in mild cognitive impairment: A direct assessment approach. *Neurology, 60*, 449–457.

Griffith, H. R., Stewart, C. C., Stoeckel, L. E., Okonkwo, O. C., den Hollander, J. A., Martin, R. C., et al. (2010). MRI volume of the angular gyri predicts financial skill deficits in patients with amnestic mild cognitive impairment. *Journal of the American Geriatrics Society, 58*, 265–274.

Grisso, T. (1986). *Evaluating competencies: Forensic assessments and instruments.* New York: Plenum Press.

Grisso, T. (2003). *Evaluating competencies: Forensic assessments and instruments* (2nd ed.). New York: Kluwer Academic.

Heaton, R. K., Marcotte, T. D., Mindt, M. R., Sadek, J., Moore, D. J., Bentley, H., et al. (2004). The impact of HIV-associated neuropsychological impairment on everyday functioning. *Journal of the International Neuropsychological Society, 10*, 317–331.

Kershaw, M., & Webber, L. (2008). Assessment of financial competence. *Psychiatry, Psychology, and Law, 15*, 40–55.

Lawton, M., & Brody, E. (1969). Assessment of older people: Self-maintaining and instrumental activities of daily living. *The Gerontologist, 9*, 179–185.

Loeb, P. (1996). *Independent Living Scales Manual.* San Antonio, TX: The Psychological Corporation.

Loewenstein, D., Amigo, E., Duara, R., Guterman, A., Hurwitz, D., Berkowitz, N., et al. (1989). A new scale for the assessment of functional status in Alzheimer's disease and related disorders. *Journal of Gerontology: Psychological Sciences, 44*, 114–121.

Marson, D. C. (2001). Loss of financial capacity in dementia: Conceptual and empirical approaches. *Aging, Neuropsychology and Cognition, 8*, 164–181.

Marson, D. C. (October 2002). *Assessment of civil competencies in the elderly: Theory, research, and clinical case studies.* Paper presented at the annual meeting of the National Academy of Neuropsychology, Miami, Florida.

Marson, D. C., & Hebert, K. (2008). Financial capacity. In B. L. Cutler (Ed.), *Encyclopedia of psychology and the law* (Vol. 1, pp. 313–316). Thousand Oaks, CA: Sage.

Marson, D. C., Hebert, K., & Solomon, A. (2011). Assessing civil competencies in older adults with dementia: Consent capacity, financial capacity, and testamentary capacity. In G. J. Larrabee (Ed.), *Forensic neuropsychology: A scientific approach* (2nd ed., pp. 334–377). New York: Oxford University Press.

Marson, D. C., Martin, R. C., Wadley, V., Griffith, H. R., Snyder, S., Belue, K., et al. (2009). Clinical interview assessment of financial capacity in older adults with mild cognitive impairment and dementia. *Journal of the American Geriatric Society, 54*, 806–814.

Marson, D. C., Sawrie, S. M., Snyder, S., McInturff, B., Stalvey, T., Boothe, A., et al. (2000). Assessing financial capacity in patients with Alzheimer disease: A conceptual model and prototype instrument. *Archives of Neurology, 57*, 877–884.

Martin, R., Griffith, H. R., Belue, K., Harrell, L., Zamrini, E., Anderson, B., et al. (2008). Declining financial capacity in patients with mild Alzheimer disease: A one-year longitudinal study. *American Journal of Geriatric Psychiatry, 16*, 209–219.

McDougall, G. J., Becker, H., Vaughan, P. W., Acee, T. W., & Delville, C. L. (2010). The revised direct assessment of functional status for independent older adults. *Gerontologist, 50*, 363–370.

Moore, D. J., Palmer, B. W., Patterson, T. L., & Jeste, D. V. (2007). A review of performance-based measures of functional living skills. *Journal of Psychiatry Research, 41*, 97–118.

Patterson, T., Goldman, S., McKibbon, C., Hughes, T., & Jeste, D. (2001). UCSD performance-based skills assessment: Development of a new measure of everyday functioning for severely mentally ill adults. *Schizophrenia Bulletin, 27*, 235–245.

Petersen, R. C., Doody, R., Kurz, A., Mohs, R. C., Morris, J. C., Rabins, P. V., et al. (2001). Current concepts in mild cognitive impairment. *Archives of Neurology, 58*, 1985–1992.

Ritchie, K., Artero, S., & Touchon, J. (2001). Classification criteria for mild cognitive impairment: A population based validation study. *Neurology, 56*, 37–42.

Rombouts, S. A., Barkhof, F., Goekoop, R., Stam, C. J., & Scheltens, P. (2005). Altered resting state networks in mild cognitive impairment and mild Alzheimer's disease: An fMRI study. *Human Brain Mapping, 26*, 231–239.

Seeley, W. W., Crawford, R. K., Zhou, J., Miller, B. L., & Greicius, M. D. (2009). Neurodegenerative diseases target large-scale human brain networks. *Neuron, 62*, 42–52.

Sherod, M. G., Griffith, H. R., Copeland, J., Belue, K., Krzywanski, S., Zamrini, E. Y., et al. (2009). Neurocognitive predictors of financial capacity across the dementia spectrum: Normal aging, mild cognitive impairment, and Alzheimer's disease. *Journal of the International Neuropsychological Society, 15*, 258–267.

Sikkes, S. A., de Lange-de Klerk, E. S., Pijnenburg, Y. A., Scheltens, P., & Uitdehaag, B. M. (2009). A systematic review of instrumental activities of daily living scales in dementia: Room for improvement. *Journal of Neurology, Neurosurgery, and Psychiatry, 80*, 7–12.

Sobel, M. E. (1982). Asymptotic intervals for indirect effects in structural equations models. In S. Leinhart (Ed.), *Social methodology* (pp. 290–312). San Francisco: Jossey-Bass.

Triebel, K., Martin, R., Griffith, H. R., Marceaux, J., Okonkwo, O., Harrell, L., et al. (2009). Declining financial capacity in mild cognitive impairment: A one-year longitudinal study. *Neurology, 73*, 928–934.

Uniform Guardianship and Protective Proceedings Act § 102(5) (1997). Retrieved on March 1, 2011, from http://www.law.upenn.edu/bll/ulc/fnact99/1990s/ugppa97.htm.

Wadley, V. G., Harrell, L. E., & Marson, D. C. (2003). Self- and informant report of financial abilities in patients with Alzheimer's disease: Reliable and valid? *Journal of American Geriatrics Society, 51*, 1621–1626.

Wechsler, D. (1997). *Wechsler Memory Scale–Third Edition*. San Antonio, TX: The Psychological Corporation.

Widera, E., Steenpass, V., Marson, D., & Sudore, R. (2011). Finances in the older patient with cognitive impairment. *Journal of the American Medical Association, 305*, 698–706.

Wilkinson, G. S. (1993). *The Wide Range Achievement Test–Third Edition: Administration Manual*. Wilmington, DE: JASTAK.

Wolinsky, F., & Johnson, R. (1991). The use of health services by older adults. *The Journals of Gerontology, Series B: Psychological Sciences, 46*, 345–357.

4

Healthcare Decision-Making Capacity

BARTON W. PALMER, GAURI N. SAVLA, AND ALEXANDREA L. HARMELL

Neuropsychologists and other clinicians are sometimes asked to evaluate whether a patient has sufficient decisional capacity to consent or refuse a recommended medical or mental health intervention. As with evaluations of competency in other domains, determination of capacity to consent to treatment requires balancing two fundamental ethical concerns: (1) respect for individual autonomy and (2) protection of those vulnerable with impaired capacity for autonomous decision making (Beauchamp & Childress, 2001; Faden, Beauchamp, & King, 1986; Grisso & Appelbaum, 1998a). However, where other domains of competency may most directly affect control of property or other environmental factors, the potential conflict between autonomy and protective considerations is particularly salient in the context of capacity to consent to treatment because the outcome of the decision has direct implications for what happens to the individual's body. The professional charged with evaluating a person's capacity to make a choice about treatment is thus faced with an important, but frequently difficult and subjective task.

The focus of this chapter is to provide an overview of the nature of capacity to consent to treatment and its assessment. [Strictly speaking, the term "competence" refers to the dichotomous decision (competent/not competent) made by a court, whereas the term "decision-making capacity" or "decisional capacity" describes a construct that may differ by degrees and is assessed by the clinician.] Capacity to consent to treatment is closely related to several other forms of capacity addressed in other chapters in this volume. Capacity to appoint a proxy for healthcare or to issue an advance directive is a form of testamentary capacity (Chapter 5). Capacity to manage one's overall healthcare (i.e., beyond consent/dissent for a particular treatment) is a broader form of capacity for independent living (Chapter 7).

CONCEPTUAL ISSUES IN THE CAPACITY TO CONSENT TO TREATMENT

The general consensus among contemporary bioethicists and other relevant experts is that capacity to consent to treatment involves four functional components: understanding, appreciation, reasoning, and expression of a choice (Appelbaum & Grisso, 1988; Grisso & Appelbaum, 1998a; Roth, Meisel, & Lidz, 1977). These components (described in detail below) were originally identified through review of court decisions, and where present, statutes, regarding competence to consent or refuse treatment (Roth et al., 1977). The four components were initially described by Roth et al. (1977) as different standards of varying stringency (e.g., with the ability to express a choice being the least stringent criterion), but they have since come to be regarded as different defining aspects of competent decision making [American Bar Association (ABA)/American Psychological Association (APA), 2008; Grisso & Appelbaum, 1998a]. Bioethicists have played a key role in synthesizing the published relevant legal decisions into a bioethical framework (Appelbaum & Roth, 1982; Beauchamp & Childress, 2001; Faden et al., 1986; Grisso & Appelbaum, 1998a), but the core contemporary construct remains one rooted in legal tradition (and primarily case law) rather than from psychological or other behavioral science theories, models, or empirical data about how people actually make decisions about their own healthcare.

A key characteristic of the construct of capacity to consent to treatment is its context- or task-specific nature (ABA/APA, 2008; Berg, Appelbaum, & Grisso, 1996; Faden et al., 1986). The question at hand is not a patient's general ability to make healthcare decisions, but rather his or her ability to make a competent choice about a particular decision. For example, a given person with moderately severe dementia may lack competence regarding a treatment decision with a complex array of procedures and risk and benefit considerations, but may very well retain sufficient capacity to validly consent to or refuse treatment with more straightforward procedures and risk–benefit considerations (Ganzini, Volicer, Nelson, Fox, & Derse, 2004; Grisso & Appelbaum, 1998a).

With the context-specific nature of decisional capacity noted above, it is important to consider definitions of the four functional components of decisional capacity in more detail. Understanding refers to a person's ability to comprehend the disclosed information relevant to his or her choice, such as the nature of his or her condition, the proposed treatment, and viable alternatives (including no treatment) and their associated risks and benefits (Appelbaum & Grisso, 1988; Grisso & Appelbaum, 1998a; Roth et al., 1977). It is important to note that a key aspect to consider in conducting the consent procedure, as well as any assessment of decisional capacity, is that understanding refers to genuine comprehension beyond the ability to repeat the words used by the clinician or others during the consent process. Fostering and ensuring such comprehension usually require an interactive discourse, not merely reading through an information sheet or consent form (Palmer, Cassidy, Dunn, Spira, & Sheikh, 2008).

Appreciation is closely related to understanding, but involves application of the disclosed information to one's own situation or condition (Appelbaum & Grisso, 1988; Grisso & Appelbaum, 1998a; Roth et al., 1977). As a hypothetical example, consider a person experiencing an acute manic episode as part of bipolar disorder. Bipolar disorder is sometimes associated with impaired awareness/insight regarding the illness (Cassidy, 2010; Varga, Magnusson, Flekkøy, Rønneberg, & Opjordsmoen, 2006). An individual might demonstrate adequate intellectual understanding of what bipolar disorder is, as well as the nature, risks, and benefits of a particularly proposed pharmacological treatment relative to viable alternatives including no treatment. Yet if that individual is experiencing poor insight about his or her condition, he or she may not believe that he or she is personally experiencing bipolar disorder or manic symptoms, or more commonly, may minimize their severity or importance. Diminished insight might thereby impair the individual's capacity to appreciate the risks that would be assumed by refusing treatment even if he or she understood the risks to someone recognized as having bipolar disorder (Cairns et al., 2005; Gruber & Persons, 2010).

Reasoning refers to using the information to think through to a decision (Appelbaum & Grisso, 1988; Grisso & Appelbaum, 1998a; Roth et al., 1977). The key of this standard is not on the quality, weight, or value one puts on the consequences that the patient generates, but rather on whether the patient evidences that a process of reasoning in fact underlies his or her stated choice. Such evidence would include the ability to generate potential consequences, as well as the ability to compare potential consequences of the available options.

Expression of a choice refers to the ability to communicate a choice (Appelbaum & Grisso, 1988; Grisso & Appelbaum, 1998a; Roth et al., 1977). In addition to the expressive language functions of this dimension (via speech, writing, gesture, or other means), this component also includes the requirement that the patient be capable of actually coming to and making a decision (Appelbaum & Grisso, 1988). A highly ambivalent person might be able to engage in the understanding, appreciation, and reasoning components of decision making, yet still be unable to make and therefore communicate a clear or temporally consistent decision. If a patient quickly vacillated between choices, the validity of his or her transient consent for treatment may be questioned.

The above four functional components of decisional capacity are not necessarily independent or orthogonal dimensions. For instance, in the absence of a basic understanding of disclosed information, it may be difficult to appreciate or reason with that information. Moreover, although there does seem to be consensus that decisional capacity involves the above four components, there has not been full consensus on the specific distinctions among these subcomponents as they have been operationalized, particularly appreciation and reasoning (Moye, Karel, Azar, & Gurrera, 2004; Saks & Jeste, 2006).

In application, it may not be essential to specify whether a patient lacks capacity due to appreciation or reasoning, as long as both elements have been evaluated. Nonetheless, one way to think about the distinction between these two components is in reference to the ability to generate and compare potential consequences of the various treatment options (reasoning) versus the degree to which one believes the identified consequences (whether personally generated or generated by the examiner) have potential relevance to one's own situation (appreciation). For example, consider the potential consequences of no treatment for the person with bipolar disorder in the hypothetical scenario described above. One of these consequences may be prolonged acute manic symptoms and therefore a need for extended inpatient treatment. If the person is able to generate those potential consequences, then he or she has evidenced capacity for consequential reasoning, and possibly comparative reasoning if he or she can contrast that to the consequences of receiving effective treatment (Grisso & Appelbaum, 1998a). The person lacking insight into his or her own illness may be able to generate such consequences for a hypothetical person whom he or she grants has bipolar disorder, but may not believe or fully appreciate that is a risk for himself or herself (cf. Misra & Ganzini, 2004). Another patient might be able to recite potential consequences that are disclosed or suggested by the examiner, but be unable to reason about those potential consequences.

PSYCHOLOGICAL INSTRUMENTS DESIGNED TO EVALUATE MEDICAL DECISION MAKING

Empirical studies of concordance rates among experts indicate low interrater reliability in regard to determinations about capacity to consent to treatment (Kitamura & Kitamura, 2000; Marson, McInturff, Hawkins, Bartolucci, & Harrell, 1997; Parker, 2008). For example, Marson et al. (1997) had five board certified physicians with "extensive clinical experience with both dementia and competency assessment" classify 16 normal comparison subjects (NCs) and 29 patients with Alzheimer's disease in terms of competence/incompetence to consent to medical treatment. Although the physicians had near perfect agreement (98%; $k = 1.00$) in regard to the competency status of the NCs, the agreement rate on competency classifications for the patients with Alzheimer's disease was only 56% ($k = 0.14$). Moreover, these classifications were based on the judges' observations of pre-recorded assessments, including clinical interview, Mini-Mental State Examination (MMSE; Folstein, Folstein, & McHugh, 1975), and patients' responses to questions in a standardized hypothetical scenario. It seems quite likely that concordance rates would have been even worse had the judgments been based on the physicians conducting their own independent interviews and assessments.

In a follow-up to the above described study, Marson, Earnst, Jamil, Bartolucci, and Harrell (2000) provided five physicians instruction about the functional components of decisional capacity, and provided them with training videos with which the physicians practiced making competency judgments relative to each of the functional components. They then each rated videos of 21 patients with mild to moderate Alzheimer's disease being interviewed with the Capacity to Consent to Treatment Instrument (Marson, Ingram, Cody, & Harrell, 1995). With this training and more focused structured assessment, overall agreement of the patients' competency status improved to 76%, $k = 0.46$. Similar results were also reported in a study by Etchells et al. (1999), together suggesting that reliability (and thus validity) can be improved when clinicians are provided with training about the functional components of decisional capacity, and their assessment, and when interviews are conducted with structured instruments that ensure systematic coverage of the relevant domains.

Given that structured instruments can be a useful component in ensuring a systematic approach to the assessment of decisional capacity, the clinician is still faced with the somewhat daunting task of choosing an appropriate instrument for their specific need. In this regard, one useful resource is a comprehensive critical review of instruments for the assessment of capacity to consent to treatment or research provided by Dunn, Nowrangi, Palmer, Jeste, and Saks (2006). Additional useful reviews of many of these instruments have been provided by Sturman (2005) and the ABA/APA Assessment of Capacity in Older Adults Project Working Group (ABA/APA, 2008). Over these three reviews there were 11 published instruments or other structured tools identified that provide for the assessment of all four components of capacity to consent to treatment. As part of preparing the present chapter we conducted an updated search in November 2010; however, no additional comprehensive instruments for assessment of capacity to consent to treatment were identified.

Four of the 11 comprehensive scales for assessing capacity to consent to treatment do so in reference to the treatment decision each patient is actually facing. These four scales are the following:

- Competency Interview Schedule (Bean, Nishisato, Rector, & Glancy, 1994);
- Structured Interview for Competency and Incompetency Assessment Testing and Ranking Inventory (Tomoda et al., 1997);
- MacArthur Competence Assessment Tool for Treatment (MacCAT-T; Grisso & Appelbaum, 1998a, 1998b; Grisso, Appelbaum, & Hill-Fotouhi, 1997); and the
- Capacity Assessment Tool (Carney, Neugroschl, Morrison, Marin, & Siu, 2001).

Of the above four instruments, the MacCAT-T appears to be the most widely used and well validated (Dunn, Nowrangi et al., 2006; Sturman, 2005). The MacCAT-T is administered as a 15- to 20-minute semi-structured interview. In the first section the interviewer informs the patient about his or her actual diagnosis, including the features of the disorders and natural course. The patient is then asked to explain that information back in his or her own words. This is followed by a series of specific follow-up questions to assess the patient's understanding about specific aspects of the disorder. In the next section of the MacCAT-T, which provides part of the assessment of appreciation, the patient is asked to consider a particular description and to explain any doubts he or she has about whether that description is actually applicable to him or her, followed, again by specific follow-up questions. Other sections of the MacCAT-T deal with understanding and appreciation of the nature and risks or benefits of the actual treatment alternatives with which the patient is faced, and still others provide for a structured assessment of reasoning and expression of a choice.

The other seven comprehensive scales assess patients' capacity to consent to treatment in reference to one or more hypothetical treatment vignettes or scenarios. These seven instruments and the nature of the hypothetical scenarios include the following:

- Competency to Consent to Treatment Instrument (CCTI; Marson, Ingram et al., 1995). The CCTI has two scenarios (brain tumor and heart blockage) that are administered to all examinees;
- MacArthur Treatment Competency Study Battery (Understanding Treatment Disclosures, Perceptions of Disorder, and Thinking Rationally About Treatment) (Grisso, Appelbaum, Mulvey, & Fletcher, 1995). Three scenarios are available (treatment for schizophrenia, major depression, or ischemic heart disease), but the patient receives only one of the three depending on his or her diagnosis;
- Schmand, Gouwenberg, Smit, and Jonker (1999) provided no formal title for their instrument, but developed and employed a vignette involving treatment of a hip fracture;
- Hopemont Capacity Assessment Interview (HCAI; Edelstein, 2000) has separate health and financial decision-making sections, but the health section has two scenarios [eye infection, cardiopulmonary resuscitation (CPR)];
- Assessment of Consent Capacity–Treatment (Cea & Fisher, 2003) has three vignettes (psychopharmacological treatment for behavioral outbursts, orthodontic work for misaligned teeth, and injections to prevent allergic reactions to dust and pollen);
- Vellinga, Smit, Van Leeuwen, Van Tilburg, and Jonker (2004) had no formal title for their instrument but developed and employed two standardized treatment vignettes (gastrointestinal endoscopy to diagnose anemia and a colon cancer surgery scenario); and
- Assessment of Capacity to Consent to Treatment Interview (ACCTI; Moye, Karel, Edelstein, Hicken, Armesto, & Gurrera, 2008) has three vignettes (a choice of whether to use medication to treat rheumatoid arthritis, a choice of whether to use CPR for a stroke patient with severe functional limitations, and a choice of toe amputation versus femoral popliteal bypass for a nonhealing toe ulcer). The patient is presented with only one of the three vignettes selected by the clinician based on relevance to the patient's situation.

Among the seven instruments employing hypothetical vignettes, the CCTI appears to be the most widely used and well validated. It was originally developed to study capacity to consent to treatment among patients with Alzheimer's disease (Marson, Ingram et al., 1995), but has since been successfully used to study consent capacity in a variety of other patient populations (Bambara et al., 2007; Dreer, Devivo, Novack, Krzywanski, & , Ingram, 2008; Griffith et al., 2010; Martin et al., 2008; Okonkwo et al., 2007; Triebel, Martin, Nabors, & Marson, 2009). Similar to the MacCAT-T, the CCTI is a 20- to 25-minute structured interview (Marson et al., 1995). However, with the CCTI scenarios the examinee is asked to *imagine* that he or she is a patient with the condition specified in the scenario, and is then asked a series of questions to assess understanding, appreciation, reasoning, and expression of a choice in regard to that hypothetical choice.

As noted above, capacity to consent to treatment is an inherently context/situation-specific construct (ABA/APA, 2008; Berg et al., 1996; Faden et al., 1986). Outside the context of general competency, the ethically relevant question of decisional capacity is not usually "Does this patient have the capacity to make treatment decisions," but rather "Does this patient presently have the capacity to make this particular treatment decision?" The nature of this construct might preclude use of any of the seven instruments that base the assessment of decisional capacity on hypothetical scenarios, except when the nature of the scenario sufficiently matches the decision for which the patient's actual decisional capacity is being evaluated. On the other hand, there is a trade-off when the item content must be tailored to each specific situation. In the absence of standardized content, it is difficult to be certain that the psychometric properties of an instrument such as the MacCAT-T, including basic characteristics such as reliability and criterion validity, generalize to the specific situation in which it is being employed. Use of standardized but hypothetical vignettes also fosters comparison of results from different sites making such instruments particularly useful for use in research on decisional capacity. In fact, many of the instruments employing hypothetical vignettes, including the CCTI, were originally developed in the context of studies of decisional capacity, rather than for clinical application with patients.

Dunn et al. (2006) noted that ". . . . every instrument has limitations. As a general recommendation, however, the best choices for measuring capacity to consent to research and treatment, given their comprehensiveness and supporting psychometric data, will frequently be the MacArthur Competence Assessment Tools for Clinical Research (MacCAT-CR) and for Treatment (MacCAT-T), respectively" (p. 1331). On the other hand, as Dunn et al. (2006) also noted that the choice of the "best instrument" depends on the specific context in which it is applied. In regard to the latter, Dunn et al. provided a table with specific recommendations (Table 3, p. 1330), and a summary of the strengths and limitations, among the various instruments for different uses, such as initial screening, comprehensive follow-up assessment, research on capacity to consent to treatment, as well as for specific patient populations. Readers are encouraged to consult that report for further guidance on instrument selection for specific purposes.

Beyond the question of which instrument(s) to employ, another difficult issue is how precisely to use the information collected through the instruments to make a determination about an individual patient's capacity. For example, the authors of the MacCAT-T intentionally did not provide either a total score reflecting performance across the entire instrument or cut-scores defining the line between capacity/incapacity overall or within the four subscales (Grisso & Appelbaum, 1998a). This absence of a priori cut-scores reflects the fact that, ultimately, determinations of decisional capacity cannot be made by an instrument alone. These instruments provide a method to systematically disclose information and to query patients in a manner that ensures coverage of all four functional components of decisional capacity. However, given the context-specific nature of the construct, no "cookbook" algorithm or cut-score can suit all situations. Beyond the information obtained from the clinical interview, chart review, and use of structured instruments to assess understanding, appreciation, reasoning, and expression of a choice, one of the key pieces of information in the clinical management of persons with potentially impaired decisional capacity is their level and pattern of cognitive strengths or weaknesses as determined through neuropsychological assessment (Moberg & Kniele, 2006; Moberg & Rick, 2008; Sullivan, 2004). The association of specific cognitive abilities with capacity to consent to treatment is presented in the next section.

NEUROPSYCHOLOGY AND CAPACITY TO CONSENT TO TREATMENT

In this section we consider the association of neuropsychological abilities to the functional components of capacity to consent to research in two ways. First, we consider the extant published empirical data on this topic. As will be summarized below, however, the definitive conclusions that can be drawn from this relatively new line of research are limited. Thus, we follow the empirical overview with a rational (nonempirical) consideration of what specific cognitive processes might reasonably be expected to underlie each of the functional components of decisional capacity. (In preparing this chapter, we considered presenting the rational expectations before presenting the empirical data. We ultimately decided on the present sequence, however, because the existing empirical reports have been largely exploratory in nature, rather than being designed to test a priori hypotheses, grounded in a clear conceptual model about differential associations between specific cognitive processes and decisional capacity. It is our hope that our speculations about such associations may help catalyze a second generation of hypothesis-driven research on this topic.)

Although clinicians might sometimes use cognitive screens such as the MMSE to assess for the presence of impaired versus intact decisional capacity, such measures lack content validity and, except in cases in which impaired decisional capacity may be obvious in the absence of formal testing, lack adequate sensitivity and specificity (Kim & Caine, 2002). Even formal neuropsychological tests do not, in themselves, have an obvious one-to-one correspondence with decisional capacity as a context-specific construct, but they may have a useful role in clarifying the specific cognitive processes that underlie deficits in one or more of the functional components of decisional capacity.

We previously conducted a comprehensive critical review of empirical studies investigating the association between cognitive functioning and capacity to consent to treatment or research (Palmer & Savla, 2007). In addition to other reports relevant to the broader topic of cognitive aspects of capacity to consent to research or treatment, we identified four studies that described the bivariate associations between specific cognitive tests or abilities and each of the functional components of capacity to consent to treatment. These studies included one focused on patients with mild to moderate Alzheimer's disease (Marson, Cody, Ingram, & Harrell, 1995; Marson, Chatterjee, Ingram, & Harrell, 1996) (these two reports are based on the same sample, but the 1995 report focused on cognitive predictors of reasoning and the 1996 report focused on cognitive predictors of understanding, appreciation, and expression of a choice), a second study focused on patients with Parkinson's disease with cognitive impairment (Dymek, Atchison, Harrell, & Marson, 2001), a third study focused on nondemented nursing home residents with a variety of medical conditions requiring placement in a skilled nursing facility (Moye & Karel, 1999), and a fourth report focused on middle-aged and older patients with schizophrenia (Palmer, Dunn, Appelbaum, & Jeste, 2004). Subsequent to publication of our review, an additional relevant study was published by Okonkwo et al. (2008) that described the cognitive correlates in two separate samples, patients with mild cognitive impairment (MCI) and a separate sample of patients with mild Alzheimer's disease. Given the well-established limitations of stepwise regression as the basis for inferences about the relative importance of correlates as potential determinants of a dependent variable (Mundry & Nunn, 2009; Thompson, 1995; Wang, Wan, & Wang, 2008; Whittingham, Stephens, Bradbury, & Freckleton, 2006), we excluded such studies from the present review unless bivariate correlations were also provided in the published report. Except for the nursing home study, each of these studies also included an NC group. However, due to constricted variance in decisional capacity in the NC samples, the bivariate correlations between cognitive functioning and decisional capacity scores were generally minimal. Thus, the present review focuses on summarizing the pattern of results for the patient samples of each study.

The bivariate association between each cognitive test score and understanding, appreciation, and reasoning, as assessed with the MacCAT-T or CCTI and reported in the five relevant studies described earlier, are summarized in Table 4.1. (Results for expression of a choice are not shown as most patients in the sampled diagnostic groups have intact capacity to express a choice.) Note that within each study there is a triad of correlations between each neuropsychological score and understanding, appreciation, and reasoning. Some of the reports did not include the correlation magnitudes for results that did not reach statistical significance. However, to the degree that can be discerned from the information provided, the highest magnitude bivariate correlation within each triad occurred for understanding in 26 triads, for appreciation in eight triads, and for reasoning in two triads. By "highest" we simply mean any difference in magnitude; an assertion about whether the magnitudes were reliably different would require a test of differences among dependent *r*s. That is, the significance values provided for the bivariate correlations are generally in reference to the null hypothesis that $r = 0$, whereas assertions of statistically significant differences between such correlations would require testing a null hypotheses of the form $r_{xy} - r_{xz} = 0$ (see Cohen, Cohen, West, & Aiken, 2003).

Table 4.1 Correlations between Neuropsychological Scores and Understanding, Appreciation, and Reasoning Scores

Authors (publication year)	**Palmer et al. (2004)**			**Marson et al. (1995/96)**			**Dymek et al. (2001)**			**Moye and Karel (1999)**			**Okonkwo et al. (2008)**			**Okonkwo et al. (2008)**		
Capacity Instrument	MacCAT-T			CCTI			CCTI			MacCAT-T			CCTI			CCTI		
Sample (*n*)	Schizophrenia (49–59)			Alzheimer's (29)			Parkinson's (20)			Nursing Home (16)			MCI (60)			Alzheimer's (31)		
	U	A	R	U	A	R	U	A	R	U	A	R	U	A	R	U	A	R
General/Global Cognition																		
MMSE Total				0.62**	0.49*	0.55*												
DRS Total	0.49**	0.27[a]	0.44**															
Receptive Language and Semantic Knowledge																		
Auditory Comprehension Screen				0.63**	0.45*	NR	NR	NR	NR									
GEMS Command Comprehension										−0.03	0.11	0.30						
Reading Comprehension Screen				NR	NR	NR												
Token Test				0.61**	0.44*	0.58*	NR	NR	NR									
WAIS-R Comprehension				0.72**	0.56*	NR	0.70**	NR	NR									
Verbal Composite	0.35[a]	0.08	0.45*															
Expressive Language																		
Animal Fluency				NR	NR	0.44*	NR	NR	NR									
Letter Fluency				NR	0.48*	0.57*	NR	NR	NR									
Semantic Fluency													NR	NR	NR	NR	NR	0.50*
Boston Naming Test				0.72**	0.43*	NR	NR	NR	NR				NR	NR	NR	NR	NR	NR
GEMS Sentence Repetition										−0.14	−0.18	−0.03						

GEMS Confrontation Naming										0.25	0.31	0.18						
GEMS Generative Naming										0.24	0.34	0.37						
Attention/Working Memory																		
DRS Attention	0.25	0.15	0.33[a]	NR	NR	0.46*	NR	NR	0.58*				NR	NR	NR	NR	NR	NR
GEMS Digits Forward										−0.11	0.49*	0.25						
GEMS Digits Backward										−0.11	0.55*	0.48*						
WAIS-R Digit Span				NR	NR	0.44*	NR	NR	NR									
WMS-R Information/ Orientation							NR	NR	NR									
WMS-R Mental Control							NR	NR	NR									
Working Memory Composite	0.38*	0.37*	0.54**															
Spatial Span													NR	NR	NR	NR	NR	NR
CPT Omission errors													NR	NR	−0.34*	NR	NR	NR
CPT Commission errors													NR	NR	NR	NR	NR	NR
Processing Speed (Composite)	0.30*	0.11	0.43*															
Trail Making—Part A				−0.56*	−0.58**	−0.45*	NR	NR	NR				NR	NR	NR	−0.71*	−0.58*	−0.46*
Digit Symbol													NR	NR	NR	NR	NR	NR
CPT Hit Reaction Time													NR	NR	NR	NR	NR	NR
Visuospatial/Constructional																		
DRS Construction	−0.02	−0.03	0.16	NR	NR	NR	NR	NR	NR				NR	NR	NR	NR	0.53*	NR
CLOX 2													NR	NR	NR	NR	NR	NR
Perceptual Organization Composite	0.31[a]	0.22	0.47**															

Table 4.1 CORRELATIONS BETWEEN NEUROPSYCHOLOGICAL SCORES AND UNDERSTANDING, APPRECIATION, AND REASONING SCORES (CONT'D)

Authors (publication year)	**Palmer et al. (2004)**			**Marson et al. (1995/96)**			**Dymek et al. (2001)**			**Moye and Karel (1999)**			**Okonkwo et al. (2008)**			**Okonkwo et al. (2008)**		
Capacity Instrument	MacCAT-T			CCTI			CCTI			MacCAT-T			CCTI			CCTI		
Sample (*n*)	Schizophrenia (49–59)			Alzheimer's (29)			Parkinson's (20)			Nursing Home (16)			MCI (60)			Alzheimer's (31)		
	U	A	R	U	A	R	U	A	R	U	A	R	U	A	R	U	A	R
Executive Functioning																		
DRS Conceptualization	0.30[a]	0.17	0.45**	0.81**	0.50*	NR							NR	NR	NR	NR	NR	NR
DRS Initiation/ Perseveration	0.35*	0.14	0.16	0.64**	NR	0.60**							NR	NR	NR	NR	NR	NR
EXIT 25							−0.75**	NR	−0.67*									
Trail Making—Part B				NR	NR	NR	NR	NR	−0.60*				−0.57*	NR	NR	NR	NR	NR
WAIS-R Similarities				0.67**	NR	NR	NR	NR	NR									
Cognitive Competency Test—Verbal Reasoning													NR	NR	NR	NR	0.54*	NR
CPT Perseveration errors													NR	NR	NR	NR	NR	NR
CLOX 1													NR	NR	NR	NR	NR	NR
Executive Composite	0.41*	0.24	0.39															
Episodic Learning/Memory																		
DRS Memory	0.54**	0.27[a]	0.46**	0.60**	NR	NR	0.71**	NR	NR				NR	NR	NR	0.71*	NR	NR
Logical Memory I				0.55*	NR	NR	NR	NR	NR				0.59*	0.39*	NR	0.69*	NR	NR
Logical Memory II				NR	NR	NR	0.65*	NR	0.48*				0.69*	0.40*	0.42*	NR	NR	NR
Verbal Paired Associates I				NR	NR	NR												
Verbal Paired Associates II				NR	NR	NR												
GEMS List Learning										0.09	0.16	−0.13						
GEMS List Recall										−0.15	0.37	0.32						

CVLT-2 Total				0.58*	0.35*	0.46*	NR	NR	NR
Visual Reproduction I				NR	NR	NR	NR	NR	NR
Visual Reproduction II				0.53*	NR	NR	NR	NR	NR
Learning Composite	0.47*	0.34*	0.45*						
10/36 Spatial Recall—Immediate				NR	NR	NR	NR	NR	NR
10/36 Spatial Recall—Delayed				NR	NR	NR	NR	NR	0.49*

* $p < 0.05$ for Palmer et al. (2004), and Moser et al. (2002), $p < 0.01$; ** $p < 0.001$.

[a] Palmer et al. (2004) used a nontraditional alpha of $p < 0.01$; the correlations indicated from this study had $p < 0.05$ but $p > 0.01$; NR reported as nonsignificant, but the precise magnitude of the correlation was not provided.

Abbreviations: DRS, Mattis Dementia Rating Scale; GEMS, Geriatric Evaluation of Mental Status; GORT, Grey Oral Reading Test; MaCAT-T, MacArthur Competence Assessment Tool for Treatment; RBANS, Repeatable Battery for the Assessment of Neuropsychological Status; WAIS-III, Wechsler Adult Intelligence Scale–Third Edition; WRAT-III, Wide Range Achievement Test—Third Edition; CPT, Connor's Continuous Performance Test; CVLT-2, California Verbal Learning Test—Second Edition.

Table 4.1 adapted, with update, from Tables originally published in The association of specific neuropsychological deficits with capacity to consent to research or treatment, by Barton W. Palmer and Gauri N. Savla, Journal of the International Neuropsychological Society, Vol. 13, No. 6 (October 2007), pp. 1047–1059

Another way of considering the within-study patterns is by the columns in Table 4.1. For instance, for the understanding component, the highest bivariate correlate was a measure of episodic memory in two samples [Okonkwo et al., 2008 (MCI sample); Palmer et al., 2004], a measure of executive functioning in two other samples (Dymek et al., 2001; Marson et al., 1996), and essentially a tie between processing speed and episodic memory in another sample [Okonkwo et al., 2008 (Alzheimer's disease sample)]. For appreciation, the strongest correlate was a measure of working memory for two samples (Moye & Karel, 1999; Palmer et al., 2004), processing speed for two samples [Marson et al., 1996; Okonkwo et al., 2008 (Alzheimer's sample)], and episodic memory for one sample [Okonkwo et al., 2008 (MCI sample)]. [The strongest bivariate correlate of appreciation could not be determined from the published results for one sample (Dymek et al., 2001).] For the reasoning component, the strongest correlate was a measure of working memory for two samples (Moye & Karel, 1999; Palmer et al., 2004), executive function for two samples (Dymek et al., 2001; Marson, Cody et al., 1995), and episodic memory and expressive language in Okonkwo et al.'s (2007) MCI and mild Alzheimer's disease samples, respectively.

Overall, the published empirical data show that cognitive abilities frequently have strong correlations with the functional components of capacity to consent to treatment, but there is no clear pattern of differential associations between specific cognitive abilities with functional components. Although the strongest correlations between cognitive test scores and the functional components of decisional capacity varied across studies, the strongest correlations tended to be those involving the understanding component. As we have discussed in detail elsewhere (Palmer & Jeste, 2006; Palmer & Savla, 2007), this may simply reflect the fact that the understanding subscale of most decisional capacity instruments (including the MacCAT-T and CCTI) tends to have the most items and to be the most psychometrically reliable. In terms of the cognitive domains, the strongest correlations with the specific domains tended to be with tests of working memory, episodic memory, executive function, and processing speed, but there is no clear pattern of systematic differential associations consistent with a conceptual model of how the various cognitive processes might differentially relate to the specific components of decisional capacity.

Although the above observations are tempered by a relatively small number of published studies, the overall pattern is consistent with that found in the Palmer and Savla (2007) review that included five additional studies focused on capacity to consent to research (Carpenter et al., 2000; Casarett, Karlawish, & Hirschman, 2003; Moser et al., 2002; Palmer & Jeste, 2006; Stroup et al., 2005) and also reviewed studies in which the association between cognition and decisional capacity was examined with stepwise regression analyses rather than bivariate correlations (Earnst, Marson, & Harrell, 2000; Gurrera, Moye, Karel, Azar, & Armesto, 2006; Marson, Hawkins, McInturff, & Harrell, 1997; Moye, Karel, Gurrera, & Azar, 2006). Because of the limitations of stepwise regression mentioned above, we decided not to include the latter studies in the present review, but a summary of those studies is available in Palmer and Savla (2007).

In short, the empirical data published have not established the presence of differential associations between specific cognitive constructs and specific functional components of decisional capacity. An obvious question is the following: Does the absence of such supporting empirical data reflect insufficiencies in the available data or an actual absence of such differential associations among the constructs in nature? We believe the extant published data provide an insufficient basis on which to accept the null hypothesis. That is, it is too early in this line of research to definitively conclude that no such specific associations exist. In part, our hesitation in concluding that there are no such associations is based on the lack of psychometric equivalence among the subscales for measuring the different functional components of decisional capacity. For instance, the understanding subscale of the MacCAT-T has 13 items, whereas the appreciation, reasoning, and expression of a choice subscales are comprised of only two, four, and one items, respectively (Grisso & Appelbaum, 1998b). Similar differences in subscale length are also present in other measures such as the CCTI and HCAI. Such basic differences in scale length tend to affect reliability as well as the sensitivity of measures (Anastasi & Urbina, 1997). In the absence of psychometrically equivalent measures of each construct, it is difficult to draw definitive conclusions about the presence or absence of differential associations (cf. Chapman & Chapman, 1973).

Despite the limitations in the empirical data noted above, valid consent (or refusal) of a proposed treatment appears to be an inherently cognitive task, and different cognitive abilities seem likely to be differentially important to the various components of decisional capacity (Marson, 2001). The following possibilities are offered as reasoned hypotheses for how we might at least expect, a priori, particular cognitive domains to be important to each of the four functional components of decisional capacity.

- Understanding: To understand information, one must be able to receive it (attention and receptive language) and hold it in mind (working memory) for processing. Crystallized verbal knowledge in general, and health literacy in particular, seem likely to be important to understanding treatment disclosures and options (Nutbeam, 2008). To the degree that one has a preexisting schema or knowledge structure, processing of treatment-specific information may be less dependent on active processing (Bransford & Johnson, 1972; Norman & Shallice, 1980; Schank, 1980).
- Appreciation: To the degree that appreciation is construed as realizing the significance of information for oneself (Grisso & Appelbaum, 1998a; Roth et al., 1977), this component may be most closely related to social cognition, particularly self-referential cognitive/psychological processes. Such self-referential processes can themselves be construed as a form of "executive functioning," at least to the degree that the latter construct includes self-management and self-regulatory processes. But the term "executive functions" itself refers to a diverse array of processes, and so it would be important to consider whether the specific test(s) selected to

operationalize executive functions is in fact a good measure of the specific type of executive functioning that would be expected to underlie appreciation.

- Reasoning: To the degree that reasoning is construed as the presence of consequential and comparative reasoning processes (Grisso & Appelbaum, 1998a; Roth et al., 1977), this component would seem to depend most directly upon working memory (information must be held "on line" for conscious comparison), and certain executive functions such as abstraction, and planning or foresight for envisioning consequences.
- Expression of a choice: To make a final choice one must be able to disengage from information processing and comparison, and actually decide. That ability to disengage seems, at least superficially, to most resemble the "mental flexibility"/"shifting" aspects of executive functions (Miyake et al., 2000; Savla et al., 2010). Once the decision is made, the primary required cognitive processes seem to be expressive language functions (vocal, written, or physical gesturing).

The above hypotheses regarding the cognitive functions that may be of prime relevance to each of the functional components of decisional capacity are not intended as a complete or definitive model. But hopefully, these illustrate the type of reasoned analysis in which clinicians can engage as they endeavor to uncover the cognitive processes that underlie apparent deficits.

NONCOGNITIVE INFLUENCES ON DECISIONAL CAPACITY

An individual's manifest ability to make a valid decision about a proposed treatment is the resulting outcome of at least three factors: (1) the inherent complexity of the decision at hand, (2) the quality of the consent process, and (3) intrapersonal factors (Dunn, Palmer, & Karlawish, 2007). Cognition is a key intrapersonal factor, with overall neurocognitive functioning consistently emerging as the strongest predictor of decisional capacity in empirical studies of this construct (reviewed in Palmer & Savla, 2007). For instance, in studies of persons with schizophrenia or bipolar disorder, cognitive test scores are stronger predictors of capacity to consent to treatment or research than are the primary psychopathological symptoms of this disorder including positive symptoms (such as hallucinations and delusions), negative symptoms (such as apathy, social withdrawal), or depressive symptoms. On the other hand, it is important to note that much of the research on which the above conclusions are based has been conducted with relatively stable outpatients. Correlations between severity of psychopathological symptoms and decisional capacity do appear somewhat higher in studies sampling more acutely psychotic inpatients relative to those seen among outpatient samples (Carpenter et al., 2000). Psychopathology, therefore, is hardly unimportant when considering decisional capacity, but it appears that cognition (which is not always the first dimension considered in reference to mental illness) is a more consistent correlate of decisional capacity across patient populations and severity of illness. This finding is commensurate with the larger empirical literature on predictors of everyday functioning (i.e., functional outcome) in schizophrenia as cognitive deficits, rather than psychopathological symptoms, are the strongest and most consistently observed predictors of functional outcome (Green, 1996; Kurtz, 2006).

In addition to the primary importance of cognitive functions noted, however, we strongly encourage clinicians to consider the potential influence of other factors on the manifest understanding of individual patients, as some of these other factors may be more directly malleable than overall cognitive skill. As an obvious example, if a patient is having difficulty attending to disclosed information due to anxiety or fatigue, then efforts to address those factors should be undertaken before deeming an individual incapable of meaningful consent or dissent. But even more stable factors such as health literacy may be modifiable. For instance, among people with schizophrenia, there is evidence that educational sessions that include explaining the basic concepts of clinical research can improve patients' capacity to consent to research (Wirshing, Wirshing, Marder, Liberman, & Mintz, 1998).

PRACTICAL GUIDELINES AND RECOMMENDATIONS

Although we provide a brief set of guidelines and recommendations below, there are several resources with more detail than is practical in this chapter. In particular, interested readers are encouraged to consult the handbook prepared and published by the ABA/APA Assessment of Capacity in Older Adults Project Working Group entitled *Assessment of Older Adults with Diminished Capacity: A Handbook for Psychologists* (ABA/APA, 2008). Although the title emphasizes assessment of older adults, the content is relevant to the assessment of adults at any age, as well as practical guidelines and useful worksheets that can be applied in decisional capacity assessments. A second resource is Grisso and Appelbaum's (1998a) guidebook for assessing capacity to consent to treatment. Among other contributions, Grisso and Appelbaum (1995) conducted the MacArthur Treatment Competence Study, which was among the first and most influential comprehensive studies of capacity to consent to treatment from an empirical perspective. They also developed the MacCAT-T and MacCAT-CR, which, as noted above, Sturman (2005) described as the "gold standard" instruments for assessment of capacity to consent to treatment or research, respectively. Their guidebook, focused on capacity to consent to treatment, includes the MacCAT-T and MacCAT-T manual in the appendix. The following is not intended as an exhaustive list, but highlights some of the points we believe warrant consideration:

Clarify the referral question and context. As reported in a survey by Ganzini et al. (2003), the two most common and important errors in decisional capacity evaluations identified by experts are "the failure to distinguish general competence from specific capacity, including the lack of understanding that capacity or incapacity is not 'all or nothing' but is specific to a decision . . .[and] the assumption that if the patient lacks capacity for one type of medical decision, the patient lacks capacity for all medical decisions" (p. 241). With that finding in mind, it is critically important that the clinician charged with evaluating a patient's capacity to consent to or refuse a recommended treatment makes himself or herself fully familiar with the nature and context of the decision at question. Doing so will involve the usual array of clinical and investigatory skills and methods that permeate good clinical assessment and practice in other domains, including talking with the referral source and reviewing available records to understand the history and context of the referral, interviewing the patient and appropriate collateral informants, as well as a review of available records and prior assessments. This process will help the clinician evaluating decisional capacity to understand the specific situation, the factors underlying any expressed concern that decisional capacity may be suboptimal, as well as in determining whether prior efforts to explain the information to the patient have been inadequate.

Consider the factors potentially affecting manifest capacity. As noted above, a patient's manifest level of decisional capacity is in part affected by the inherent complexity of the relevant information and decision to be made, such as the nature of his or her condition, the proposed treatment and alternatives, and the nature of the risks and benefits associated with each potential choice. These contextual elements may not be modifiable in any one situation, but there are other factors that influence the patient's understanding that may be modifiable. It is important to determine what modifications in the consent process have been attempted already, so that other viable options may be identified. For instance, one of the simplest yet most effective means to ensure and improve comprehension is to conduct the consent process as an iterative discussion, with explanation, query to evaluate the patient's comprehension, and re-explanation of initially misunderstood components (Palmer et al., 2008). Presentation of the text in bullet format, as well as use of pictures, graphs, and audiovisual aids, may also be helpful (Dunn & Jeste, 2001). Beyond how the consent process is conducted, there is also potential value in considering the timing of when the consent discussion occurs. For example, by addressing potentially transient intrapersonal factors such as delirium, fatigue, sleepiness, or overmedication, an initially "incapable" patient may be helped to become decisionally capable. In regard to stable intrapersonal factors, underlying cognitive functioning may not be a probable candidate for rapid modification, but educational efforts might be a means to improve health literacy.

Include a structured assessment of decisional capacity. Although none of the available instruments for assessing capacity to consent to treatment can provide the definitive answer about whether a patient does or does not have sufficient capacity to consent, these instruments are invaluable in ensuring systematic coverage of the four components of decisional capacity. Given that it was designed to be tailored to the actual decision that a patient is being asked to make, as well as the degree of supporting empirical data on its reliability and validity, the MacCAT-T may presently be the best choice for many situations to ensure systematic assessment of an individual's capacity to consent to treatment. But the needs of a specific situation may make one of the other available instruments a better option in some situations. Thus, as noted above, readers are encouraged to study the specific recommendations provided by Dunn et al. (2006) (Table 3, p. 1330), as their table summarizes the strengths and limitations among the various instruments for different uses.

CASE STUDY

Mr. X is a 28-year-old man with a 9-year history of paranoid schizophrenia. Mr. X is stable on his medications (clozapine) and has not had an acute psychotic episode for at least 3 years. He occasionally has breakthrough psychotic symptoms, especially delusions of reference (the most typical of which is that people on the television are directly talking to him). Mr. X is physically healthy and lives in an apartment with a roommate. He recently underwent work rehabilitation and is employed as a stocker and bagger in a supermarket. This is the longest paid job he has held (1 year) and his supervisor says that he is a good worker. However, Mr. X takes a long time to learn new things on the job, and it took nearly 3 months for him to master his job duties. The supermarket manager has also been putting off giving Mr. X any new duties because he says that Mr. X tends to be distractible during training and needs to be given simple, concrete instructions repeatedly, which is time-consuming for his supervisor. Mr. X is also not able to "think on his feet" and solve problems as they arise. Mr. X has been asking his psychiatrist, Dr. A, about a new medication that the TV ads say has been shown to "decrease emotional problems and improve attention in some people with schizophrenia." Mr. X is convinced that this new medication was developed especially to "cure" him because the TV announcer "looked directly at him." The medication has side effects such as weight gain, dizziness, and drowsiness. There are no studies on the long-term effects of the drug.

Mr. X has previously failed multiple trials of both conventional and atypical antipsychotics, but has so far tolerated clozapine well. With the help of his phone calendar, he is adherent to the medication and has never missed an appointment with his psychiatrist or his routine 2-week blood test to check for agranulocytosis. Dr. A thinks that given his past treatment failures, Mr. X is not a good candidate for the new drug and does not understand that the positive effects of the drug on mood and cognition were seen only in a small proportion of patients. Dr. A thinks that Mr. X's delusional belief that the medication will "cure" him complicates his ability to make an informed decision about the new treatment. Dr. A does not think that Mr. X appreciates the risks of starting a new medication and how it could affect his current functioning. Dr. A also thinks that Mr. X does not understand that the new medication may or may not help him, and that it may have risks that could interfere with his functioning. However, Mr. X's direct request to change his medication and his recent history of being able to follow the complicated treatment protocol for a drug such as clozapine seem to suggest that he may in fact have the capacity to consent to the new medication with some intervention from his psychiatrist.

Dr. A prepares a MacCAT-T written in short sentences with simple and concrete language that is tailored to the new drug and clozapine, and sets up a time to meet with Mr. X. Mr. X shows inadequate comprehension on the first trial, but Dr. A repeats the information, using flash cards to help explain certain concepts, and Mr. X does show some improvement, although still less than ideal understanding.

Dr. A then asks Dr. C, the neuropsychologist on the treatment team, to conduct an evaluation to further clarify the nature of any cognitive impairments underlying Mr. X's understanding deficits. Dr. C's evaluation suggests that Mr. X's primary impairments are in attention and learning on episodic memory tests. Once learned, however, Mr. X seems capable of retaining information. Based on these findings, Dr. C suggest that Dr. A use visual aids (including bullet-pointed text of key points) and an iterative process of disclosure, query, and re-explanation during his discussions with Mr. X about the risks and benefits of clozapine versus the new medication. He notes bullet points facilitate processing because the relevant information is made salient. Moreover, the iterative disclosure process will help compensate for Mr. X's deficits in information acquisition.

Dr. A follows Dr. C's advice and readministers the MacCAT-T, finding significant improvements. He found that once Mr. X was able to understand the information, his appreciation, reasoning, as well as expression of a choice were all appropriate. Mr. X, at this time, had adequate capacity to make a decision about his treatment.

The above vignette highlights a few important points about the capacity to consent to healthcare:

1. *Capacity to consent was established for a specific context and may not be generalized to other types of capacity or capacity to consent in any other healthcare context.*
2. *Neuropsychological testing can assist in determining the reasons for poor decision-making capacity and targets for intervention.*
3. *Certain aspects of capacity to consent, especially understanding, are teachable, which can further enhance appreciation, reasoning, and the ability to state a choice. Capacity, therefore, is malleable in some cases.*
4. *Instruments to assess capacity to consent may also be effectively used as interventions for improving capacity to consent.*

CONCLUSIONS/DIRECTIONS FOR FURTHER RESEARCH

Assessment of the capacity to consent to treatment is an ethically important task, but one that remains challenging, in part due to the context-specific nature of the construct. A neuropsychological perspective is helpful in considering decisional capacity (Moberg & Kniele, 2006; Moberg & Rick, 2008; Sullivan, 2004), but there are still many questions that remain to be answered or addressed through empirical research. High on the list for further research are (1) the ongoing need for improved instruments for assessing capacity to consent to treatment, as even the best of the available instruments remain suboptimal (Dunn et al., 2006;

Sturman, 2005), and (2) further efforts to discern the role of specific cognitive processes and other participant characteristics in specific functional components of capacity to consent to treatment (Palmer & Savla, 2007). Empirical advances on those two points would also facilitate the development of conceptually and empirically grounded methods of improving the consent process itself (Eyler & Jeste, 2006).

References

American Bar Association Commission on Law and Aging & American Psychological Association (2008). *Assessment of older adults with diminished capacity: A handbook for psychologists.* Washington, D.C.: American Bar Association Commission on Law and Aging—American Psychological Association.

Anastasi, A., & Urbina, S. (1997). *Psychological testing* (7th ed.). Upper Saddle River, NJ: Prentice Hall.

Appelbaum, P. S., & Grisso, T. (1988). Assessing patients' capacities to consent to treatment. *New England Journal of Medicine, 319,* 1635–1638.

Appelbaum, P. S., & Roth, L. H. (1982). Competency to consent to research: A psychiatric overview. *Archives of General Psychiatry, 39,* 951–958.

Bambara, J. K., Griffith, H. R., Martin, R. C., Faught, E., Wadley, V. G., & Marson, D. C. (2007). Medical decision-making abilities in older adults with chronic partial epilepsy. *Epilepsy Behavior, 10,* 63–68.

Barlow, D. H., & Nock, M. K. (2009). Why can't we be more idiographic in our research? *Perspectives on Psychological Science, 4,* 19–21.

Bean, G., Nishisato, S., Rector, N. A., & Glancy, G. (1994). The psychometric properties of the competency interview schedule. *Canadian Journal of Psychiatry, 39,* 368–376.

Beauchamp, T., & Childress, J. (2001). *Principles of biomedical ethics* (5th ed.). New York: Oxford University Press.

Berg, J. W., Appelbaum, P. S., & Grisso, T. (1996). Constructing competence: Formulating standards of legal competence to make medical decisions. *Rutgers Law Review, 48,* 345–396.

Bransford, J. D., & Johnson, M. K. (1972). Contextual prerequisites for understanding: Some investigations of comprehension and recall. *Journal of Verbal Learning and Verbal Behavior, 11,* 717–726.

Cairns, R., Maddock, C., Buchanan, A., David, A. S., Hayward, P., Richardson, G., & Hotopf, M. (2005). Prevalence and predictors of mental incapacity in psychiatric in-patients. *British Journal of Psychiatry, 187,* 379–385.

Carney, M. T., Neugroschl, J., Morrison, R. S., Marin, D., & Siu, A. L. (2001). The development and piloting of a capacity assessment tool. *Journal of Clinical Ethics, 12,* 17–23.

Carpenter, W. T., Gold, J. M., Lahti, A. C., Queern, C. A., Conley, R. R., Bartko, J. J., & Appelbaum, P. S. (2000). Decisional capacity for informed consent in schizophrenia research. *Archives of General Psychiatry, 57,* 533–538.

Casarett, D. J., Karlawish, J. H., & Hirschman, K. B. (2003). Identifying ambulatory cancer patients at risk of impaired capacity to consent to research. *Journal of Pain and Symptom Management, 26,* 615–624.

Cassidy, F. (2010). Insight in bipolar disorder: Relationship to episode subtypes and symptom dimensions. *Neuropsychiatric Disease and Treatment, 6,* 627–631.

Cea, C. D., & Fisher, C. B. (2003). Health care decision-making by adults with mental retardation. *Mental Retardation, 41*, 78–87.

Chapman, L. J., & Chapman, J. P. (1973). Problems in the measurement of cognitive deficit. *Psychological Bulletin, 79*, 380–385.

Cohen, J., Cohen, P., West, S., & Aiken, L. (2003). *Applied multiple regression/correlation analysis for the behavioral sciences* (3rd ed.). Hillsdale, NJ: Lawrence Erlbaum Associates.

Dreer, L. E., Devivo, M. J., Novack, T. A., Krzywanski, S., & Marson, D. C. (2008). Cognitive predictors of medical decision-making capacity in traumatic brain injury. *Rehabilitation Psychology, 53*, 486–497.

Dunn, L. B., & Jeste, D. V. (2001). Enhancing informed consent for research and treatment. *Neuropsychopharmacology, 24*, 595–607.

Dunn, L. B., Nowrangi, M., Palmer, B. W., Jeste, D. V., & Saks, E. (2006). Assessing capacity to consent to treatment and research: A review of instruments. *American Journal of Psychiatry, 163*, 1323–1334.

Dunn, L. B., Palmer, B. W., & Karlawish, J. H. (2007). Frontal dysfunction and capacity to consent to treatment or research: Conceptual considerations and empirical evidence. In B. Miller & J. L. Cummings (Eds.), *The human frontal lobes: Functions and disorders–second edition* (pp. 335–344). New York: Guilford Press.

Dunn, L. B., Palmer, B. W., Keehan, M., Jeste, D. V., & Appelbaum, P. S. (2006). Assessment of therapeutic misconception in older schizophrenia patients with a brief instrument. *American Journal of Psychiatry, 163*, 500–506.

Dymek, M. P., Atchison, P., Harrell, L., & Marson, D. C. (2001). Competency to consent to medical treatment in cognitively impaired patients with Parkinson's disease. *Neurology, 56*, 17–24.

Earnst, K. S., Marson, D. C., & Harrell, L. E. (2000). Cognitive models of physicians' legal standard and personal judgments of competency in patients with Alzheimer's disease. *Journal of the American Geriatrics Society, 48*, 919–927.

Edelstein, B. (2000). Challenges in the assessment of decision-making capacity. *Journal of Aging Studies, 14*, 423–437.

Etchells, E., Darzins, P., Silberfeld, M., Singer, P. A., McKenny, J., Naglie, G., & Strang, D. (1999). Assessment of patient capacity to consent to treatment. *Journal of General Internal Medicine, 14*, 27–34.

Eyler, L. T., & Jeste, D. V. (2006). Enhancing the informed consent process: A conceptual overview. *Behavioral Sciences and the Law, 24*, 553–568.

Faden, R., Beauchamp, T., & King, N. (1986). *A history and theory of informed consent.* New York: Oxford University Press.

Folstein, M. F., Folstein, S. E., & McHugh, P. R. (1975). "Mini-Mental State": A practical method for grading the cognitive state of patients for the clinician. *Journal of Psychiatric Research, 12*, 189–198.

Ganzini, L., Volicer, L., Nelson, W., & Derse, A. (2003). Pitfalls in assessment of decision-making capacity. *Psychosomatics, 44*, 237–243.

Ganzini, L., Volicer, L., Nelson, W. A., Fox, E., & Derse, A. R. (2004). Ten myths about decision-making capacity. *Journal of the American Medical Directors Association, 5*, 263–267.

Green, M. F. (1996). What are the functional consequences of neurocognitive deficits in schizophrenia? *American Journal of Psychiatry, 153*, 321–330.

Griffith, H. R., Okonkwo, O. C., den Hollander, J. A., Belue, K., Copeland, J., Harrell, L. E., & Marson, D. C. (2010). Brain metabolic correlates of decision making in amnestic mild cognitive impairment. *Neuropsychology, Development, and Cognition. Section B, Aging, Neuropsychology and Cognition, 17*, 492–504.

Grisso, T., & Appelbaum, P. S. (1995). The Macarthur treatment competence study. III: Abilities of patients to consent to psychiatric and medical treatments. *Law and Human Behavior, 19*, 149–174.

Grisso, T., & Appelbaum, P. S. (1998a). *Assessing competence to consent to treatment: A guide for physicians and other health professionals*. New York: Oxford University Press.

Grisso, T., & Appelbaum, P. S. (1998b). *MacArthur Competence Assessment Tool for Treatment (MacCAT-T)*. Sarasota, FL: Professional Resource Press.

Grisso, T., Appelbaum, P. S., & Hill-Fotouhi, C. (1997). The MacCAT-T: A clinical tool to assess patients' capacities to make treatment decisions. *Psychiatric Services, 48*, 1415–1419.

Grisso, T., Appelbaum, P. S., Mulvey, E. P., & Fletcher, K. (1995). The MacArthur Treatment Competence Study. II: Measures of abilities related to competence to consent to treatment. *Law and Human Behavior, 19*, 127–148.

Gruber, J., & Persons, J. B. (2010). Unquiet treatment: Handling treatment refusal in bipolar disorder. *Journal of Cognitive Psychotherapy, 24*, 16–25.

Gurrera, R. J., Moye, J., Karel, M. J., Azar, A. R., & Armesto, J. C. (2006). Cognitive performance predicts treatment decisional abilities in mild to moderate dementia. *Neurology, 66*, 1367–1372.

Heaton, R. K., & Marcotte, T. D. (2000). Clinical neuropsychological tests and assessment techniques. In F. Boller, J. Grafman, & G. Rizzolatti (Eds.), *Handbook of neuropsychology* (2nd ed., Vol. 1, pp. 27–52). New York: Elsevier Science, B.V.

Kaplan, E. (1988). A process approach to neuropsychological assessment. In M. Dennis, E. Kaplan, M. I. Posner, D. G. Stein, & R. F. Thompson (Eds.), *Clinical neuropsychology and brain function: Research, measurement, and practice* (pp. 129–167). Washington, D.C.: American Psychological Association.

Kim, S. Y., & Caine, E. D. (2002). Utility and limits of the Mini Mental State Examination in evaluating consent capacity in Alzheimer's disease. *Psychiatric Services, 53*, 1322–1324.

Kitamura, T., & Kitamura, F. (2000). Reliability of clinical judgment of patients' competency to give informed consent: A case vignette study. *Psychiatry and Clinical Neurosciences, 54*, 245–247.

Kurtz, M. M. (2006). Symptoms versus neurocognitive skills as correlates of everyday functioning in severe mental illness. *Expert Review of Neurotherapeutics, 6*, 47–56.

Marson, D. C. (2001). Loss of competency in Alzheimer's disease: Conceptual and psychometric approaches. *International Journal of Law and Psychiatry, 24*, 267–283.

Marson, D. C., Chatterjee, A., Ingram, K. K., & Harrell, L. E. (1996). Toward a neurologic model of competency: Cognitive predictors of capacity to consent in Alzheimer's disease using three different legal standards. *Neurology, 46*, 666–672.

Marson, D. C., Cody, H. A., Ingram, K. K., & Harrell, L. E. (1995). Neuropsychologic predictors of competency in Alzheimer's disease using a rational reasons legal standard. *Archives of Neurology, 52*, 955–959.

Marson, D. C., Earnst, K. S., Jamil, F., Bartolucci, A., & Harrell, L. E. (2000). Consistency of physicians' legal standard and personal judgments of competency in patients with Alzheimer's disease. *Journal of the American Geriatrics Society, 48*, 911–918.

Marson, D. C., Hawkins, L., McInturff, B., & Harrell, L. E. (1997). Cognitive models that predict physician judgments of capacity to consent in mild Alzheimer's disease. *Journal of the American Geriatrics Society, 45*, 458–464.

Marson, D. C., Ingram, K. K., Cody, H. A., & Harrell, L. E. (1995). Assessing the competency of patients with Alzheimer's disease under different legal standards. A prototype instrument. *Archives of Neurology, 52*, 949–954.

Marson, D. C., McInturff, B., Hawkins, L., Bartolucci, A., & Harrell, L. E. (1997). Consistency of physician judgments of capacity to consent in mild Alzheimer's disease. *Journal of the American Geriatrics Society, 45*, 453–457.

Martin, R. C., Okonkwo, O. C., Hill, J., Griffith, H. R., Triebel, K., Bartolucci, A., & Marson, D. C. (2008). Medical decision-making capacity in cognitively impaired Parkinson's disease patients without dementia. *Movement Disorders, 23*, 1867–1874.

Misra, S., & Ganzini, L. (2004). Capacity to consent to research among patients with bipolar disorder. *Journal of Affective Disorders, 80*, 115–123.

Miyake, A., Friedman, N. P., Emerson, M. J., Witzki, A. H., Howerter, A., & Wager, T. D. (2000). The unity and diversity of executive functions and their contributions to complex "frontal lobe" tasks: A latent variable analysis. *Cognitive Psychology, 41*, 49–100.

Moberg, P. J., & Kniele, K. (2006). Evaluation of competency: Ethical considerations for neuropsychologists. *Applied Neuropsychology, 13*, 101–114.

Moberg, P. J., & Rick, J. H. (2008). Decision-making capacity and competency in the elderly: A clinical and neuropsychological perspective. *NeuroRehabilitation, 23*, 403–413.

Moser, D. J., Schultz, S. K., Arndt, S., Benjamin, M. L., Fleming, F. W., Brems, C. S., & Andreasen, N. C. (2002). Capacity to provide informed consent for participation in schizophrenia and HIV research. *American Journal of Psychiatry, 159*, 1201–1207.

Moye, J., & Karel, M. J. (1999). Evaluating decisional capacities in older adults: Results of two clinical studies. *Advances in Medical Psychotherapy, 10*, 71–84.

Moye, J., Karel, M. J., Azar, A. R., & Gurrera, R. J. (2004). Capacity to consent to treatment: Empirical comparison of three instruments in older adults with and without dementia. *Gerontologist, 44*, 166–175.

Moye, J., Karel, M. J., Edelstein, B., Hicken, B., Armesto, J. C., & Gurrera, R. J. (2008). Assessment of capacity to consent to treatment: Challenges, the "ACCT" approach, future directions. *Clinical Gerontologist, 31*, 37–66.

Moye, J., Karel, M. J., Gurrera, R. J., & Azar, A. R. (2006). Neuropsychological predictors of decision-making capacity over 9 months in mild-to-moderate dementia. *Journal of General Internal Medicine, 21*, 78–83.

Mundry, R., & Nunn, C. L. (2009). Stepwise model fitting and statistical inference: Turning noise into signal pollution. *American Naturalist, 173*, 119–123.

Norman, D. A., & Shallice, T. (1980). *Attention to action: Willed and automatic control of behavior*. La Jolla, CA: Center for Human Information Processing, University of California, San Diego.

Nutbeam, D. (2008). The evolving concept of health literacy. *Social Science & Medicine, 67*, 2072–2078.

Okonkwo, O. C., Griffith, H. R., Belue, K., Lanza, S., Zamrini, E. Y., Harrell, L. E., & Marson, D. C. (2007). Medical decision-making capacity in patients with mild cognitive impairment. *Neurology, 69*, 1528–1535.

Okonkwo, O. C., Griffith, H. R., Belue, K., Lanza, S., Zamrini, E. Y., Harrell, L. E., & Marson, D. C. (2008). Cognitive models of medical decision-making capacity in patients with mild cognitive impairment. *Journal of the International Neuropsychological Society, 14*, 297–308.

Palmer, B. W., Cassidy, E. L., Dunn, L. B., Spira, A. P., & Sheikh, J. I. (2008). Effective use of consent forms and interactive questions in the consent process. *IRB: Ethics & Human Research, 30*, 8–12.

Palmer, B. W., Dunn, L. B., Appelbaum, P. S., & Jeste, D. V. (2004). Correlates of treatment-related decision-making capacity among middle-aged and older patients with schizophrenia. *Archives of General Psychiatry, 61*, 230–236.

Palmer, B. W., & Jeste, D. V. (2006). Relationship of individual cognitive abilities to specific components of decisional capacity among middle-aged and older patients with schizophrenia. *Schizophrenia Bulletin, 32*, 98–106.

Palmer, B. W., & Savla, G. N. (2007). The association of specific neuropsychological deficits with capacity to consent to research or treatment. *Journal of the International Neuropsychological Society, 13*, 1047–1059.

Parker, M. (2008). Patient competence and professional incompetence: Disagreements in capacity assessments in one Australian jurisdiction, and their educational implications. *Journal of Law and Medicine, 16*, 25–35.

Roth, L. H., Meisel, A., & Lidz, C. W. (1977). Tests of competency to consent to treatment. *American Journal of Psychiatry, 134*, 279–284.

Saks, E. R., & Jeste, D. V. (2006). Capacity to consent to or refuse treatment and/or research: Theoretical considerations. *Behavioral Sciences and the Law, 24*, 411–429.

Savla, G. N., Twamley, E. W., Delis, D. C., Roesch, S. C., Jeste, D. V., & Palmer, B. W. (2010). Dimensions of executive functioning in schizophrenia and their relationship with processing speed. *Schizophrenia Bulletin*. Advance online publication. DOI: 10.1093/schbul/sbq149

Schank, R. C. (1980). What's a schema anyway? *Contemporary psychology: APA Review of Books, 25*, 814–816.

Schmand, B., Gouwenberg, B., Smit, J. H., & Jonker, C. (1999). Assessment of mental competency in community-dwelling elderly. *Alzheimer Disease and Associated Disorders, 13*, 80–87.

Stroup, S., Appelbaum, P., Swartz, M., Patel, M., Davis, S., Jeste, D., & Lieberman, J. (2005). Decision-making capacity for research participation among individuals in the Catie schizophrenia trial. *Schizophrenia Research, 80*, 1–8.

Sturman, E. D. (2005). The capacity to consent to treatment and research: A review of standardized assessment tools. *Clinical Psychology Review, 25*, 954–974.

Sullivan, K. (2004). Neuropsychological assessment of mental capacity. *Neuropsychology Review, 14*, 131–142.

Thompson, B. (1995). Stepwise regression and stepwise discriminant analysis need not apply here: A guidelines editorial. *Educational and Psychological Measurement, 55*, 525–534.

Tomoda, A., Yasumiya, R., Sumiyama, T., Tsukada, K., Hayakawa, T., Matsubara, K., & Kitamura, T. (1997). Validity and reliability of structured interview for competency incompetency assessment testing and ranking inventory. *Journal of Clinical Psychology, 53*, 443–450.

Triebel, K. L., Martin, R. C., Nabors, L. B., & Marson, D. C. (2009). Medical decision-making capacity in patients with malignant glioma. *Neurology, 73*, 2086–2092.

Varga, M., Magnusson, A., Flekkøy, K., Rønneberg, U., & Opjordsmoen, S. (2006). Insight, symptoms and neurocognition in bipolar I patients. *Journal of Affective Disorders, 91*, 1–9.

Vellinga, A., Smit, J. H., Van Leeuwen, E., Van Tilburg, W., & Jonker, C. (2004). Competence to consent to treatment of geriatric patients: Judgments of physicians, family members and the vignette method. *International Journal of Geriatric Psychiatry, 19*, 645–654.

Wang, X., Wan, F., & Wang, J. J. (2008). A common misuse of stepwise regression in studies of ratio of metastatic lymph nodes for gastric cancer. *Annals of Surgical Oncology, 15*, 1805–1806.

Whittingham, M. J., Stephens, P. A., Bradbury, R. B., & Freckleton, R. P. (2006). Why do we still use stepwise modelling in ecology and behaviour? *Journal of Animal Ecology, 75*, 1182–1189.

Wirshing, D. A., Wirshing, W. C., Marder, S. R., Liberman, R. P., & Mintz, J. (1998). Informed consent: Assessment of comprehension. *American Journal of Psychiatry, 155*, 1508–1511.

5

Testamentary Capacity

CARMELLE PEISAH AND KENNETH I. SHULMAN

In this chapter, we review the medical, neuropsychological, and legal aspects of testamentary capacity including the related concept of undue influence. We will present an approach to the contemporaneous as well as retrospective assessment of testamentary capacity and vulnerability to undue influence based on the limited literature available. A case illustration of a retrospective assessment will highlight many of the issues discussed in this chapter.

Challenges to wills on the basis of testamentary capacity are likely to increase significantly in the coming decades as a result of a number of confluent factors. The dramatic increase in the number of old adults, especially the very old, will result in a higher prevalence of cognitive impairment, dementia, and associated behavioral and psychiatric disorders. At the same time that this vulnerable population is growing, modern families are becoming more complex and asset disposition more complicated and sensitive. This can lead to feelings of rejection and injustice, which can fuel the impulse to challenge wills that are perceived to be unfair (Shulman, Cohen, Kirsh, Hull, & Champine, 2007). Moreover, we are about to see the greatest intergenerational exchange of wealth in the history of humanity. Prior to the recent economic downturn, it was estimated that $41 trillion of wealth would be transferred before 2050 via inheritance (Hall, Hall, Myers, & Chapman, 2009). All of these trends conspire to produce a significant, if not dramatic, increase in will challenges and concomitant requests for capacity assessments both contemporaneous and retrospective.

Although the court remains the final arbiter in will challenges, the evidence to support such a challenge is often informed by the assessment of a medical or psychological expert. Thus, testamentary capacity is a construct that crosses both the legal and medical domains inviting a collaborative approach to both its definition and its assessment. It behooves medical and psychological experts to be aware of the legal, medical, and psychiatric issues that underlie the assessment of testamentary capacity as well as the inextricably linked role of undue influence.

THE ROLE OF THE EXPERT

In all legal jurisdictions, rules apply to expert evidence. Increasingly, the courts are concerned about the impartiality and validity of expert evidence and thus have moved to a more rigorous approach to expert testimony. One of the earliest judgments that outlined the role and responsibilities of experts in civil cases was tried before Justice Creswell in the Queen's Bench Division Commercial Court in London, England (Lloyd's Law Reports, 1993). In the case known as "the Ikarian Reefer," Justice Creswell outlined a number of key components for expert witnesses in civil cases. (1) "An expert witness should provide independent assistance to the court by a way of objective unbiased opinion in relation to matters within his expertise . . . . An expert in the high court should never assume the role of advocate." (2) "The expert should outline the facts and assumptions on which his opinion is based. Moreover, the expert should not omit to consider material facts which may detract from his concluded opinion." (3) "An expert witness should confine themselves to areas that fall only within their area of expertise." Gutheil (2007) emphasizes that the expert must be prepared to say "I do not know" when the evidence is insufficient to yield an opinion to a reasonable degree of certainty.

The Province of Ontario, like many jurisdictions, recently amended its Rules of Civil Procedure to clarify the rules that apply to expert evidence (Province of Ontario, 1990). The new rules (1) emphasize that experts have an overriding duty to the court and (2) direct that experts on opposite sides of a case may be required to meet prior to trial to settle issues on which they agree and to set out issues on which they disagree. Rule 4.1.01 states that it is the duty of experts to provide opinions that are fair, objective, and nonpartisan, as well as opinions related only to matters within the expert's expertise. Duty to the court prevails over any obligation to the party by whom or on whose behalf he or she is retained. The courts appear to be increasingly intolerant of any hint that the expert has adopted an advocacy role on behalf of the person or persons who have engaged them. Australian Courts have adopted similar rules for experts (e.g., the Uniform Civil Procedure Rules Amendment No. 12, 2006).

O'Neill and Peisah (2011) considered the kind of experts that are appropriate in various circumstances. Cases in which there is a clear psychiatric disorder or psychotic symptoms may be more suited to psychiatrists. Cases that may be better handled by a neurologist or a geriatric internist involve patients with delirium and complex underlying medical conditions. The neuropsychologist may be the best choice when there is little formal medical documentation of dementia and it is necessary to rely on the extrapolation of behavioral disturbances in order to prove cognitive impairment. Neuropsychologists may also assist when an objective measure of cognitive function is desired. In practice, there is a great deal of overlap between experts from these disciplines.

RELEVANT CASE LAW

The assessment of testamentary capacity, as with any capacity task, must be framed in the context of the relevant legal test or criteria. The test for will-making capacity in common law countries was established in 1870, when Chief Justice (CJ) Cockburn gave the judgment of the Court of Queens Bench in *Banks v. Goodfellow*. This test has been reaffirmed many times in the twentieth and twenty-first centuries (O'Neill & Peisah, 2011). Cockburn wrote that in relation to the capacity or power to make a will:

> It is essential to the exercise of such a power that a testator shall understand the nature of the act and its effects; shall understand the extent of the property of which he is disposing; shall be able to comprehend and appreciate the claims to which he ought to give effect; and, with a view to the latter object, that no disorder of mind shall poison his affections, pervert his sense of right, or prevent the exercise of his natural faculties—that no insane delusions shall influence his will in disposing of his property and bring about a disposal of it which, if the mind had been sound, would not have been made.

In modern language an additional stipulation has evolved, namely the ability to express wishes clearly and consistently in an orderly plan of disposition (Shulman et al., 2007).

In *Banks v. Goodfellow* it was held that the maker of the will, John Banks, was suffering from insane delusions. Nevertheless, his capacity and right to make a will were upheld. Cockburn counseled:

> No doubt, where the fact that the testator has been subject to any insane delusion is established, a will should be regarded with great distrust, and every presumption should in the first instance be made against it. Where insane delusion has once been shown to have existed, it may be difficult to say whether the mental disorder may not possibly have extended beyond the particular form or instance in which it manifested itself. It may be equally difficult to say how far the delusion may not have influenced the testator in the particular disposal of his property. And the presumption against a will made under such circumstances becomes additionally strong where the will is . . . one in which natural affection and claims of near relationship have been disregarded.

Cockburn noted that neither of the delusions from which Banks suffered, namely that he was pursued by spirits and that a man long since dead came to molest him, had "affected the general faculties of his mind, and could have no affect upon the will" and held that there was "no sufficient reason why the testator should be held to have lost his right to make a will, or why a will made under these circumstances should not be upheld."

Consequently, *Banks v. Goodfellow* not only laid down the test for will-making capacity, but also acknowledged that "unsoundness of mind" may be circumscribed and not impact testamentary disposition, and thus should not necessarily result in deprivation of the person's power to dispose of his or her property in a will. This reasoning presaged modern day thinking that capacity is task specific and not diagnosis bound (Peisah et al., 2009; Katona et al., 2009). Despite the insights demonstrated in *Banks v. Goodfellow*, modern case law has been accused, even by a member of the judiciary, of "marching with medicine but in the rear and limping a little" (*Mount Isa Mines Ltd v. Pusey*, 1970). How far has medicine and mental health progressed in the area of testamentary capacity? This chapter addresses research findings in the area of testamentary capacity and the practical relevance of such findings.

The assessment of testamentary capacity, like all capacities, is task specific and is related to the specific case law as defined above. *Banks v. Goodfellow* (1870) firmly established the task-specific criteria for testamentary capacity. Less well developed is the notion of situation-specific factors that are relevant to the ultimate determination of capacity. All complex capacities must incorporate an environmental component; perhaps nowhere is this more relevant than in will disputes in which the testator finds himself in the midst of a complicated and conflictual family milieu in which competing claims are being made from potential beneficiaries. Figure 5.1 illustrates the nature of the relationship between cognitive and emotional stability and the complexity or conflictual nature of the testator's milieu. In this model, a high level of conflict or complexity requires a higher level of cognitive and emotional stability compared to a testator in an uncomplicated milieu. The fundamental question posed to the court as well as to experts is whether an individual has the task-specific capacity to execute a will in the context of his or her situation-specific environment. It should be the interrelationship of mental state and environment that is the focus of the assessment. The same individual

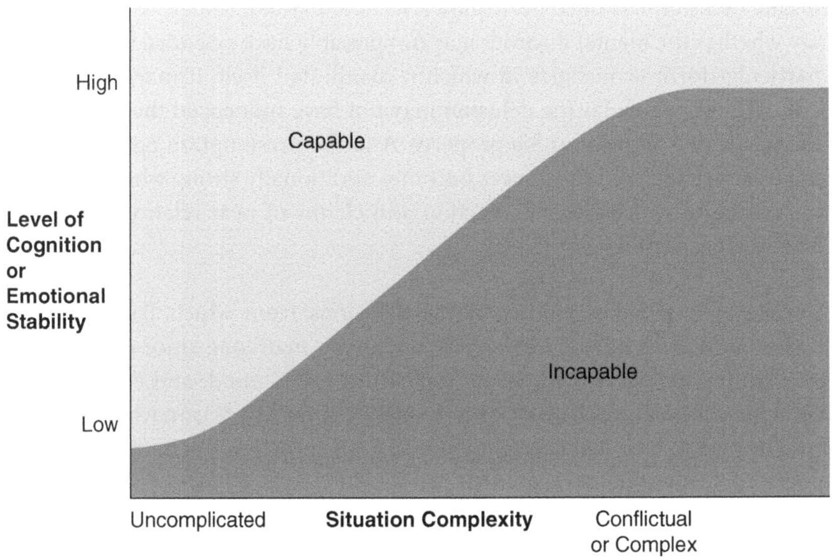

Figure 5.1 Cognition, Emotions, and Situation-Specific Capacity. (Adapted from Shulman et al., 2007.)

may be capable in a stable environment and yet is incapable in a complicated and conflictual environment that overwhelms his or her capacity to understand and appreciate the relevant issues and competing claims.

Pamela Champine (2006) assiduously reviewed extensive case law on challenges to wills based on the lack of testamentary capacity. She notes that "two centuries of experience adjudicating will contests might have produced a well accepted standard to determine the relevant roles of expert evidence. It has not." She concludes that the "sole certainty in testamentary capacity case law is unpredictability." It may be that the individualistic focus of the testamentary capacity standard (that includes situation-specific factors) allows by its very nature a great range of discretion to consider all relevant facts and circumstances in reaching the ultimate conclusion about testamentary capacity. It is this very element of discretion that may produce the unpredictability referred to above. However, Champine argues that the existence of a standard that would guide the decision maker's discretion would produce a more consistent pattern in case law.

RELEVANT NEUROPSYCHOLOGICAL RESEARCH

Testamentary Capacity and Neuroscience

There have been many attempts to define the neuropsychological or neurobiological correlates of the legal elements of will making, namely, understanding the nature of the will-making act and the extent of one's property, and understanding and appreciating the claims of beneficiaries. Yet understanding of these elements remains more theoretical than empirical, and is drawn from the area of medical decision-making capacity, where there has been an attempt to explore the neuropsychological and neurobiological bases of the legal standards that define the construct. Some 15 years ago, Grisso and Appelbaum (1995a,b,c,d) identified four of the commonly applied legal standards in courts in the United States for determining medical decision-making competence. These standards are as follows:

1. Ability to communicate a choice
2. Ability to understand relevant information
3. Ability to appreciate the situation and its likely consequence
4. Ability to manipulate information rationally (or reason about it) in a manner that allows one to make comparisons and weigh options.

A large body of research based on these constructs and applied to medical capacity in patients with a range of neuropsychiatric and medical conditions has since emerged (Dunn, Palmer, & Karlawish, 2007). Yet only one study has explored the specific brain regions involved in medical capacity, which might have theoretical application to will making. In a study of patients with schizophrenia, Eyler et al. (2007) found that understanding of a consent form correlated with activation of the right hippocampus, bilateral parahippocampus, cerebellum, and thalamus. These findings were consistent with their assumption that understanding of a consent form is related to an individual's ability to learn and remember information. Although medical capacity may be more reliant on verbal learning due to the importance of factual understanding of treatment, verbal learning is still relevant to will making as the testator may need to be informed of the value of the estate prior to disposition.

Other than the latter study on medical decision-making capacity, most of our understanding regarding brain regions and the neuropsychology of capacity has been extrapolated from functional neuroanatomy and cognitive neuroscience. For example, considering the second and third of the Grisso and Applebaum abilities, appreciation and reasoning, there is general consensus that "frontal executive functions" are involved (Dunn et al., 2007). The corollary for these functions in testamentary capacity is the understanding and appreciation of claims of potential beneficiaries. However, it is important to note that recent work has suggested that this often-used concept of "frontal executive function," thought to underlie most decision making, is overly simplistic. Not all executive functions are frontal and not all frontal functions are executive (Shulman & Feinstein, 2006).

Specifically, at least three frontal-subcortical circuits (dorsolateral prefrontal, orbitofrontal, and anterior cingulate) serve the affective, behavioral, and cognitive functions that appear to have a direct relevance to understanding, appreciation, and reasoning (Dunn et al., 2007). The dorsolateral prefrontal circuit has been implicated in many of the functions classically ascribed to the concept of "executive function," such as problem solving, planning, goal selection, self-monitoring, working memory, shifting of set, and, possibly, self-awareness and insight (Royall et al., 2002; Dunn et al., 2007). The anterior cingulate circuit and its limbic connections are involved in affect regulation, motivation, and placing valence on present and future outcomes (Dunn et al., 2007), as well as conflict monitoring and considering choice alternatives, reward, and pay-off (with some involvement of the lateral prefrontal and the orbitofrontal cortices) (Botvinick, 2007; Kennerley, Dahmubed, Lara, & Wallis, 2009). Finally, trust reciprocity (a concept with theoretical relevance to weighing beneficiaries, particularly "new found friends") has been associated with neural responses in the dorsal striatum (King-Casas et al., 2005).

It has been theorized that decision making is a dual process involving rapid intuitive/emotional processes (and probably involving ventromedial, basal ganglia, and limbic regions), and higher cognitive "executive" functions involved in the conscious weighing of pros and cons (probably related to dorsolateral regions) (Sanfey, Lowenstein, McClure, & Cohen, 2006; Kahneman, 2003). In particular, the role of emotions and affective signals in healthy decision making has been emphasized (Damasio 1994; Wood & Tanius, 2007; Bechara, Damasio, Tranel, & Damasio, 1997) and is probably important for the appraisal of relationships that are unique to the testamentary capacity task.

Autobiographical memory is another important and complex cognitive function that has relevance not only to weighing the claims of beneficiaries, but also for knowledge of the value of the estate. Autobiographical memory involves a distributed network of brain regions, including the ventrolateral and medial prefrontal cortex, the lateral and medial temporal regions, the temporoparietal cortex, the posterior cingulate/retrospinal regions, and the cerebellum, with secondary involvement of the lateral and orbital prefrontal cortices (McKinnon, Svoboda, & Levine, 2007). Autobiographical memory emerges from an interaction among episodic, semantic, and working memory processes. Episodic autobiographical memory involves the conscious recollection of temporally and spatially specific events from one's past, including event details, thoughts, and feelings, and is heavily reliant on prefrontal functions (McKinnon et al., 2007). Semantic memory comprises both public (world knowledge) and personal factual information such as identity, historical data, and the facts supporting awareness of personal events, including knowledge that an event has occurred, and is less dependent on prefrontal function (McKinnon et al., 2007). It is thus probably important for the appraisal of personal relationships and knowledge of assets. Recent studies have focused on the contribution of emotions to autobiographical memory recollection, suggesting intimate connections between prefrontal and limbic cortices in emotional processing and moral reasoning (McKinnon et al., 2007). Other cortical regions linked to decision making include the parietal lobe for calculation (Wood & Tanius, 2007), essential for the disposition of complex assets and fractional distribution. Clearly, the range of neuropsychological functions and brain candidate regions potentially involved in testamentary capacity is myriad. As stated by Wood and Tanius (2007, p. 95): "There can be no capacimeter that can tap into one localized brain region involved in decision making."

The actual recruitment of brain regions will probably vary with each will. Intuitively, the disposition of the family home to a spouse of 40 years might involve different neurocognitive processes than disposition of a complex art and jewelry collection divided among 12 cousins, sisters-in-law, and nieces who are in conflict and bargaining with the testator over who is the most deserving recipient. However, this remains speculative and not empirically established. In Table 5.1 we have outlined a range of candidate neuropsychological functions involved in the testamentary task.

In addition to the variation conferred by the complexity of the person's social environment and assets on the neuropsychological processes involved in testamentary capacity, there may be variation conferred by the novelty of the task. Are different cognitive demands involved in endorsing a previously expressed testamentary disposition compared with a novel disposition? Functional brain magnetic resonance imaging studies of the medial temporal lobe and the amygdala indicate greater activation by novel rather than familiar stimuli (Hashimoto et al., 2010). Novelty differentially engages other affective brain areas including those involved in controlling and regulating amygdala responses (e.g., orbitofrontal cortex), as well as those transmitting sensory signals that the amygdala modulates (e.g., occipitotemporal visual cortex) (Weierich, Wright, Negreira, Dickerson, & Barrett, 2010). Hypothetically, a familiar disposition devised before the onset of neurodegenerative disorder and merely endorsed during the disorder might thus be less taxing for the testator than a novel testamentary task executed during the neurodegenerative disorder.

Table 5.1 Criteria and Proposed Cognitive Functions for Testamentary Capacity

Criteria	Proposed Cognitive Function
Understanding the nature of the act and its effects	• Crystallized semantic knowledge
Understanding the extent of the property	• Long-term semantic and autobiographical memory regarding assets • Recent episodic and working memory if there has been recent changes to the estate (e.g., sale of the family home) • Verbal learning if the testator has been informed about the extent of the estate by the instructing solicitor • Calculia
Understanding and appreciating the claims to which the testator ought to give effect	• Long-term autobiographical/episodic memory to recall relationships, conflicts, and previous gifting • Executive functions of planning, judgment, and reasoning to weigh and consider • Conflict monitoring, choice evaluation • Working memory to hold potential beneficiaries in mind and consider them
Communicating the decision	• Expressive and receptive language

Development of Capacity Assessment Instruments

Champine (2006) highlighted the importance of a contemporaneous assessment of testamentary capacity in predicting the outcome of judicial cases. She also argued that the unpredictability of outcomes in testamentary cases could be mitigated by the development of a forensic assessment instrument for such cases. The development and ultimate adoption of such an assessment instrument have the potential to improve the quality of testamentary capacity determinations. However, this would be the case only if such instruments are soundly designed and utilized in a proper fashion. A forensic assessment instrument can function only in relation to a particular legal test reflecting the task-specific nature of all capacities. The development of such an instrument calls for a collaborative approach between lawyers and psychologists or other cognate experts. Lawyers must be knowledgeable about the legal test to which the instrument will relate and psychologists or other experts must design their questions so that the fact finder will have information about the cognitive functions that are relevant to the legal standards. The gold standard for such instruments is derived from the MacArthur Treatment Competence Study (Grisso & Applebaum, 1995b). This study developed a reliable and valid instrument to address questions regarding the abilities of mentally ill individuals to make decisions about psychiatric treatment. This led to the notion that decision makers must have the ability to work rationally with information that bears on their decisions and to appreciate their impact. It is precisely this high level "executive function" that is difficult to operationalize into a standardized test. The challenge is to isolate the cognitive component of an abstract concept such as "appreciation" and separate it from value judgments. Translating the concept of appreciation and the notion of rational manipulation of relevant information are at the core of the design of such assessment instruments.

Forensic instruments, if developed, would not substitute for the legal adjudications of capacity (Champine, 2006). Rather, they are designed to supply the fact finders with information that might not otherwise be available. The instrument could serve a "gate-keeping function" that would isolate borderline cases and channel those without clear-cut capacity to alternative procedures for adjudication. If a forensic assessment instrument was developed for testamentary capacity, it would not be subject to the concern that has been expressed in "consent to treatment" regarding the need for multiple administrations. This is because in the execution of a will, a single transaction occurs at a particular moment in time. The instrument would thus need to be validated only on that particular occasion. A testamentary capacity assessment instrument that clearly identifies the testator's capacity should be able to protect such testators against future lawsuits. Champine (2006) and Marson and Briggs (2001) make the case that a contemporaneous assessment instrument could help to develop a coherent body of law in place of the unpredictable morass of current testamentary capacity decisions.

Recent research on the refinement of capacity assessment instruments has addressed consent to treatment and financial decision making (Applebaum & Grisso 2001; Marson, Earnst, Jamil, Bartolucci, & Harrell, 2000). The knowledge gained in these areas has yet to be applied to testamentary capacity. These capacity assessment instruments may help to standardize judicial decisions and to improve the extremely low reliability of general clinical examinations as demonstrated by Marson et al. (2000) with respect to the consistency of physicians' judgments of legal standards. Previous work (Marson, Cody, Ingram, & Harrell, 1995) has found a lack of agreement between physicians in assessing patients with mild Alzheimer's disease. Moreover, physicians tend to base their capacity judgments on different cognitive skills of patients. However, with the development of legal standards and associated training, this could be improved.

Marson et al. (2000) developed legal standards for use in "consent to treatment" by extracting variables from relevant case law and culling information from the forensic psychiatry literature. This resulted in five progressively more complex legal standards that could be applied to a testamentary instrument:

LS 1: Evidence a treatment choice.
LS 2: Make the reasonable treatment choice when the alternative is manifestly unreasonable.[1]

1. Though this is not an accepted legal standard for judging consent capacity because of concerns about possible arbitrariness and questions about determining what constitutes a

LS 3: Appreciate the consequences of a treatment choice.
LS 4: Provide rational reasons for a treatment choice.
LS 5: Understand the treatment situation and choices.

Marson et al. (2000) found that personal competency judgments were most closely associated with the higher legal standards LS 4 and LS 5, reflecting a more sophisticated cognitive approach to decision making. Their research has also shown a correlation between specific neurocognitive abilities and the tasks necessary for consent to treatment. Specifically, as reflected in legal standard LS 5, the understanding of relevant material is best reflected by tests of verbal conceptionalization, verbal recall, and semantic memory. On the other hand, reasoning is correlated with verbal fluency. Understanding and reasoning are considered most clinically relevant and appropriate for deciding competency in consent to treatment cases and may be generalizable to other complex capacities such as testamentary capacity.

Earnst, Marson, and Harrell (2000) studied cognitive models of physicians' judgments of competency in patients suffering from Alzheimer's disease. They concluded that the assessment of competency should include an evaluation of semantic knowledge, verbal recall, and simple reasoning abilities. In previous work, Marson, Hawkins, McInturff, and Harrell, (1997) isolated those cognitive models that predicted physician judgments of capacity to consent to treatment in patients with Alzheimer's disease. For example, "conservative" physicians were most sensitive to a memory model of capacity emphasizing verbal recall. In cases in which they found impaired memory, they judged the patient to be incompetent. In contrast, "liberal" physicians depended on an executive model in which competent patients were found to have intact higher level functioning and information processing. These findings continue to support the use of a standardized competency instrument that could incorporate specific legal standards and cognitive functions and hence reduce the unpredictability of clinician judgments and ultimately judicial decisions.

Although not explicitly stated, these legal standards take into account situation-specific complexity that may be helpful in determining whether a testator's cognitive function is adequate to deal with his or her situation. For example, in mild to moderate Alzheimer's disease, there is still a preservation of communication. Therefore in a relatively non-conflictual and uncomplicated milieu, a lower threshold such as legal standard LS 1 (evidencing a choice) may still meet the standard for competence. In contrast, a complex and a conflictual environment would require a higher legal standard involving the appreciation of the consequences of specific choices, the provision of rational reasons for a change in disposition, and an ability to understand their milieu and the impact of their decision. However, in a severe dementia, receptive aphasia and impaired semantic memory impair the ability of individuals to express themselves clearly. Even for evidencing a simple choice, they would not meet the lowest legal standard threshold, and thus would not be considered capable.

"reasonable choice," it has been found to be useful in understanding treatment preferences of patients with neurocognitive impairment (see Marson & Herbert, 2008).

Marson and Briggs (2001) crystallized the research on cognitive models and decision making by posing the ultimate question regarding capacity: "Is he/she competent to do X in the context of Y?" This incorporates both task-specific and situation-specific factors. Grisso (1986) had already highlighted the fact that clinical findings, including test results, need to be linked to the specific capacities with which the law is concerned. Such individuals must be able to process relevant information at different levels (dependent on the specifics and complexity of their situation) and then integrate this information with established knowledge incorporating their personal values and beliefs. Ultimately, they need to be able to weigh all the information in a rational manner to arrive at a decision or choice and then must have the capacity to communicate that decision in an understandable fashion. Cognitive functions that are required to perform these important tasks include short-term and long-term memory, receptive and expressive language, and conceptualization as well as executive function such as judgment and reasoning, especially in complex situations or milieus (see Table 5.1).

Thus, the challenge in developing a testamentary capacity assessment instrument is to incorporate the relevant conceptual models specific to the legal test of testamentary capacity with related cognitive functions based on empirical findings. Whether this is feasible remains to be seen; the unpredictability and variability of physician judgments and legal decisions make this a compelling challenge.

COMMON MEDICAL CONDITIONS THAT MAY AFFECT TESTAMENTARY CAPACITY

Banks v. Goodfellow (1870) was based on a case of psychosis. In modern times, cases of dementia far outnumber cases of psychosis as the basis for will challenges. In a case series of 25 challenges to testamentary capacity, 40% were based on dementia, 28% were alcohol related, 28% were based on a neurological (nondementia) or psychiatric disorder, 20% were due to personality disorder, and 12% were related to suicide (Shulman, Cohen, & Hull, 2005). Another series of will challenges in Australia reflected a similar, albeit greater, preponderance of dementia among a heterogeneous group of syndromes. In a series of 41 will challenges, 78% were based on dementia, 7% on delirium or complex medical conditions, 5% on schizophrenia or paranoid states, and 2.5% each on alcohol, personality disorder, bipolar disorder, and depression/suicide (O'Neill & Peisah, 2011). Although not as frequently represented as the primary condition, alcohol abuse was the most common comorbid condition. Clearly this pattern will vary according to the specialty of the expert and the patterns of referral to neuropsychologists or geriatricians may differ from that of psychiatrists.

Dementia and Testamentary Capacity

Etiology: Dementia is a heterogeneous condition, the causes of which are dominated by Alzheimer's disease, mixed vascular dementia and Alzheimer's disease, vascular dementia, and Lewy Body dementia (Mendez & Cummings, 2003). Distinguishing the cause of dementia in a person whose testamentary capacity is in question may help predict the likelihood of certain deficits at different stages of the disease, although there is still much variation between individuals. For example, an individual with vascular dementia may have early loss of frontal, "executive" functions such as judgment and reasoning and accordingly have difficulties weighing the claims of beneficiaries.

Severity: Few conclusions about testamentary capacity can be drawn from a knowledge of the severity of dementia alone. It has been suggested that an estimate of severity is relevant only at the extremes of dementia, such that a person with severe dementia lacks testamentary capacity whereas a person with mild dementia or mild cognitive impairment retains capacity (Shulman et al., 2007). However, such assumptions do not take into account the complexity of the testamentary task. An assessment of the severity of dementia merely provides a context for the understanding of the person's mental abilities to deal with the testamentary task. Importantly, dementia does not have to be severe to affect a person's capacity for highly complex reasoning such as appraisal of family members

Furthermore, the threshold concept relies on more than simply a rating of severity of cognitive impairment. Rather, severity is part of "vulnerability load" comprising emotional factors, cognition, mental disorder, personality, and psychosocial situations that interact with the complexity of the will in the determination of testamentary capacity (Shulman et al., 2007). For example, an individual with mild global cognitive impairment, but with significant frontal lobe deficits affecting reasoning and judgment or with comorbid emotional/mental disorder or adverse psychosocial circumstances, may not be able to handle a simple will.

Lucidity: Although the courts have long held the idea that those with mental illnesses may be able to make wills during lucid periods (a period of clarity or temporary improvement in mental state), lucidity is a concept that confounds the understanding of dementia and testamentary capacity, and has more relevance to delirium (see below). Certainly, persons with dementia will often fluctuate and may have better days or better times of the day, such that the person may be able to converse to some extent or carry out activities of daily living some days whereas on other days the person may urinate in a wastepaper basket or shout at the staff. The issue for consideration is the fit between the task and the cognitive abilities of the testator at the time of the evaluation. Having said that, although much has been made of the determination of mental capacity at the precise moment the will is made, it is often difficult to ignore the "before and after evidence" (Sprehe & Kerr, 1996). For example, although accepting evidence as to "good days and bad days," an Australian judge, Windyer, noted in *Robinson v. Spratt*:

> The clear psychiatric evidence is that the deceased was on a downhill path from 1989 onwards as a result of dementia. There were some better periods but the path was always downwards. [2002; NSWSC 426, [43]; also see *Estate of Harms* 149 P. 2d 557 (2006)]

Other Conditions That May Affect Testamentary Capacity

Aphasia: One of the hallmarks of capacity is the ability to communicate a preference or a decision, which makes it dependent on language ability. The presence of aphasia may thus hamper the assessment of both capacity and overall cognitive function. The challenge for the clinician is to determine the extent of cognitive impairment, if any, accompanying aphasia (Ferguson et al., 2003). Indeed, there is mounting evidence to suggest that it is impossible to predict the status of other aspects of cognition on the basis of language skills alone (Helm-Estabrooks, 2002). Higher level executive skills such as judgment, flexibility, planning, and foresight are the most vulnerable to the type of brain damage associated with aphasia and must be carefully screened in such patients (Helm-Estabrooks, 2002). Therefore, previous suggestions of using prompted recall and recognition memory with cues (e.g., identifying the correct response from a list of correct and incorrect answers) to maximize communication with an aphasic will-maker will provide a fairly gross estimation of understanding and should ideally be interpreted by a speech-language pathologist (Spar & Grab, 1992).

Delirium: Delirium is a transient, usually fluctuating impairment in consciousness, attention, and cognition, most commonly due to a chest or urinary tract infection, electrolyte disturbance, or drug toxicity. It is usually reversible once the underlying cause is treated. The issue of delirium is often relevant when instructions for a will are taken in the hospital setting, particularly when someone decides, or is prompted, to write or change a will on their "death bed" or when they are extremely ill. Delirium may affect testamentary capacity due to its global effects on cognition, and particularly its effects on concentration, perception of reality, memory, and reasoning, although the effect on will-making will depend largely on the severity of the delirium, its fluctuation, and the complexity of the will-making task (Liptzin et al., 2010). The fluctuating nature of delirium including the possibility of lucid intervals has led to rulings such as *O'Rourke v. Hunter* (2006) in which the following was held:

> The critical question is whether the testator was of sound mind at the time the will was executed. It has been held that "a person . . . may possess testamentary capacity at any given time and lack it at all other times."

This explicitly acknowledges that if an individual was experiencing a lucid interval when he or she signed the will, then it is valid, particularly if there is consistency over time (hours, days, weeks, or months) in the person's expressed wishes (Liptzin, Peisah, Shulman, & Finkel, 2010). This is more difficult in the case of delirium complicating dementia, where the underlying dementia makes it unlikely that a person can be "lucid enough" to have testamentary capacity even during lucid intervals (Sprehe & Kerr, 1996).

Alcohol and drug-related disorders: Alcohol-related disorder is an important comorbid condition in documented will challenges, comprising 28% of the challenges in one small series (Shulman et al., 2005). Regardless of whether the will maker suffered habitual intoxication, abuse, or dependence, the effect of alcohol abuse is relevant only if the person was intoxicated, withdrawing from alcohol, or suffering other consequences of alcohol abuse, such as paranoid ideation, at the time of making the will and only if such mental disorder rendered the individual incapable of performing one or more of the mental functions necessary to make a valid will (Shulman, Hull, & Cohen, 2003; Shulman et al., 2007). This is the case with any drug-related disorder. Drugs or withdrawal from them can cause changes in consciousness, perception of reality, and reasoning, all of which can impact the will-making process. Drug effects can vary between subtly altering the way complex decisions are made at one extreme and rendering a patient unconscious at the other (Ferner, 1997).

Psychotic conditions: Psychotic symptoms include delusions and hallucinations. They may occur in the context of illnesses such as schizophrenia or bipolar disorder, either of which may be present and continue into old age or present for the first time in old age (late onset). Dementia is complicated by delusions in 20–73% of cases and hallucinations in 15–49% of cases (Mizrahi, Starkstein, Jorge, & Robinson, 2006; Hart et al., 2003).

The task of the capacity assessor in regards to psychosis is twofold: First, to distinguish whether beliefs are psychotic and, if so, to ascertain if they affect testamentary capacity. The law places some importance on distinguishing between "mere antipathy" or capriciousness, albeit unreasonable, toward a beneficiary, and psychotic, or more specifically, paranoid beliefs. Paranoia has, in fact, been the basis of many will changes in common law countries [*Re Estate of Griffith; Easter v. Griffith* (1995) 217 ALR 284; for a U.S. statement of the insane delusion test see *Breeden v. Stone* 922 P.2d 1167 (2006) and for a U.S. example of an insane delusion leading to the setting aside of a will see *Miami Rescue Mission Inc. v. Roberts* 943 So. 2d 274, 2006].

Mood disorders and suicide: Mood disorders such as depression may have an impact on the will-making process if they are accompanied by symptoms of hopelessness or delusions of persecution, poverty, or sin, which might affect the will maker's perception of his or her assets or relationships. As already noted, the act of suicide is not regarded as evidence per se of incapacity (e.g., *Re Hodges; Shorter v. Hodges,* 1988). Suicide usually occurs in the context of psychiatric disorders such as depression, alcohol abuse, and psychosis and its relevance to capacity must be interpreted in the light of these contextual psychiatric disorders as well as the nature of gifting set out in the will (i.e., whether it was expected or rational or otherwise) and the proximity of the making of the will to the writing of the suicide note and the suicide itself (Shulman et al., 2003).

Personality disorders: As stated previously, the law draws a distinction between mere antipathy, albeit unreasonable, and judgment affected by psychosis. The "mere antipathy" referred to in legal cases usually arises in the context of personality disorders and there has been some debate as to whether personality disorder constitutes a disorder of mind [*Re Estate of Griffith; Easter v. Griffith* (1995) 217 ALR Gleeson CJ and Handley JA; Kirby in dissent 293]. In specific cases personality disorders might have an effect on testamentary capacity just as distorting as frank psychotic symptoms (O'Neill & Peisah, 2011).

Some personality disorders, such as paranoid, borderline, and narcissistic can present as serious disorders, associated with abnormalities in mood, ideation, and object relations (i.e., relations with loved ones). In severe cases, symptoms such as (1) splitting (e.g., the good wife, the good son versus the bad son and the bad wife), (2) idealization, (3) devaluation, and (4) paranoid ideation with or without accompanying mood disturbance may poison affections toward beneficiaries and render a will maker unable to adequately weigh the claims of potential beneficiaries (O'Neill & Peisah, 2011). However, caution is advised when suggesting that personality disorder is incompatible with will making because the diagnosis of personality disorder is based on a life-long and enduring pattern of behavior and relating to others. It is probably incompatible with sound disposition only in severe cases or during times of crisis or decompensation (i.e., when under stress, the person with personality disorder becomes particularly disturbed).

ROLE OF UNDUE INFLUENCE

Another basis of will challenges is undue influence. For a court to make a finding of undue influence, it must first have found that the person possessed testamentary capacity. Perhaps the most succinct description of undue influence in relation to will making was given by Sir James Hannen in 1885 as follows:

> To be undue influence in the eye of the law there must be—to sum it up in a word—coercion. (*Wingrove* v. *Wingrove*, 1885)

Sir James Hannen elaborated:

> The coercion may of course be of different kinds, it may be in the grossest form, such as actual confinement or violence, or a person in the last days or hours of life may have become so weak and feeble that very little pressure will be sufficient to bring about the desired result. (*Wingrove v. Wingrove*, 1885)

The clinician expert's evidence should deal with the question of the will maker's vulnerability to undue influence. It is for the court to decide whether influence was exercised or not. To that end, a recent international task force has outlined the kind of risk factors that make a will maker vulnerable to undue influence (Peisah et al., 2006, 2009). These include the following:

(1) Relationship risk factors, namely "confidential" or close relationships between vulnerable will makers and a range of family members, friends, associates, or carers;
(2) Social or environmental risk factors such as psychological and or physical dependency on a carer, sequestration and isolation, family

conflict, being of migrant background, and unable to converse in the language of the new country;

(3) Psychological factors such as delirium; emotional vulnerability conferred by grief, loneliness, death bed situations, and sexual bargaining; personality traits such as dependency; psychiatric illnesses such as depression, psychosis, and anxiety; and cognitive impairment. With regards to cognitive impairment, a range of neuropsychological factors associated with dementia may confer vulnerability to undue influence. These include impairments in judgment and reasoning, and deficits in autobiographical and working memory. Additionally, personality changes such as increased passivity and paranoid ideation regarding previously favored loved ones may enhance vulnerability (Peisah, Brodaty, & Quadrio, 2006; Peisah et al., 2009).

(4) Legal risk factors such as the procurement of the will by the beneficiary who is favored in the will, unnatural provisions, which exclude natural beneficiaries, and a will that is inconsistent with previous wishes (Spar & Garb, 1992).

CONTEMPORANEOUS ASSESSMENT OF TESTAMENTARY CAPACITY

Despite indications that a contemporaneous assessment instrument can be of significant value, there is still a current need to provide direction and guidelines for those clinicians conducting assessments of testamentary capacity for the benefit of the courts. Shulman et al. (2009) on behalf of the International Psychogeriatric Association Task Force provided guidelines for clinicians/experts performing testamentary capacity assessments. Common reasons for retaining an expert opinion include the following:

1. Suspicious circumstances (Hull & Hull 1996)—especially where there has been a dramatic change from previous wills or previously expressed wishes with respect to estate distribution.
2. Presumptive evidence of a concurrent mental or neurological disorder.
3. Circumstances that suggest a challenge to the will is very likely by aggrieved potential beneficiaries.
4. Extreme frailty or advanced age.

A contemporaneous assessment of testamentary capacity, if done properly, may provide protection for the testator against future challenges. However, Jacoby and Steer (2007) raise a concern with respect to the possible increase in requests for contemporaneous assessments. They note that many clinicians do not have the requisite knowledge and skills necessary for the assessment of testamentary capacity. This includes a lack of understanding of the legal test that speaks to the recently accepted codes of conduct for expert evidence highlighting the fact that the clinician must give opinions only within his or her area of expertise.

Prior to undertaking an assessment of testamentary capacity the assessor should ensure that he or she has sufficient clinical expertise to provide such an assessment including adequate knowledge of the legal test and the medicolegal literature related to testamentary capacity.

The following materials, where available, should be reviewed by the assessor: prior wills as well as the specific will in question, other related legal documents such as Powers of Attorney, a list of the testator's assets from a reliable source, and all relevant medical records.

In addition to the specific criteria of *Banks v. Goodfellow*, Shulman et al. (2007) highlighted areas for probing and documentation that would ultimately assess whether the testator can formulate a coherent testamentary disposition that links prior beliefs, values, and relationships with the proposed distribution. Specific issues that require attention in a contemporaneous assessment include the documentation of a clear and consistent rationale for any dramatic changes or significant deviations from prior wills or previously expressed wishes regarding the estate. One of the advantages conferred by a contemporaneous assessment is the ability of a clinician to cue testators in order to determine whether they show an awareness of their prior beliefs, wishes, or prior wills. Similarly, the exploration of knowledge of assets may require cuing in some vulnerable individuals. However, given the consensus that only a general knowledge of the extent and nature of assets is required, such contemporaneous cuing may reveal that a testator with some help can still provide a consistent understanding of the nature and extent of assets that he or she wishes to distribute. Contemporaneous exploration should include the following situation-specific and task-specific factors (Shulman et al., 2009):

- Testators' understanding and appreciation of conflicts or tensions in their environment or milieu.
- Especially in a distribution that deviates from prior wills or excludes "natural" beneficiaries such as close family members or spouses, an appreciation of the consequences and impact of such distributions in addition to the rationale.
- Identifying those potential beneficiaries who are excluded from the will or who are bequeathed lower amounts than might be expected and clarifying the specific concerns that led to that distribution. The clinician conducting a contemporaneous assessment is in a position to rule out the presence of a delusion or overvalued idea or cognitive impairment that may influence such distribution.
- The clinician can document evidence of behavioral or psychiatric symptoms associated with dementia or other mental disorders to understand the connection between mental and cognitive functioning and the proposed disposition.
- Establish whether testators can communicate a clear and consistent choice with respect to their asset distribution. This may require assessment on more than one occasion to demonstrate consistency of thinking over time.

Without the benefit of a standardized forensic assessment instrument, Shulman et al. (2007) have recommended a semi-structured approach to mental status and cognitive examination. This includes an assessment of sensory or language impairment that may affect the perception of capacity. The assessor should ensure that an adequate means of communication has been established to determine whether comprehension or communication is the primary deficit. The mental status examination should include appearance and behavior; speech; mood and affect; thought process and content; and perceptual abnormalities, insight, and judgment. With respect to cognitive functioning, it is recommended that the assessor use validated cognitive screening instruments such as the Mini-Mental Status Examination (MMSE) (Folstein et al., 1975), the Clock Drawing test (Shulman, 2000), as well as frontal and executive tests that include verbal fluency and abstract ability. Examples include the Frontal Assessment Battery (FAB) (Dubois, Slachevsky, Litvan, & Pillon, 2000), which includes the three-step Luria test and the Go/No-Go test. Consistent with the work of Earnst et al. (2000), it may be helpful to correlate neuropsychological findings on specific tasks to an individual's capacity. Ultimately, the findings on mental status and cognitive testing should support a diagnosis that connects the expert's opinion on capacity to the specific legal test.

Although the MMSE correlates with testamentary capacity (Roked & Patel, 2008) we caution against generalizing these findings to the task and situation specifics of each case. Although it is true that most individuals with high MMSE scores will have capacity and most individuals with low MMSE scores will be incapable, there are many examples of cases in which this does not apply. In a highly complex and conflictual environment even mild cognitive impairment may be sufficient to overwhelm the capacity of a testator. Conversely, a moderately impaired individual may be capable of giving direction for a will where values and wishes have been consistently held over many years in an uncomplicated situation.

RETROSPECTIVE ASSESSMENT OF TESTAMENTARY CAPACITY

Contemporaneous assessment has many clear advantages including the opportunity to probe and cue the testator to determine whether a clear consistent wish is evident in relation to the legal test for testamentary capacity. However, a retrospective assessment has some advantages, especially in situations in which the level of the testator's cognitive and psychiatric status is not clear at the time of the execution of the will. There may be more documentation available than was the case at the time the will was executed (O'Neill & Peisah, 2011). Documentation should include the following where available:

- Full medical records including hospital records
- Notes of the general practitioner are especially helpful or those of psychiatrists, neurologists, or geriatricians
- Nursing home records
- Community health practitioner assessments

- Lawyer's notes regarding the execution of the will
- Affidavits of people who had a close relationship with the testator
- Prior wills and other relevant legal documents such as Powers of Attorney reflecting the nature of key relationships and pattern of prior wishes with respect to the assets of the testator

The ability to look retrospectively and determine the long-term course of a dementing illness may cast a different light on the testator's concerns and beliefs at the time the will was executed (see case below). Changes in attitude, behavior and suspiciousness common in the early stages of dementia may be easier to assess in the context of 20/20 hindsight. Preservation of social graces is a common confounding phenomenon in the early and middle stages of dementia. The courts need to have the input of expert assessors to interpret the behavioral and psychological symptoms of dementia such as paranoid ideation and suspiciousness that may be influencing the disposition. In most other respects, the retrospective assessment of testamentary capacity involves the same issues that have been highlighted in contemporaneous assessments. However, the inability to examine the testator directly is a significant limitation of the retrospective assessment, but in many cases, the courts must rely on these assessments when there has been no contemporaneous assessment. Where there has been a contemporaneous assessment, the court may benefit from an expert evaluation of the quality and relevance of such an assessment.

CASE STUDY OF RETROSPECTIVE ASSESSMENT OF TESTAMENTARY CAPACITY

W. executed her last will on March 12, 2002 at age 85. She never married and had no children and lived alone for most of her life. Alice was a long-time friend and fellow Community Club member. Linda was also a long-time friend, but the evidence suggests that she was not especially close to W. until the events of the last 2 years of her life. W. along with friends established the Community Club that became central to this will dispute. At the heart of the dispute was W.'s intention with respect to the property that she owned on which the Social Club was located. The will of 2002 (her last will) bequeathed the property to Linda and the Community Club whereas her previous will had bequeathed her entire estate, including the property, to her friend Alice.

Prior Wills and Other Legal Documents

The 1980 will was divided into 10 equal shares. Five of those 10 shares were allocated to Alice. Only one share was assigned to the Community Club. A second will was executed in 1997, but this was a hand-written "drugstore will" apparently drafted by W. without the knowledge of Alice. This will bequeathed W.'s entire estate to Alice and her husband. The assumption is that in 1997 W. was still a capable and fiercely independent individual and took it upon herself to draft this will. An earlier Power of Attorney designated Alice and shortly thereafter a Transfer of Title for the property was made to Alice.

Assumptions Until 2001

1. *The documentation strongly supports the notion that until 1999, a strong and sustained personal and trusting relationship existed between W. and Alice.*
2. *There is no evidence that Alice exerted significant pressure or influence on W. nor did they act improperly in the legal transactions involving earlier wills, Power of Attorney or Transfer of Title.*
3. *W. remained fiercely independent and mentally capable in all spheres until approximately 2001 when overt signs of significant cognitive impairment became evident.*
4. *The relationship between Alice and W. was a mutually trusting relationship until approximately late fall 2001, coincident with the onset of W.'s dementia.*

Cognitive Changes from 2001 Onward and Related Developments

Community assessments: *In the summer of 2001, community nurses became involved with W. because of concerns regarding her ability to function independently. A MMSE was done in the summer of 2001. W. scored 20/30 reflecting a moderately severe level of cognitive impairment given her high premorbid level of intelligence.*

The concern about financial abuse was raised by a number of individuals who knew W. in January 2002. Linda and others reported that W. was apparently surprised and upset to hear that her previous will had left all of her properties and belongings to Alice. This led Linda and others to conclude that Alice had acted improperly or had exerted undue influence on W. However, W. was unable to recall significant events from the past in which she was directly involved including the previous wills five and ten years earlier, the earlier Power of Attorney, and the Transfer of Title. This seems to be the state in which W. wanted to change her will in March 2002 when a community care nurse assessed W. at her home just 2 days after the execution of the last will. Her Mini-Mental State score was 12/30 on that date and the Clock Drawing test revealed right/left reversal and severe visuospatial organizational difficulties, reflecting a moderately severe level of cognitive impairment.

In May 2002, 2 months after the execution of the last will, a community care nurse assessed W. at her home in the company of her friend, Linda. The community nurse reports what appeared to be W.'s impression that checks were being written from her bank account without her knowledge. W. also reported that several items went missing from her home and that it was her impression that Alice was "feigning friendship."

Linda's new relationship with W: *Linda became much more involved with W. in December 2001. At that time, the earlier Transfer of Title to Alice was discovered and concerns were raised regarding the possibility of financial abuse. These concerns were based on the statements made by W., which were taken at face value by Linda and others including the lawyer who helped prepare the 2002 will. W. believed that she had been abandoned by Alice and began to seek help from Linda and others as she was feeling overwhelmed and agitated about her situation. She developed an increasingly strong antipathy toward Alice based on a number of paranoid beliefs. She became convinced that Alice had stolen property from her and was threatening to harm her. It appeared that W. had completely forgotten about the transfer of Title that occurred several years earlier. Linda reports W.'s feelings: "I need you to help me, I want to get rid of Alice." All she could think about was getting rid of Alice. She was terrified of Alice. Linda reports that W. had police phone numbers on the wall, reflecting her level of fearfulness and distress.*

Evaluation by psychiatrist Dr. A: *Dr. A noted that the Mini-Mental State scores in March and April 2002 ranging from 12 to 16 out of 30 reflected consistently and severely impaired cognitive functioning at the time she executed her will. He also confirmed W.'s lack of insight as a result of her dementia as well as her vulnerability to influence at that time. Dr. A completed a capacity assessment on April 24, 2002 (1 month after the execution of her last will) in which he concluded that she had dementia of the Alzheimer type of moderate severity. He also concluded in that document that "this lady is vulnerable and it is highly likely that she was abused financially." This was based on input from her new friend Linda. Dr. A assessed W. again in September 2002 at the long-term care facility where she was transferred. The documentation confirms evidence for a progressive dementia, which was already well advanced by 2002 at the time that the last will was executed.*

W.'s lawyer: *A lawyer was involved in advising W. and her friends regarding the March 2002 will. He did not discuss the content with W. or even the existence of the previous legal documents including the earlier wills, Power of Attorney, and Title transfer. He based his conclusion that W. was capable of executing a will in March 2002 on her repeated "clear statements" that she wanted the Community Club property to go to the Club and not to Alice, who she now vilified. It appears that W. may still have had preserved social graces that gave the appearance of being intact unless probed or challenged. Moreover, it cannot be assumed that her clear or emphatic statements imply capacity.*

Summary of Case

W. was suffering from a dementing illness that became clearly manifest in 2001 and progressed until her death in 2003. Certainly by 2002, the evidence is overwhelming that W. was in an advanced stage of dementia. It would appear that her friend Linda and others, including her lawyer, interpreted W.'s concerns on the basis of the faulty assumption that she was cognitively intact and without the benefit of a detailed mental status examination or probing of rationale. Dementia can be easily missed unless it is specifically evaluated (O'Neill & Peisah, 2011). The belief that Alice had abandoned W. and had stolen items from her was in all probability based on paranoid misperceptions/delusions secondary to W.'s cognitive impairment. In dementia, paranoid ideation is commonly a compensatory mechanism for memory loss and may result in alienation of previously trusted family or friends (Peisah et al., 2006). Certainly when items went missing, W. did not have insight that she was impaired. As she became more suspicious and paranoid about Alice, the focus of her delusions was sharpened primarily onto Alice. She based her subsequent actions (with the misguided help of her friends) on these false beliefs. Furthermore, her memory impairment as a result of the dementia in 2002 precluded her recollection of her past actions. This made her incapable of understanding and appreciating the relevant issues involved in the 2002 changes to the will. If she had no recollection that she had bequeathed significant amounts of her estate to Alice and had no recollection of appointing her as Power of Attorney or transferring her Land Title, then she was not capable of giving legal directions in 2002. She lacked the capacity to appreciate the rationale for her previous actions and falsely assumed that Alice had somehow cheated her way into becoming the chief beneficiary. Her lawyer, her friends, and even some of the mental health professionals mistakenly assumed that financial abuse had been taking place and that the legal documents that had been executed in the past were obtained by fraudulent or coercive means.

From a clinical perspective, W. was not capable of understanding and appreciating the consequences of the will that was executed in March 2002. Moreover, her decision to change her will was based on delusional beliefs about Alice, which were a result of her cognitive impairment. By 2002, the combination of delusions and memory impairment also made her extremely vulnerable to undue influence.

FUTURE CONSIDERATIONS IN TESTAMENTARY CAPACITY ASSESSMENTS

The unpredictability of judicial opinions related to testamentary capacity and undue influence makes this a pressing societal concern. The lack of consistency in physician judgments and the variability in the quality of reports by experts only exacerbate this unpredictability. Hopefully, the new codes of conduct for experts will help to produce greater consistency in the approach to the evaluation of testamentary capacity. Additionally, new instruments can be developed that incorporate the necessary legal standards and situation-specific factors that are critical to testamentary capacity (Champine, 2006; Marson et al., 2004). Such instruments must connect relevant cognitive functions and models to the testamentary test and incorporate them into a standardized instrument. This will require a collaborative effort of lawyers, physicians, psychologists, and even ethicists.

Banks v. Goodfellow (1870) remains the predominant legal standard for testamentary capacity and, almost a century and a half later, this remains a landmark English case (O'Neill & Peisah, 2011). However, society and will makers have evolved in a dramatic way as has our understanding of cognition. The new demographic has created a cohort of older and often cognitively compromised will makers. Wills will be challenged not as much on the basis of schizophrenic delusions (such as John Banks) but more commonly on the basis of deficits in cognition, memory, judgment, and reasoning. For a compromised testator, the task of weighing and discriminating between the various claims of potential beneficiaries is a difficult one, especially when faced with a complicated wealth portfolio and complex family dynamics. This is not necessarily what the law makers and testators faced in the nineteenth century, but what they certainly face now in the twenty-first century.

References

Applebaum, P. S., & Grisso, T. (2001). *MacArthur Competence Assessment Tool for Clinical research (MacCAT-CR)*. Sarasota, FL: Professional Resource Press.

Banks v. Goodfellow (1870). LR 5 QB 549.

Bechara, A., Damasio, H., Tranel, D., & Damasio, A. (1997). Deciding advantageously before knowing the advantageous strategy. *Science, 275,* 1293–1295.

Botvinick, M. M. (2007). Conflict monitoring and decision making: Reconciling two perspectives on anterior cingulate function. *Cognitive, Affective and Behavioural Neuroscience, 7,* 356–366.

Champine, P. (2006). Expertise and instinct in the assessment of testamentary capacity. *Villanova Law Review, 51,* 25–94.

Damasio, A. (1994). *Descartes error: Emotion, reason and the human brain*. New York: Avon Books.

Dubois, B., Slachevsky, A., Litvan, I., & Pillon, B. (2000). The FAB: A Frontal Assessment Battery at bedside. *Neurology, 16,* 21–26.

Dunn, L. B., Palmer, B. W., & Karlawish, J. H. T. (2007). Frontal dysfunction and capacity to consent to treatment of research. In R. L. Miller & J. L. Cummings (Eds.), *The human frontal lobes* (pp. 335–344). New York: Guilford Press.

Earnst, K. S., Marson, D. C., & Harrell, L. E. (2000). Cognitive model of physicians' legal standard and personal judgments of competency in patients with Alzheimer's disease. *Journal of the American Geriatric Society, 48,* 919–927.

Estate of Harms 149 P. 2d 557 (2006).

Eyler, L. T., Olsen, R. K., Nayak, G. V., Mirzakhanian, H., Brown, G. G., & Jeste, D. V. (2007). Brain response correlates of decisional capacity in schizophrenia: A preliminary fMRI study. *Journal of Neuropsychiatry and Clinical Neurosciences, 19,* 137–144.

Ferguson, A., Worrall, L., McPhee, J., Buskell, R., Armstrong, E., & Togher, L. (2003). Testamentary capacity and aphasia: A descriptive case report with implications for clinical practice. *Aphasiology, 17,* 965–980.

Ferner, R. E. (1997). Drugs and testamentary capacity. *Journal of Clinical Forensic Medicine, 4,* 185–187.

Folstein, M. F., Folstein, S. E., & McHugh, P. R. (1975). "Mini-Mental State": A practical method for grading the cognitive state of patients for the clinician. *Journal of Psychiatric Research, 12,* 189–198.

Grisso, T. (1986). *Evaluating competencies: Forensic assessments and instruments.* New York: Plenum Press.

Grisso, T., & Appelbaum, P. S. (1995a). Comparison of standards for assessing patients' capacities to make treatment decisions. *American Journal of Psychiatry, 152,* 1033–1037.

Grisso, T., & Applebaum, P. S. (1995b). The MacArthur Treatment Competence Study. I: Mental illness and competence to consent to treatment. *Law & Human Behavior, 19,* 105–126.

Grisso, T., & Applebaum, P. S. (1995c). The MacArthur Treatment Competence Study. II: Measures of abilities related to competence to consent to treatment. *Law & Human Behavior, 19,* 127–148.

Grisso, T., & Applebaum, P. S. (1995d). The MacArthur Treatment Competence Study. III: Abilities of patients to consent to psychiatric and medical treatments. *Law & Human Behavior, 19,* 149–174.

Gutheil, T. G. (2007). Common pitfalls in the evaluation of testamentary capacity. *Journal of the American Academy of Psychiatry and the Law, 35,* 514–517.

Hall, R. C. W., Hall, R. C. W., Myers, W. C., & Chapman, M. J. (2009). Testamentary capacity: History, physician's role, requirements, and why wills are challenged. *Clinical Geriatrics, 17,* 18–24.

Hart, D. J., Craig, D., Compton, S. A., Critchlow, S., Kerrigan, B. M., McIlroy, S. P., & Passmore, A. P. (2003). A retrospective study of the behavioural and psychological symptoms of mid and late phase Alzheimer's disease. *International Journal of Geriatric Psychiatry, 18,* 1037–1042.

Hashimoto, R., Abe, N., Ueno, A., Fujii, T., Takahashi, S., & Mori, E. (2010 Changing the criteria for old/new recognition judgments can modulate activity in the anterior hippocampus. *Hippocampus.* Sep 29. doi: 10.1002/hipo.20878. [Epub ahead of print]

Helm-Estabrooks, N. (2002). Cognition and aphasia: A discussion and a study. *Journal of Communication Disorders, 35,* 171–186.

Hull, R., and Hull, I. (1996). Suspicious circumstances in relation to testamentary capacity and undue influence. In *Estates: Planning, Administration, and Litigation* (pp. 77–87). Law Society of Upper Canada, Special Lectures. Toronto, Canada: Carswell.

Jacoby, R., and Steer, P. (2007). How to assess capacity to make a will. *British Medical Journal, 335,* 155–157.

Kahneman, D. (2003). A perspective on judgment and choice: Mapping bounded rationality. *American Psychologist, 58,* 697–720.

Katona, C., Chiu, E., Adelman, S., Baloyannis, S., Camus, V., Firmino, H., et al. (2009) World Psychiatric Association Section of Old Age Psychiatry Consensus Conference on Ethics and Capacity in old people with mental disorders. *International Journal Geriatric Psychiatry, 24,* 1319–1324.

Kennerley, S. W., Dahmubed, A. F., Lara, A. H., & Wallis, J. D. (2009). Neurons in the frontal lobe encode the value of multiple decision variables. *Journal of Cognitive Neuroscience, 21,* 1162–1178.

King-Casas, B., Tomlin, D., Anen, C., Camerer, C. F., Quartz, S. R., & Montague, P. R. (2005). Getting to know you: Reputation and trust in a two-person economic exchange. *Science, 1,* 308 (5718), 78–83.

Liptzin, B., Peisah, C., Shulman, K., & Finkel, S. for the International Psychogeriatric Association Task Force on Wills, Testamentary Capacity. (2010). Testamentary capacity and delirium. *International Psychogeriatrics, 22,* 950–956.

Lloyd's Law Reports. (1993). Q.B. (Com. Ct.) vol. 2, p. 69.

Marson, D. C., & Briggs, S. S. (2001). Assessing competency in Alzheimer's disease: Treatment consent capacity and financial capacity. In S. Gauthier & J. Cummings (Eds.), *Alzheimer's disease* (pp. 165–192). New York: Martin Dunitz.

Marson, D. C., Cody, H. A., Ingram, K. K., & Harrell, L. E. (1995). Neuropsychological predictors of competency in Alzheimer's disease using a rational reasons legal standard. *Archives of Neurology, 52*, 955–959.

Marson, D. C., Earnst, K., Jamil, F., Bartolucci, A., & Harrell, L. E. (2000). Consistency of physician's legal standard and personal judgments of competency in patients with Alzheimer's disease. *Journal of the American Geriatrics Society, 48*, 911–918.

Marson, D. C., Hawkins, L., McInturff, B., & Harrell, L. E. (1997). Cognitive models that predict physician judgment of capacity to consent in mild Alzheimer's disease. *Journal of the American Geriatrics Society, 45*, 458–464.

Marson, D. C., & Hebert, K. (1995). Assessing civil competencies in older adults with dementia: Consent capacity, financial capacity, and testamentary capacity. In G. J. Larrabee (Ed.), *Forensic neuropsychology: A scientific approach* (pp. 334–377). New York: Oxford.

Marson, D. C., & Hebert, K. R. (2008). Testamentary capacity. In B. L. Cutler (Ed.), *Encyclopedia of psychology and law* (pp. 798–801). Los Angeles: Sage Publications.

Marson, D. C., Huthwaite, J., & Hebert, K. (2004). Testamentary capacity and undue influence in the elderly: A jurisprudent therapy perspective. *Law and Psychology Review, 28*, 71–97.

McKinnon, M. C., Svoboda, E., & Levine, B. (2007). The frontal lobes and autobiographical memory. In R. L. Miller & J. L. Cummings (Eds.), *The human frontal lobes.* (pp. 227–248). New York: Guilford Press,

Mendez, M. F., & Cummings, J. L. (2003). *Dementia: A clinical approach* (3rd ed.). Philadelphia: Butterworth Heinemann.

Mizrahi, R., Starkstein, S. E., Jorge, R., & Robinson, R. G. (2006). Phenomenology and clinical correlates of delusions in Alzheimer disease. *American Journal of Geriatric Psychiatry, 14*, 573–581.

Mount Isa Mines Ltd v. *Pusey* (1970). 125 CLR 383, 395.

O'Neill, N., & Peisah, C. (2011, in press). Capacity to make a will. In *Capacity and the Law*. Published online by the Australian Institute of Legal Information (AustLII), August 2011.

O'Rourke v. *Hunter* (2006). 446 Mass. 814, 826–827.

Peisah, C., Brodaty, H., & Quadrio, C. (2006). Family conflict in dementia: Prodigal sons & black sheep. *International Journal of Geriatric Psychiatry, 21*, 485–492.

Peisah, C., Finkel, S., Shulman, K., Melding, P., Luxenberg, J., Heinik, J., Jacoby, R., Reisberg, B., Stoppe, G., Barker, A., Firmino, H., & Bennett, H. (2009). International Psychogeriatric Association Task Force on Wills and Undue Influence. The wills of older people: Risk factors for undue influence. *International Psychogeriatrics, 21*, 7–15.

Province of Ontario. RRO, 1990. Regulation 194. Last amendment: 0.Reg. 186/10.

Roked, F., & Patel, A. (2008). Which aspects of cognitive function are best associated with testamentary capacity in patients with Alzheimer's disease? *International Journal of Geriatric Psychiatry, 23*, 552–553.

Royall, D. R., Lauterback, E. C., Cummings, J. L., Reeve, A., Rummans, T. A., Kaufer D. L., LaFrance, W. C., Jr., & Coffey, C. E. (2002). Executive control function: A review of its promise and challenges for clinical research: Report from the Committee on Research of the American Neuropsychiatric Association. *Journal of Neuropsychiatry and Clinical Neurosciences, 14*, 377–405.

Sanfey, A., Lowenstein, G., McClure, S. M., & Cohen J. D. (2006). Neuroeconomics: Cross currents in research on decision-making. *Trends in Cognitive Sciences, 10*, 108–116.

Shorter v. Hodges (1988). 14 NSWLR 689.

Shulman, K. I. (2000). Clock-drawing: Is it the ideal cognitive screening test? *International Journal of Geriatric Psychiatry, 15*, 548–561.

Shulman, K., Cohen, C., & Hull, I. (2005). Psychiatric issues in retrospective challenges of testamentary capacity. *International Journal of Geriatric Psychiatry, 20*, 63–69.

Shulman, K., Cohen, C. A., Kirsh F. C., Hull, I. M., & Champine, P. R. (2007). Assessment of testamentary capacity and vulnerability to undue influence. *American Journal of Psychiatry, 164*, 722–727.

Shulman, K., & Feinstein, A. (2006). *Quick cognitive screening for clinicians*. London, UK: Informa Healthcare.

Shulman, K. I., Hull, I., & Cohen, C. A. (2003). Testamentary capacity and suicide: An overview of legal and psychiatric issues." *International Journal of Law & Psychiatry, 26*, 403–415.

Shulman, K. I., Peisah, C., Jacoby, R., Heinik, J., & Finkel, S. (2009). Contemporaneous assessment of testamentary capacity. *International Psychogeriatrics, 21*, 433–439.

Spar, J. E., & Garb, A. S. (1992). Assessing competency to make a will. *American Journal of Psychiatry, 149*, 169–174.

Sprehe, D. J., & Kerr, A. L. (1996). Use of legal terms in will contests: Implications for psychiatrist. *Bulletin of the American Academy of Psychiatry and Law, 24*, 255–265.

Uniform Civil Procedure Rules (Amendment No. 12) 2006, under the Civil Procedure Act 2005, New South Wales, Australia.

Weierich, M. R., Wright, C. I., Negreira, A., Dickerson, B. C., & Barrett, L. F. (2010). Novelty as a dimension in the affective brain. *Neuroimage, 49*, 2871–2878.

Wingrove v. Wingrove (1885). LR11PD 81 at 82–83.

Wood, S., & Tanius, B. E. (2007). Impact of dementia on decision making abilities. In S. H. Qualls & M. A. Smyer (Eds.), *Changes in decision making capacity in older adults.* Wiley Series in Clinical Geropsychology (pp. 91–106). Hoboken, NJ: John Wiley & Sons.

6

Driving Capacity

PENNY L. WOLFE AND JESSICA A. CLARK

The independence that driving affords is often taken for granted until that freedom is lost. After an individual experiences a change in cognitive status or has certain medical conditions, he or she may have to cease driving either temporarily or permanently. The purpose of this chapter is to provide an overview of evidence-based information about assessment of driving capacity, legal and ethical considerations, practical guidelines, resources, and brief case examples.

LEGAL AND ETHICAL CONSIDERATIONS

Galski and McDonald (2009) describe driving as a privilege granted by the states as part of our pursuit of life, liberty, and happiness. However, they also point out that the privilege must be weighed against the rights of the public to be protected from potential dangers by persons whose impairments may interfere with their ability to safely operate a motor vehicle. An individual may obtain the privilege of driving by meeting the standards set forth by the individual states' regulatory division, such as the Division of Motor Vehicles (DMV). Although specific requirements vary from state to state, there are common standards that are used to determine an individual's competency to drive: An individual must meet the minimum age for driving, have sufficient vision, and be able to pass both the written and on-road examinations.

As the specific standards for obtaining a driver's license vary from state to state, so do the laws pertaining to determining and reporting unsafe drivers (Galski & McDonald, 2009). The type of conditions that may lead to unsafe driving, and how they are defined, also varies. For example, in Washington, D.C. if a driver has a seizure disorder/loss of consciousness, he or she must be seizure free for 12 months before a license may be reinstated. In other states, there is no specific condition or timeline provided and the decision as to whether a medical condition may lead to problems with driving is left to the physician. In some states, an individual's physician is required by law to report when a patient has an impairment or a condition that could lead to the unsafe operation of a motor vehicle. However, in other states, reporting medical information to a DMV is a violation of a patient's confidentiality. Another complicating factor is that other healthcare providers, including psychologists, may become aware of an individual's impairment in the course of assessment and/or treatment. Again, the rules for reporting such information vary depending on the state. Physicians, psychologists, and other clinicians should familiarize themselves with the pertinent laws governing the definitions of unsafe drivers and the reporting laws in their particular jurisdiction. Specifically, this information may be obtained on the website of the state's Department of Motor Vehicles, Department of Transportation, and/or Department of Public Safety. For a general overview of State licensing and reporting laws, an excellent resource is the American Medical Association's (AMA; 2010) online document, *Physician's Guide to Assessing and Counseling Older Drivers, Chapter 8: State Licensing and Reporting Laws.* If the information provided on the website is insufficient, or if one does not fully understand the information provided, he or she should contact the department directly and ask for clarification.

In addition to the legal issues highlighted above, clinicians must also consider the ethical issues that arise in the assessment of driving capacity. As described by Marottoli and colleagues (1997), losing the ability to drive can be perceived as a great loss and may lead to increased mental health problems. Freund and Colgrove (2008) point out that access to friends, family, work, cultural opportunities, and religious affiliation often necessitates transportation. Restriction of transportation may lead to isolation and cultural impoverishment. Another ethical consideration is whether one should include details in one's informed consent that explains that the neuropsychological evaluation may be used in decisions about the loss of driving capacity (M. J. O'Connell, personal communication, January 4, 2011). If one's practice involves a large client base of older adults, persons with brain injury, or other potentially disabling conditions, one should consider how to incorporate such a statement in the informed consent form.

FACTORS AFFECTING THE ABILITY TO OPERATE A MOTOR VEHICLE

According to the National Highway Traffic Safety Administration (NHTSA), older persons accounted for 15% of all traffic fatalities and 18% of all pedestrian fatalities in 2008. The majority of traffic fatalities involving older drivers occurred during the daytime (80%), on weekdays (72%), and involved other vehicles (69%). Aging, injury, and certain medical conditions may impact the ability to have sufficient visual and perceptual abilities to drive safely. A report published by the U.S. Department of Transportation NHTSA (September 2005) provides an extensive review of the literature regarding medical conditions and driving. A brief summary of these major areas is presented below.

Visual Conditions. Conditions affecting vision that may impede driving ability include low vision (ranging from 20/200 to 20/50), cataracts, glaucoma, diabetic retinopathy, retinitis pigmentosa, monocular vision (especially right eye blindness), macular degeneration, nystagmus, and visual field deficits (Carr & Ott, 2010; National Highway Traffic Safety Administration, 2005).

Physical Conditions. Because of the significant motor component of driving a vehicle, it is necessary to consider the physical capabilities of the driver. Conditions or illnesses that limit the ability to move freely (flexibility), quickly, and even with sufficient strength may result in decreased driving safety (Carr & Ott, 2010). For example, individuals who have orthopedic injuries affecting their upper or lower extremities may have difficulty managing a steering wheel or pushing the brake pedal. An individual with severe arthritis in the hands may be unable to grip the steering wheel with enough strength to make proper and safe turns or lane changes.

Psychiatric Conditions. As with certain medical conditions, psychiatric conditions have been shown to have a possible impact on the ability to safely operate a motor vehicle (National Highway Traffic Safety Administration, 2005). The studies that were reviewed in this area are dated and have methodological issues. However, the general findings were that persons with psychiatric disorders such as schizophrenia, personality disorders, untreated psychosis, and untreated alcoholism were more at risk for crashes. Furthermore, the report reflected conflicting studies about the role of suicidal ideation and suicide attempts in the rate of crashes.

Medications. The NHTSA review (2005) reported that a number of medications have been examined in terms of potentially adversely affecting driving performance. In particular, medications alone, or in the context of interaction effects, that have sedating properties are most problematic. NHTSA (2005) and the American Medical Association (2010) indicate that use of the following medications should be considered to assist in the determination of driving safety: antidepressants, antipsychotics, antihistamines, benzodiazepines, anticonvulsants, and analgesics/narcotics. The use of these medications alone does not preclude driving; however, the medication side-effect profile and possible abuse should be considered to determine the potential impact on driving.

DRIVER EVALUATION AND TRAINING

Once an individual is identified as having one of the aforementioned problems, or has been reported to the state licensing agency, further evaluation can be initiated. In addition, results from a neuropsychological evaluation often elicit a further, driving-specific evaluation. Though the subsequent evaluation process varies from state to state, this may involve an interview, a medical questionnaire, a medical evaluation by a physician, vision testing (possibly including night vision and depth perception), motor testing, and/or a driving test (American Bar Association Commission on Law and Aging & American Psychological Association, 2008; ABA/APA). This driving evaluation might involve a written, on-road, or simulated driving assessment. Based upon the results of this evaluation, recommendations might include driving restrictions (e.g., daytime driving only, use of adaptive equipment), suspension or revocation of a license, or a recommendation for driving training. Driver training courses are available for older drivers and drivers recovering from injury and/or disability, and programs are frequently available through state licensing agencies, hospitals, or driving clubs [i.e., the American Automobile Association (AAA)]. For instance, the driver's training program at the hospital with which the authors are affiliated offers services such as predriving assessment (e.g., of vision, strength, coordination, reaction time, and knowledge of current driving laws), driving education for those recovering from neurological insult, on-road driving evaluation/training, training on the use of up-to-date adaptive equipment (e.g., hand controls, ramps, lifts) when necessary, and preparation for state road tests. Of note, some of these programs may require a physician's order. A major aspect of some training programs includes driving training in a simulator, in the hope of improving reaction time, stopping distance, useful field of view, and driver's confidence, as well as reducing the risk of accidents. Although the use of driving simulators for both training and assessment is beyond the scope of this chapter, there is a wealth of research on the topic.

NEUROPSYCHOLOGICAL ASSESSMENT OF DRIVING CAPACITY

The process of evaluating driving capacity varies in terms of the domains assessed, and may require a multidisciplinary approach to assessment. This may include physicians, psychologists/neuropsychologists, occupational therapists, and driving specialists. The role neuropsychologists typically play is to assess an individual's cognitive and psychological functioning. Importantly, the referral question for neuropsychologists is rarely to assess just the individual's driving capacity. Instead, the clinician may be asked to characterize a patient's cognitive functioning to answer a variety of questions such as, for example, the presence or extent of cognitive impairment in an older individual, or the assessment of strengths/weaknesses in an individual recovering from traumatic brain injury (TBI) who wants to return to work or school. Driving capacity may thus arise as an area of clinical importance when answering the main referral question. Therefore, it makes sense to address each cognitive domain in terms of its utility in determining driving capacity and to highlight any "red flags" that may indicate impaired driving abilities.

The possible cognitive domains related to driving include mental status, attention/concentration, visual perception and visual spatial abilities, processing speed, language, memory, executive functions (e.g., divided attention/dual processing, inhibition, initiation/perseveration, switching), and awareness of deficits. However, a number of methodological issues exist that affect the ability to assess the relationship between neuropsychological testing and driving capacity. First, there is variability in the specific neuropsychological tests used to tap the previously mentioned cognitive domains. Second, the dependent measures used to establish this relationship vary widely. For example, some studies use prediction of real-world vehicle collisions or traffic citations, whereas others use performance on driving simulators (e.g., simulated crashes, number of times participant crossed a double line) to assess this relationship. Third, most studies confine their sample to only those with Alzheimer's disease, other types of dementia, mild cognitive impairment (MCI), TBI, stroke, or multiple sclerosis (MS), thus making it difficult to generalize test utility across populations. A final consideration when reviewing studies of driving capacity is whether a study compares patient group scores with a control group. As exemplified in a meta-analysis of neuropsychological testing and driving capacity by Reger and colleagues (2004), comparison with a control group may overinflate the ability of cognitive tests to predict driving ability. For instance, in their study, between-groups analyses indicate that the dementia group did worse than the control group, without necessarily looking at the ability of neuropsychological tests to predict driving performance within the patient group, which is the question that neuropsychologists are typically asked to answer clinically. Reger et al. (2004) suggest that removal of a control group to examine the correlation of cognitive tests to driving performance *within* a patient group is necessary to obtain the most clinically relevant data.

Given the limitations in the literature, it can be difficult to address the extent to which neuropsychological testing predicts on-road driving capacity. With the exception of cases in which profound impairment is identified, neuropsychological testing alone may often elicit a referral for a more comprehensive, driving-specific assessment. Despite these limitations, what follows is an overview of pertinent cognitive domains, with an emphasis on the rationale for assessing each domain, research findings regarding the utility of assessing each domain, and specific tests that have shown particular promise in predicting driving capacity.

Brief Mental Status Examinations. Mental status examinations are simple to administer and provide valuable information regarding a patient's basic level of cognitive functioning. Although these measures have a low ceiling (i.e., they are relatively easy to pass and a failing score indicates significant impairment), they serve as a screening measure to capture individuals with clear cognitive problems. The most commonly administered measure of mental status is the Mini-Mental State Examination (MMSE; Folstein, Folstein, & McHugh, 1975), but other measures may include the Mattis Dementia Rating Scale (MDRS; Mattis, 1976), Dementia Rating Scale, Second Edition (DRS-2; Jurica, Leittenn, & Mattis, 2001), Blessed Dementia Rating Scale (Blessed, Tomlinson, & Roth, 1968), and the Montreal Cognitive Assessment (MoCA; Nasreddine et al., 2005).

Studies of mental status and driving capacity are generally inconsistent. A review of studies by Anstey, Wood, Lord, and Walker (2005) suggests that the MMSE is not associated with self-reported or state-recorded crashes, but is associated with on-road driving performance in older adults. A meta-analytic study of individuals with dementia found that mental status examinations showed a moderate relationship to on-road driving performance when a control group was utilized; however, when control groups were removed, there was no significant relationship with road tests, but a moderate relationship with non-road tests and a small relationship with caregiver reports of driving ability (Reger et al., 2004). Stated another way, mental status examinations were not predictive of on-road driving performance, but were predictive of how patients with dementia performed on non-road tests and how their caregivers rated their driving. A retrospective study comparing older drivers deemed as safe, restricted, or unsafe based on simulator performance found that those who were safe or restricted had better MMSE scores than those who were unsafe (Freund & Colgrove, 2008). Similarly, another study showed that MMSE scores among older adults who continued to drive were higher as compared to those who had ceased driving or those who had never driven, suggesting that older individuals who are aware of compromised mental status may cease driving (Mann, McCarthy, Wu, & Tomita, 2005). Furthermore, this study suggested that limiting an older adult's driving may result in social isolation, which can put individuals at risk for cognitive decline and subsequently affect mental status (Mann et al., 2005). Though the studies mentioned here have found some differences among groups, overall, measures of mental status for assessing driving capacity have not demonstrated consistent clinical utility in predicting driving performance.

Visual Perception and Visual Spatial Abilities. Sensory changes occurring as a result of aging or neurological dysfunction may limit driving capacity. Issues such as visual acuity, visual field integrity, and neglect should be assessed in addition to visual spatial abilities. These abilities relate to almost all aspects of driving, such as being able to see other cars and pedestrians on or near the road, perceiving safe distances from these and other obstacles, viewing road signs and signals, and route finding.

Traditional neuropsychological measures of visual perception include tests such as Block Design (from the Wechsler series; Wechsler, 2008), clock drawing tests, complex figure tests, judgment of line orientation tests, the Hooper Visual Organization Test (HVOT; Hooper, 1958), and the Motor-Free Visual Perceptual Test (MVPT; Colarusso & Hammill, 2003). Meta-analytic results found that measures of visual spatial abilities showed the highest relationship to driving capacity as compared to other cognitive domains in a sample of patients with dementia (controls excluded), with moderate effect sizes for performance on road and non-road tests, and small effect sizes for caregiver report of an individual's driving abilities (Reger et al., 2004). A meta-analysis by Mathias and Lucas (2009) found that among older drivers, clock drawing and a judgment of line orientation task were predictive of simulated driving performance, and Block Design was predictive of on-road driving problems. Likewise, clock drawing tests and the MVPT have shown utility in predicting driving capacity among older drivers (Oswanski et al., 2007), and the MVPT has been shown to be a strong predictor of on-road failures (Schultheis & Fleksher, 2009).

Studies have found that measures of visual spatial abilities are among the most predictive cognitive tests of driving abilities in individuals with Parkinson's disease (Amick, Grace, & Ott, 2007; Stolwyk, Charlton, Triggs, Iansek, & Bradshaw, 2006). Specifically, the Rey-Osterreith Complex Figure Test (ROCF; Stern et al., 1999) copy accuracy was predictive of on-road driving errors (Amick et al., 2007) and Block Design correlated with tactical errors on simulator performance (e.g., speed adaptation and complex curve navigation according to Stolwyk, 2006). The ROCF and the MVPT have also demonstrated utility in predicting fitness to drive in patients recovering from stroke (Akinwuntan et al., 2006; Mazer, Korner-Bitensky, & Sofer, 1998). A measure of visual spatial learning and recall

(7/24 Spatial Recall Test) was shown to be one of the most predictive neuropsychological tests in determining on-road driving performance among a sample of individuals with MS (Schultheis et al., 2010). Gorman and colleagues (2009) suggest that visual spatial ability is useful in predicting driving performance (both simulator and on-road) in patients with HIV, particularly in older drivers with the disease.

Although not included in most traditional neuropsychological batteries, the Useful Field of View (UFOV; Ball & Roenker, 1998) test is frequently cited in the driving literature. This measure goes beyond examining visual acuity and simply the range of an individual's visual field. Rather, it incorporates several aspects of visual attention to assess the test-taker's ability to attend to visual stimuli and inhibit distracters within their field of view. This consists of three subtests assessing basic visual attention/information processing, divided attention, and selective attention. Reaction time is measured for each subtest. Participants are first asked to identify when a vehicle appears in the center of the screen. In the second subtest, localization of a car in the participant's periphery is added to the first task. Finally, distracters are also added to the participant's periphery thus making localization of the elements of the task more difficult.

Studies indicate that the UFOV has been related to driving performance among patients with TBI (in relation to simulator crashes; Cyr et al., 2009) and HIV (in relation to real-world automobile crashes, Gorman et al., 2009), but may not be clinically useful for identifying driving performance among patients with Parkinson's disease. In fact, Amick and colleagues (2007) found that composite UFOV scores were not predictive of on-road driving performance in this population. They suggest that this measure has not been consistently associated with driving capacity in the Parkinson's disease literature and may not be appropriate for use with such patients (Amick et al., 2007). In a meta-analysis of older patients without dementia, a large effect size for the UFOV was found when differentiating those who pass or fail on-road driving tests and simulator tests, as well as predicting driving problems (Mathias & Lucas, 2009). Studies have shown that UFOV indicates poor visual attention in stroke survivors, especially among older patients (Mazer, Sofer, Korner-Bitensky, & Gelinas, 2001), and that stroke drivers perform more poorly on the UFOV than nonstroke drivers (Fisk & Mennimeier, 2006). However, as highlighted by Schultheis and Fleksher (2009), the potential application of UFOV among stroke survivors is limited by the lack of research linking performance on this measure to on-road driving measures. That said, studies have used UFOV as a proxy for driving performance in other populations. Using this methodology, MS patients with cognitive impairment performed significantly worse on the UFOV than individuals with MS who had no cognitive impairment (Schultheis, Garay, & DeLuca, 2001).

As can be seen, visual spatial and visual attentional abilities, as measured by several neuropsychological tests, are associated with driving performance in a variety of neurological samples. It is important that any assessment used to determine driving capacity include measures of visual spatial and visual attentional functioning.

Attention/Concentration. Attention includes the ability to attend to incoming information and maintain this data while filtering out distracters. Multiple meta-analyses indicate that there are more individual studies of attention and concentration of driving capacity than any other cognitive domain (Reger et al., 2004; Mathias & Lucas, 2009). This makes sense, given the importance of abilities such as paying attention to other cars and pedestrians, attending to traffic signs and signals, and filtering out distracters both outside and inside the vehicle.

When tests of attention were aggregated in a meta-analysis utilizing a dementia sample (excluding control samples), the effect sizes for correlation to on-road tests was small, and there was no significant relationship to non-road tests (Reger et al., 2004). Studies have linked basic attentional abilities to on-road performance using the Integrated Visual and Auditory Continuous Performance Test (IVA; Sandford & Turner, 2000) in a sample of older drivers (Zook, Bennett, & Lane, 2009). Attention has also been linked to driving performance in those with HIV, especially within older drivers (Gorman et al., 2009). Complex Reaction time, a measure of divided attention speed and inhibition, was the most predictive neuropsychological test in a study of stroke survivors (Lundqvist, Gerdle, & Ronnberg, 2000). Likewise, a listening span task has been shown to be predictive of driving performance in stroke patients both on-road and in a simulator (Lundqvist et al., 2000).

Although included as a measure of visual perception and visual spatial abilities, the UFOV test incorporates aspects of divided and selective attention. Results from this test may be conceptualized as more than a measure of an individual's visual field. Rather, scores from the UFOV reflect an individual's ability to process information in his or her visual field, including attending to relevant stimuli and inhibiting distracters. As the above review suggests, this test may be useful in assessing driving capacity in some neurologically impaired populations (e.g., TBI, HIV, or MS).

Clearly, attention in many forms (simple, sustained, divided, and selective) is imperative to assess when making recommendations regarding driving capacity, and attentional impairments should be cause to contemplate a more formal on-road driving evaluation.

Processing Speed. Processing speed, which may include measures of psychomotor speed and/or reaction time, is affected by many conditions, from neurological disorders to normal aging. This has clear implications for driving, such as the ability to react, break, avoid obstacles, and adapt to new driving situations. Measures of processing speed may include tests such as Trail Making Test Part A (Reitan, 1958), Symbol Digit Modalities Test (SDMT; Smith, 1982), Digit Symbol Coding and Symbol Search from the Wechsler series (Wechsler, 2008), and a number of measures of reaction time. In addition, some studies include tests such as a complex reaction time test (requiring response inhibition) or Trail Making Test Part B as measures of processing speed, whereas others may include these as measures of attention/concentration or executive functioning.

Lundqvist and colleagues concluded that measures of information processing speed and attention were the most useful tools for predicting driving performance in a sample of stroke patients (Lundqvist et al., 2000) as well as in a longitudinal study of TBI patients (Lundqvist, Alinder, & Ronnberg, 2008). They found that a brief neuropsychological battery (including Trails B, complex reaction time, and tests of focused and simultaneous attentional capacity) predicted driving performance 10 years after testing, and was even more sensitive to future impaired driving performance than on-road driving tests in patients with TBI (Lundqvist et al., 2008). However, there is some debate as to whether the speeded component or the more complex executive functioning component in these measures better accounts for impaired driving (Cyr et al., 2009). For instance, complex reaction time, more so than simple reaction time, has been associated with on-road driving performance in older adults (Anstey et al., 2005). Similar results were found in a meta-analysis of studies of older drivers as complex reaction time differentiated between drivers who passed or failed an on-road driving test (Mathias & Lucas, 2009). Still, in other samples, "pure" measures of processing speed have been implicated as key to driving capacity. For instance, processing speed as measured by the oral version of the SDMT has been shown to be the strongest predictor of on-road driving performance among a sample of individuals with MS (Schultheis et al., 2010). In summation, processing speed may predict real-world driving performance, and significant impairments within this domain may be cause for concern and referral for a further on-road evaluation of driving skills.

Language. Language functioning, such as receptive language and reading ability, is important for driving as drivers need to read signage, comprehend driving directions, read and understand driving laws, and pass written driving evaluations. A meta-analysis based on studies of individuals with dementia suggests medium to large effect sizes between tests of language functioning (e.g., confrontation naming tests, Verbal IQ) and both on-road tests and written non-road tests (Reger et al., 2004). However, this statistically significant relationship disappeared when control subjects were excluded, which suggests that language measures may have limited utility in predicting driving performance (Reger et al., 2004). In general, the relationship between language functioning and driving capacity has received less research attention than other cognitive domains and it appears as though measures of language functioning have not demonstrated clinical utility in the prediction of driving performance.

Memory. Being able to remember directions and routes are essential aspects of driving. Anecdotally, it seems as though a loved one becoming lost when driving frequently causes family members to initially question an individual's driving capacity, thereby eliciting referral for formal driving evaluation. Meta-analytic results indicate that memory functioning on measures such as Facial Recognition, Logical Memory, and Visual Reproduction from the Wechsler series (Wechsler, 1987, 1997, 2009) and on the Benton Visual Retention test (Sivan, 1992) demonstrates medium to large effect sizes in predicting both on-road and non-road test performance when control groups are included (Reger et al., 2004). Although the authors were unable to calculate on-road test performance when controls were excluded, a small effect size for non-road test performance remained even when control participants were removed. Visual Reproduction was found to have a medium to large effect size when differentiating between older drivers who passed or failed a driving evaluation in another meta-analysis as well (Mathias & Lucas, 2009). Measures such as the Hopkins Verbal Learning Test–Revised (HVLT-R; Brandt & Benedict, 2002) have demonstrated utility in older community dwelling individuals; lower scores on this measure predicted on-road driving performance such as basic vehicle operating skills (e.g., turning right at an intersection) (Zook et al., 2009). Research suggests that nonverbal memory performance in patients with HIV was predictive of various components of driving abilities within simulator studies (Gorman et al., 2009). Despite the promising results presented above, the literature is mixed with regard to memory performance and driving capacity. For instance, there are a number of studies that suggest that memory as measured by neuropsychological testing is not predictive of driving performance in those with dementia (Brown & Ott, 2004; Bieliauskas, Roper, Trobe, Green, & Lacy, 1998).

One potential reason for the lack of strong predictive relationships between memory and on-road driving capacity is that driving frequently relies heavily on overlearned, procedural memory (Bieliauskas et al., 1998). Conversely, neuropsychological tests of learning and memory typically measure explicit memory. Case studies suggest that even patients with severe amnesia due to bilateral hippocampal lesions demonstrate performance similar to healthy normal drivers on measures of vehicle control (steering, speed control, safety errors, and driving with distraction), driving rules, safety procedures, and meanings of road signs, likely due to intact procedural memory (Anderson et al., 2007). However, when the driving situation is more challenging, for example, following route directions or responding to a crash avoidance scenario on a simulator, performance is impaired in amnesia (Anderson et al., 2007). Given these mixed reviews, caution is warranted in presuming driving deficits due to impaired memory performance, but on-road driving evaluations utilizing novel driving scenarios may be warranted.

Executive Functioning. Executive functioning is one of the most frequently studied cognitive domains in the driving literature. It includes abilities such as judgment, planning, switching, mental flexibility, simultaneous processing, and response inhibition. These areas are clearly fundamental in driving, especially when presented with challenging, new, or unanticipated situations. A wealth of data suggests that executive functioning shows great utility in predicting driving capacity. Various measures of executive functioning are predictive of driving performance in older individuals (Zook et al., 2009; Mathias & Lucas, 2009) and in those with dementia (Brown & Ott, 2004), Parkinson's disease (Amick et al., 2007; Stolwyk et al., 2006), HIV (Gorman et al., 2009), TBI (Brouwer & Withaar, 1997), and stroke (Lundqvist et al., 2000).

One of the most frequently utilized and cited tool is the Trail Making Test Part B, likely due in part to its ease of administration. Trails B has been shown to be related to driving performance in a number of populations, including older drivers (Mathias & Lucas, 2009) and in those with dementia or stroke (Cyr et al., 2009). This measure was shown to successfully differentiate between safe and restricted or unsafe older drivers based on on-road performance (Freund & Colgrove, 2008). Color-word inhibition tests such as the Stroop Color-Word Test have also been shown to be related to driving skill within a sample of stroke survivors (both on-road and within a simulator; Lundqvist et al., 2000) and older drivers (negatively correlating with accident risk; Daigneault, Joly, & Frigon, 2002). Further evidence linking poor performance on color-word inhibition tasks with driving problems has been provided by meta-analytic review of studies of older drivers (Mathias & Lucas, 2009). The Wisconsin Card Sorting Test is another commonly administered neuropsychological measure. Perseverative errors on this test have been associated with increased accident risk in older drivers (Daigneault et al., 2002). Much like visual spatial perception, attention, and processing speed, measures of executive functioning should be included in any assessment that will be used to make driving recommendations, as deficits in executive functioning appear to be among the best predictors of driving problems.

Awareness. If individuals with cognitive difficulties are aware of problem areas, they will be more likely to adopt compensatory strategies to be safe on the road. Such strategies may include restricting driving to daytime, clear weather, off-peak traffic hours, familiar routes, limited distances, or only when accompanied by another adult. Ryan et al. (2009) studied the effect of awareness on driving behaviors in patients with MS. Results suggest a direct relationship between awareness of cognitive impairments (as measured by the Awareness Questionnaire) and use of compensatory strategies. Furthermore, there was an inverse relationship between the perceived need for compensatory strategies and both miles driven and driving incidents, with decreased perceived need leading to more miles driven and more on-the-road incidents (Ryan et al., 2009). A study by Scott et al. (2009) demonstrated that stroke survivors tended to overestimate their driving abilities (even more than healthy adults), but that their estimation of abilities tended to improve when they compared their abilities to someone familiar (e.g., a family member) as opposed to someone unfamiliar or abstract (e.g., the "average driver"). These results suggest that awareness of cognitive impairment may help to predict the likelihood of utilizing compensatory strategies and future accident risk. It is thus important that awareness of deficits be considered when making any driving recommendations.

Driving-Specific Measures. There are several measures designed specifically for the assessment of driving that provide more ecologically valid measurement tools. For instance, the Neurocognitive Driving Test (NDT; Schultheis & Chute, 1999) is a computer-based measure designed to assess driving skills at the strategic (route finding, costs, etc.), tactical (adjustment behaviors, on-road judgments to pass or negotiate a curve, etc.), and operational (steering, breaking, etc.) levels. It contains five subtests, including self-evaluation questions, predriving questions, simple and choice reaction time tests, driving scenarios, and a visual task. Accuracy and latency are recorded for all tasks. Significant relationships have been found between the NDT and behind-the-wheel assessment, and it has been shown to discriminate between patients with acquired brain injury who passed or failed an on-road driving evaluation (Schultheis, Hillary, & Chute, 2003).

Another measure is the Driving Scenes subtest of the Neuropsychological Assessment Battery (NAB; Stern & White, 2003), which shows participants a street scene from a driver's perspective for 30 seconds. A second similar picture is shown, and individuals are asked to indicate what is new or missing from the scene. This is done for a total of six scenes. The NAB has shown some promise in a very mildly demented sample; healthy control participants were found to perform better on the NAB Driving Scenes than those with mild dementia (Brown et al., 2005). Furthermore, test scores on this measure differentiated among participants with dementia who were classified by a driving instructor as safe, marginal, or unsafe (based on total scores from on-road driving maneuvers), therefore suggesting good ecological validity (Brown et al., 2005). A final measure is the Cognitive Behavioral Driver's Inventory (CBDI; Engum, Lambert, Womac, & Pendergrass, 1988). The measure consists of 27 computer-based and manual tests that assess a variety of neurocognitive domains such as attention, processing speed, visual scanning and perception, sequencing, and coordination (Engum et al., 1988). Although frequently cited in research studies, a recent study suggested that although the CBDI was useful for predicting on-road performance for patients with right-sided stroke and TBI, it was not predictive for patients with left-sided stroke or age-related cognitive decline, and should therefore be used only with the patient's diagnosis in mind (Bouillon, Mazer, & Gelinas, 2006).

In summary, impairments in any of the above cognitive domains may potentially negatively affect driving performance. However, impairments in specific domains, such as complex attention, visual spatial abilities, processing speed, and executive functioning, may serve as particular warning signs that further, behind-the-wheel driving assessment is necessary. Although compensatory strategies such restricting the distance or situation in which one drives may be implemented in some cases, these strategies may do more to decrease the likelihood of an accident than to truly compensate for cognitive inefficiencies. It is difficult to adequately account for impaired executive functioning, problems with visual spatial perception, poor attention, and/or slowed processing speed, and drivers may still pose a risk to others and themselves. Although additional information is necessary to address thoroughly a patient's capacity to drive, recommendations with regard to driving should be made with these concerns in mind.

CASE EXAMPLE 1

An 84-year-old woman was referred by her neurologist for differential diagnosis of dementia versus depression. According to her medical records, she had a within-normal-limits performance on the MMSE. However, collateral information from her sister and the retirement residence indicated that she had nighttime wandering, reversal of the day–night sleep cycle, and memory deficits, including sometimes forgetting to take her medication. The patient reported no recollection of such behavior and denied any cognitive decline. In addition, the patient had a medical history significant for bilateral hearing loss, cataracts, and macular degeneration. Performance on neuropsychological testing revealed significant deficits in visual acuity, executive function, memory, processing speed, and psychomotor slowness. Additionally, she presented with periods of vertigo and very poor self-awareness. Although some of her visual deficits may have been improved with cataract surgery and new eyeglasses, the vision loss from the macular degeneration would still preclude her from driving safely. Her cognitive deficits were consistent with dementia and therefore were likely to be progressive in nature. Because of the complete lack of awareness of how her physical, cognitive, and sensory deficits might potentially result in unsafe operation of a vehicle, the clinical decision to recommend cessation of driving was made. She was not referred for a driving evaluation or driver training because her medical conditions precluded safe driving, even on an on-road test, and were not able to be rehabilitated. The retirement community, in which she was living, requested that family members remove her from the residence and provide a higher level of care and supervision. The patient's sister legally acquired power of attorney and made the decision to sell the patient's car and to move her into an assisted-living facility with 24-hour supervision. The patient continues to reside in the assisted-living facility and has been participating in individual psychotherapy with this neuropsychologist for the past 3 years. Interestingly, the issue of return to driving has been raised by the patient on numerous occasions. Specifically, she indicates that she should purchase a new car and start driving herself to places, both local and cross country. She has no recollection that she has been informed several times that she should no longer drive and has no awareness of any reasons why she should not be driving. In each instance when this issue arises, the focus of the therapy session involves gently helping her to understand her situation and providing support for her loss of independence.

CASE EXAMPLE 2

A 40-year-old man who sustained a traumatic brain injury after falling about six feet from a landing and hitting his head on the pavement was referred for neuropsychological assessment. He experienced a loss of consciousness of less than 1 hour and had left frontal and parietal contusions and a small left subdural hematoma. Following acute hospitalization, he underwent relatively short comprehensive rehabilitation and was discharged home. Upon discharge from the rehabilitation facility, he and his wife were informed that he would be unable to return to driving until cleared by his physician. Furthermore, the patient's wife made the official report to the local DMV of her husband's injuries. By local law in Maryland, the patient would be unable to legally drive until he went 6 months without having a seizure and then undergoing a formal driving evaluation. He continued with outpatient rehabilitation and progressed quickly in his recovery. He was administered a brief neuropsychological battery 4 months postinjury. He showed good cognitive recovery and obtained average to high average scores on tests of attention/concentration, memory, executive function, information processing speed, and visuospatial ability. His primary deficits were in language (due to residual aphasia), mild bilateral motor slowness, and occasional fatigue. The results of the neuropsychological evaluation were provided to his neurologist who proceeded to clear the patient for driving rehabilitation. He underwent a comprehensive driver retraining program with a Driving Rehabilitation Specialist and successfully completed the program. By the time he completed the program he had met his 6-month seizure-free requirement and was allowed to undergo formal driving evaluation. He passed the driving evaluation and was given medical clearance to return to driving. He was then able to reinstate his driver's license. It should be noted that the patient was also counseled extensively about the importance of gradually increasing his driving endurance as he continued to experience intermittent fatigue. He continued in psychotherapy for approximately 2 years post-injury. During this period of his recovery and treatment, issues related to driving arose intermittently. Specifically, when medication changes were made, there were discussions about changes in his side-effects profile and how these may impact his ability to drive. Sleep disturbance and daytime fatigue were also issues that needed to be addressed during psychotherapy and in the context of operating a vehicle. The patient was receptive to suggestions and followed through with recommendations. For example, it was recommended that if he did not sleep well and experienced daytime drowsiness/fatigue, he should refrain from driving, which he did.

CONCLUSIONS

The assessment of an individual's capacity to drive requires a multidisciplinary approach. A thorough evaluation of an individual's sensory and physical functioning, medical history (including medications), psychological status, cognitive abilities and deficits, knowledge of driving rules/regulation, and an ability to operate a vehicle safely in both routine and challenging conditions is necessary. Psychologists who work with individuals who are in at-risk groups for unsafe driving should obtain relevant information pertaining to reporting requirements, the legal standards for driving, and at what point an individual is considered too impaired to operate a vehicle safely. It is also necessary to consider the ethical issues that arise when evaluating patients who may have compromised ability to operate a motor vehicle such as the impact on the individual versus the risk of harm to the general population.

Results from the neuropsychological evaluation can provide useful information in determining an individual's capacity to drive. Although impairments in any cognitive domain may be cause for concern, research has shown that deficits in complex attention, visual spatial abilities, processing speed, and executive functioning have shown the most robust link to poor driving outcomes. Individuals with impairments within these domains may pose a risk to themselves and others on or near the road if they are allowed to remain behind the wheel. However, information from the neuropsychological evaluation should be placed within the context of the previously discussed factors. In situations in which an individual's ability to drive is unclear test data can elicit a referral for a further behind-the-wheel evaluation. In this way, the neuropsychological assessment of cognition is one of several pieces of data that can contribute to determining driving capacity, and neuropsychologists serve an important role in the multidisciplinary assessment of this function.

As indicated in the chapter on driving capacity by ABA/APA (2008), as the number of older adults increases in the coming years, the involvement of neuropsychologists evaluations of driving capacity is likely to increase. Furthermore, due to advances in medicine, vehicle safety features, and protective equipment, more people are surviving what might have previously been a fatal brain injury or illness. Therefore, it is important for neuropsychologists to make themselves aware of the laws and ethical issues related to driving capacity and the process by which evaluations are conducted and to collaborate with other professionals within the context of assessing capacity to drive.

With regard to areas of future research and development of evaluative techniques for the assessment of driving capacity, several issues deserve consideration. Schultheis et al. (2010) indicate the importance of identifying adequate criteria for the determination of fitness to drive. On-road testing and frequency of motor vehicle accidents or moving violations are the two most common criteria used to define driving performance. However, on-road testing may be contaminated by subjectivity, road conditions, and nonuniformity. The frequency of motor vehicle accidents and moving violations is not always accurate as not all DMVs have specific information and not all moving violations or accidents are caught or reported. To increase the generalizability of future research, Schultheis recommends multiple driving performance measures within a study, increased length of time for follow-up of driving performance, and standardization of and objective defining of driving behaviors in the context of the on-road driving evaluation.

References

Akinwuntan, A. E., Feys, H., DeWeerdt, W., Baten, G., Arno, P., & Kiekens, C. (2006). Prediction of driving after stroke: A prospective study. *Neurorehabilitation and Neural Repair, 20,* 417–423.

American Bar Association Commission on Law and Aging & American Psychological Association. (2008). *Driving capacity. Assessment of older adults with diminished capacity: A handbook for psychologists* (pp. 91–100). Washington, D.C.: Authors.

American Medical Association. (2010). *Physician's Guide to Assessing and Counseling Older Drivers, Chapter 8: State Licensing and Reporting Laws.* (http://www.ama-assn.org/ama1/pub/upload/mm/433/older-drivers-chapter8.pdf)

Amick, M. M. Grace, J., & Ott, B. R. (2007). Visual and cognitive predictors of driving safety in Parkinson's disease patients. *Archives of Clinical Neuropsychology, 22,* 957–967.

Anderson, S. W., Rizzo, M., Skaar, N., Stierman, L., Cavaco, S., Dawson, J., & Damasio, H. (2007). Amnesia and driving. *Journal of Clinical and Experimental Neuropsychology, 29,* 1–12.

Anstey, K. J., Wood, J., Lord, S., & Walker, J. G. (2005). Cognitive, sensory and physical factors enabling driving safety in older adults. *Clinical Psychology Review, 25,* 45–65.

Ball, K., & Roenker, D. (1998). *Useful field of view*. San Antonio, TX: The Psychological Corporation.

Bieliauskas, L. A., Roper, B. R., Trobe, J., Green, P., & Lacy, M. (1998). Cognitive measures, driving safety, and Alzheimer's disease. *The Clinical Neuropsychologist, 12,* 206–212.

Blessed, G., Tomlinson, B. E., & Roth, M. (1968). The association between quantitative measures of dementia and of senile change in the cerebral grey matter of elderly subjects. *British Journal of Psychiatry, 114,* 797–811.

Bouillon, L., Mazer, B., & Gelinas, I. (2006). Validity of the Cognitive Behavioral Driver's Inventory in predicting driving outcome. *American Journal of Occupational Therapy, 60,* 420–427.

Brandt, J., & Benedict, R. H. B. (2002). *The Hopkins Verbal Learning Test Revised: Professional manual.* Odessa: Psychological Assessment Resources.

Brouwer, W. H., & Withaar, F. K. (1997). Fitness to drive after traumatic brain injury. *Neuropsychological Rehabilitation, 7,* 177–193.

Brown, L. B., & Ott, B. R. (2004). Driving and dementia: A review of the literature. *Journal of Geriatric Psychiatry and Neurology, 17,* 232–240.

Brown, L. B., Stern, R. A., Cahn-Weiner, D. A. Rigers, B., Messer, M. A., Lannon, M. C., Maxwell, C., Souza, T., White, T., & Ott, B. R. (2005). Driving scenes test of the Neuropsychological Assessment Battery (NAB) and on-road driving performance in aging and very mild dementia. *Archives of Clinical Neuropsychology, 20,* 209–215.

Carr, D. B., & Ott, B. R. (2010). The older adult driver with cognitive impairment: "It's a very frustrating life." *Journal of the American Medical Association, 303,* 1632–1641.

Colarusso, R. P., & Hammill, D. D. (2003). *Motor-Free Visual Perception Test (MVPT-3).* Los Angeles: Western Psychological Services.

Cyr, A. A., Stinchcombe, A., Gagnon, S., Marshall, S., Hing, M. M. S., & Finestone, H. (2009). Driving difficulties of brain-injured drivers in reaction to high-crash-risk simulated road events: A question of impaired divided attention? *Journal of Clinical and Experimental Neuropsychology, 31,* 472–482.

Daigneault, G., Joly, P., & Frigon, J. Y. (2002). Executive functions in the evaluation of accident risk of older drivers. *Journal of Clinical and Experimental Neuropsychology, 24,* 221–238.

Engum, E. S., Lambert, E. W., Womac, J., & Pendergrass, T. (1988). Norms and decision-making rules for the Cognitive Behavioral Driver's Inventory. *Cognitive Rehabilitation, 6,* 12–19.

Fisk, G. D., & Mennemeier, J. (2006). Common neuropsychological deficits associated with stroke survivor's impaired performance on a useful field of view test. *Perceptual Motor Skills, 102,* 387–394.

Folstein, M. F., Folstein, S. E., & McHugh, P. R. (1975). "Mini-mental state": A practical method for grading the cognitive state of patients for the clinician. *Journal of Psychiatric Research, 12,* 189–198.

Freund, B., & Colgrove, L. A. A. (2008). Error specific restrictions for older drivers: Promoting continued independence and public safety. *Accident Analysis and Prevention, 40,* 97–103.

Galski, T., & McDonald, M. A. (2009). Driving and the law. In M. T. Schultheis, J. DeLuca, & D. Chute, Eds., *Handbook for the assessment of driving capacity* (pp. 187–200). San Diego: Academic Press.

Gorman, A. A., Foley, J. M. Ettenhofer, M. L., Hinkin, C. H., & van Gorp, W. G. (2009). Functional consequences of HIV-associated neuropsychological impairment. *Neuropsychology Review, 19,* 186–203.

Hooper, H. E. (1958). *The Hooper Visual Organization Test manual.* Los Angeles: Western Psychological Services.

Jurica, P. J., Leittenn, C. L., & Mattis, S. (2001). *Dementia Rating Scale-2: Professional Manual.* Lutz, FL: Psychological Assessment Resources.

Lundqvist, A., Alinder, J., & Ronnberg, J. (2008). Factors influencing driving 10 years after brain injury. *Brain Injury, 22,* 295–304.

Lundqvist, A., Gerdle, B., & Ronnberg, J. (2000). Neuropsychological aspects of driving after a stroke–in the simulator and on the road. *Applied Cognitive Psychology, 14,* 135–150.

Mann, W. C., McCarthy, D. P., Wu, S. S., & Tomita, M. (2005). Relationship of health status, functional status, and psychosocial status to driving among elderly with disabilities. *Physical and Occupational Therapy in Geriatrics, 23,* 1–24.

Marottoli, R. A., Mendes de Leon, C. F., Glass, T. A., Williams, C. S., Cooney, L. M., Berkman, L. F., & Tinetti, M. (1997). Driving cessation and increased depressive symptoms: Prospective evidence from the New Haven EPESE. Established Populations for Epidemiologic Studies of the Elderly. *Journal of the American Geriatric Society, 45,* 202–206.

Mathias, J. L., & Lucas, L. K. (2009). Cognitive predictors of unsafe driving in older drivers: A meta-analysis. *International Psychogeriatrics, 21,* 637–653.

Mattis, S. (1976). Mental status examination for organic mental syndrome in the elderly patient. In R. Bellack & B. Karasu (Eds.), *Geriatric psychiatry* (pp. 77–121). New York: Grune & Stratton.

Mazer, B. L., Korner-Bitensky, N. A., & Sofer, S. (1998). Predicting ability to drive after stroke. *Archives of Physical Medicine & Rehabilitation, 79,* 743–750.

Mazer, B. L., Sofer, S., Korner-Bitensky, & N., Gelinas, I. (2001). Use of the UFOV to evaluate and retrain visual attention skills in clients with stroke: A pilot study. *American Journal of Occupational Therapy, 55,* 552–557.

Nasreddine, Z. S., Philips, N. A., Bedirian, V., Charbonneau, S., Whitehead, V., Collin, I., Cummings, J. L., & Chertkow, H. (2005). The Montreal Cognitive Assessment, MoCA: A brief screening tool for mild cognitive impairment. *Journal of the American Geriatrics Society, 53,* 695–699.

National Highway Traffic Safety Administration. (2008). Traffic safety facts: 2008 data. http://www-nrd.nhtsa.dot.gov/Pubs/811161.PDF.

Oswanski, M. F., Sharma, O. P., Raj, S. S., Vassar, L. A., Woods, K. L., Sargent, W. M., & Pitock, R. J. (2007). Evaluation of two assessment tools in predicting driving ability of senior drivers. *American Journal of Physical Medicine & Rehabilitation, 86,* 190–199.

Reger, M. A., Welsh, R. K., Watson, G. S., Cholerton, B., Baker, L. D., & Craft, S. (2004). The relationship between neuropsychological functioning and driving ability in dementia: A meta-analysis. *Neuropsychology, 18,* 85–93.

Reitan, R. M. (1958). Validity of the Trail Making Test as an indicator of organic brain damage. *Perceptual Motor Skills, 8,* 271–276.

Ryan, K. A., Rapport, L. J., Harper, K. T., Fuerst, D., Bieliauskas, L., Khan, O., & Lisak, R. (2009). Fitness to drive in multiple sclerosis: Awareness of deficit moderates risk. *Journal of Clinical and Experimental Neuropsychology, 31,* 126–139.

Sandford, J. A., & Turner, A. (2000). *Integrated visual and auditory continuous performance test manual.* Richmond: Braintrain, Inc.

Schultheis, M. T., & Chute, D. L. (1999). Development of an ecologically valid, computerized driving assessment program: The Neurocognitive Driving Test. *Archives of Clinical Neuropsychology, 14,* 749–795.

Schultheis, M. T., & Fleksher, C. (2009). Driving and stroke. In M. T. Schultheis, J. DeLuca, & D. Chute, Eds., *Handbook for the assessment of driving capacity* (pp. 117–130). San Diego: Academic Press.

Schultheis, M.T., Garay, E., & DeLuca, J. (2001). The influence of cognitive impairment on driving performance in multiple sclerosis. *Neurology, 56,* 1089–1094.

Schultheis, M. T., Hillary, F., & Chute, D. L. (2003). The Neurocognitive Driving Test: Applying technology to the assessment of driving ability following brain injury. *Rehabilitation Psychology, 48,* 275–280.

Schultheis, M. T., Weisser, V., Ang, J., Elovic, E., Nead, R., Sestito, N., Fleksher, C., & Millis, S. R. (2010). Examining the relationship between cognition and driving performance in multiple sclerosis. *Archives of Physical Medicine & Rehabilitation, 91,* 465–473.

Scott, C. A., Rapport, L. J., Bryer, R. C., Griffen, J., Hanks, R., & McKay, C. (2009). Self-awareness of driving ability and the decision to resume driving following stroke. *Journal of Clinical and Experimental Neuropsychology, 31,* 353–362.

Sivan, A. B. (1992). *Benton Visual Retention Test* (5th ed.). San Antonio: The Psychological Corporation.

Smith, A. (1982). *Symbol Digit Modalities Test (SDMT) manual (revised).* Los Angeles: Western Psychological Services.

Stern, R. A., Javorsky, D. J., Singer, E. A., Harris, N. G., Sommeriville, J. A., Duke, L. M., Thompson, J. A., & Kaplan, E. (1999). *Boston Qualitative Scoring System of the Rey-Osterreith Complex Figure.* Odessa: Psychological Assessment Resources.

Stern, R. A., & White, T. (2003). *Neuropsychological Assessment Battery (NAB).* Lutz, FL: Psychological Assessment Resources, Inc.

Stolwyk, R. J., Charlton, J. L., Triggs, T. J., Iansek, R., & Bradshaw, J. L. (2006). Neuropsychological function and driving ability in people with Parkinson's disease. *Journal of Clinical and Experimental Neuropsychology, 28,* 898–913.

Wechsler, D. (1987). *Wechsler Memory Scale-revised.* New York: Psychological Corporation.

Wechsler, D. (1997). *Wechsler Memory Scale–third edition.* New York: Psychological Corporation

Wechsler, D. (2008). *Wechsler Adult Intelligence Scale–fourth edition.* San Antonio: NCS Pearson, Inc.

Wechsler, D. (2009). *Wechsler Memory Scale–fourth edition.* San Antonio: NCS Pearson, Inc.

Zook, N. A., Bennett, T. L., & Lane, M. (2009). Identifying at-risk older adult community-dwelling drivers through neuropsychological evaluation. *Applied Neuropsychology, 16,* 281–287.

7

Personal Care and Independence

D. ERIK EVERHART, KATIE A. LEHOCKEY, ALICIA M. MORAN, AND JONATHAN M. HIGHSMITH

The constructs of personal care and independence fall primarily within the realm of basic activities of daily living (ADLs), which consist of a variety of self-care skills including dressing, grooming, personal hygiene, and toileting. These activities are typically distinguished from the more complex instrumental activities of daily living (IADLs) such as managing finances, using transportation, doing laundry, making healthcare decisions, and managing medications (Wolinsky, Callahan, Fitzgerald, & Johnson, 1993). Although ADLs and IADLs overlap and represent related constructs, there is a reason to consider them separately. Most importantly, the basic ADLs that are related to personal care (which is the focus of this chapter) are somewhat resilient to neurodegenerative processes, whereas a decline in IADLs is evident in preclinical and early stages of neurodegenerative disease such as Alzheimer's disease (AD) (Marson & Hebert, 2006). Given this distinction, it seems intuitive that the use of traditional neuropsychological measures for the evaluation of personal care and independence may be somewhat limiting with regard to reaching a decision about capacity within this domain of function. The incorporation of other assessment procedures, including direct observation, and collateral informants, is important for the determination of whether an individual can care for themselves independently.

This chapter focuses on the evaluation of personal care and independence. The goal of this chapter is to review the literature pertaining to the evaluation of the basic ADLs that pertain to self-care, and to provide recommendations for the evaluation of personal care among patients who may be suffering from functional decline. The chapter concludes with an illustrative case study and section on future directions, as neuropsychological research that pertains to personal care is limited.

LEGAL CONSIDERATIONS

An important legal ramification of the evaluation of capacity for personal care and independence concerns the possible denial of fundamental freedoms and basic civil liberties. The codified protection of basic liberties is afforded to all citizens of the United States in the Fifth Amendment of the U.S. Constitution, which states, "No person shall be ... deprived of life, liberty, or property, without due process of law." The Fourteenth Amendment uses almost identical wording, and restricts states from deprivation of the individual without due process. Similar protections are afforded to citizens in most other countries. Indeed, international law is committed to the protection of human rights through the United Nations Universal Declaration of Human Rights (UDHR; 1948). However, within all of these documents, the rights of the disabled were afforded no special protections. This prompted the United Nations to organize a Convention on the Rights of Persons with Disabilities (CRPD, 2006) as a legally binding set of principles and rights to protect the dignity, autonomy in decision making, and independence of individuals with disabilities. Of the articles within the CRPD, Article 19 is most applicable to personal care and independence in that it ensures "the equal right of all persons with disabilities to live in the community, with choices equal to others." Two of the specific rights provided include the right to choose their own place of residence and where and with whom they live, and access to resources to prevent isolation or segregation. Although more specific legal regulations govern how psychologists implement and make decisions regarding recommendations of independence, we must not lose sight of these fundamental principles. Moreover, the importance of these fundamental rights should be evident in careful selection of instruments and through an approach to making recommendations that ensures that the denial of liberties occurs only when there is a preponderance of clear, cogent, and convincing evidence (the standard used in North Carolina) that an individual is incompetent and needs guardianship.

The due process clauses noted above ensure that governmental entities cannot deprive an individual of basic liberties without ensuring due process. From a federal level, there currently exists no clear definition of what determines when such evidence exists as there are no federal or uniform state laws delineating the comprehensiveness or quality of the evidence needed. This is problematic when attempting to review relevant case law due to the considerable differences between the states in law and judicial makeup. We therefore focus on higher court decisions and an example of state general statutes.

One example of a higher court decision is *Olmstead, Commissioner, Georgia Department of Human Resources,* et al. *v. L. C., by Zimring, guardian ad litem and next friend,* et al. In this case, two plaintiffs were institutionalized in Georgia for schizophrenia and mental retardation. Following assessments that determined both individuals could receive appropriate treatment in a community setting, the plaintiffs successfully sued the state of Georgia for release from institutionalization. The opinion of the court held that under Title II of the Americans with Disabilities Act (ADA; 1990), a mental illness is a form of disability and is covered under ADA. Furthermore, removal of the individual from a community, when it was determined that a viable treatment that did not restrict the individual's freedom existed, violated their right to be included in community life and that any confinement "diminishes the everyday life activities of individuals, including family relations, social contacts, work options, economic independence, educational advancement, and cultural enrichment." The court upheld that limiting the independence of an individual with a disability causes undue negative effects on many aspects of the individual's life. Also, this decision implies that if no appropriate option exists to support independence, then restricting individual freedoms is appropriate. We must remain cognizant that any restrictions will cause disruption of many areas of life and cause significant harm to the individual. Again, this argues for restraint in restricting independence unless the risks of harm outweigh the substantial disruptions to the persons' lives.

When the focus shifts from disability in general to the evaluation of an individual's capacity to live independently, a number of specific statutes are important, namely guardianship statutes and any other specific state laws related to independence and capacity. However, even within these statutes there is typically little specificity to inform the assessment process and clinicians must use their judgment and focus on supporting the spirit of the above mentioned freedoms. Guardianship statutes vary widely across states in specific requirements in evaluations. One example is the North Carolina General Statue (35A-1111), which states that a Multidisciplinary Evaluation should include medical, psychological, and social work elements, both to aid determining the level of disability and to aid in the development of guardianship plans, and may be considered at the hearing for adjudication of incompetence, the hearing for appointment of a guardian, or both. However, even at the state level, no specific direction is provided regarding the type, quality, or quantity of evidence required for the adjudication of incompetence, only which services should be included within the Multidisciplinary Evaluation.

One model act that was created to aid states when revising guardianship statutes is the Uniform Guardianship and Protective Proceedings Act (UGPPA; 1997). This act identifies three separate elements necessary for evaluations: a cognitive element governing information processing, decision making, and communication; a functional element governing activities of daily living, safety, and physical health; and a necessity element governing whether independence may be maintained through the use of any type of technological assistance. However, many states have not adopted this standard and continue to require a diagnostic element, and the specific requirement of any state varies in the mix of these elements.

Thus, the specific functional areas required for the evaluation of capacity and thus the adjudication of competence vary by state and specificity of law and regulation. Although the state requirements might not require the inclusion of all of these four elements (diagnostic, cognitive, functional, and necessity), the selection of instruments and clinical interviews attempts to provide information regarding each area to inform fully the adjudication process. In addition to these, focusing on other aspects that can influence this process including interventions, individual values, advanced directives, and social history may highlight that the final recommendation concerning the capacity to live independently is not a static, but an ongoing, process that may change due to the success of rehabilitation as well as medical and/or other intervention efforts.

NEUROPSYCHOLOGICAL RESEARCH AND EVALUATION OF PERSONAL CARE

The functions that are associated with personal care and independence include basic ADLs such as dressing, bathing, feeding, and toileting. These skills are over-learned patterns of behavior that are typically learned within the first few years of development. The procedural nature of these skills likely accounts for the relative sparing of function in the beginning phases of dementia (Baum, Edwards, Yonan, & Storandt, 1996). Likewise, these skills require the use of well-learned basic motor programs (Patterson, Mack, Neundorfer, Martin, Smyth, & Whitehouse, 1992). Thus, personal care entails the use of automatic processes that require low cognitive load and little conscious attention, and that can be performed with other tasks (Jorm, 1986; Marson & Hebert, 2006). The automatic and procedural nature of these skills suggest that performance of the basic ADLs is less dependent on primary memory systems such as the hippocampus and dorsomedial nucleus of the thalamus, which may partially account for the preservation of function observed in the dementing disorders that affect these regions. Marson and Hebert (2006) suggest that frank impairment of these skills is "very often a cardinal sign of probable dementia," provided that the impairment is due to loss of cognitive function and not physical disability (Marson & Hebert, 2006; Patterson et al., 1992). Thus, the clinician must determine whether the loss of function is attributable to cognitive decline rather than to the decline in physical ability that is seen in aging.

Although the basic ADLs are typically spared early-on, the eventual loss of function during later stages of dementia results in greater caregiver burden and higher rates of institutionalization (Goode, Haley, Roth, & Ford, 1998). Likewise, the retained ability to perform personal care activities is sometimes a requirement for placement in settings that do not provide close supervision (i.e., 24-hour care).

With regard to neuropsychological testing, the ecological validity of neurocognitive tests is limited, particularly with the evaluation of personal care (Chaytor & Schmitter-Edgecombe, 2003). Indeed, much of the research that has evaluated the relationship between neurocognitive decline and function has focused on IADLs (Cahn-Weiner et al., 2007), leaving a void in the understanding of the relationship between neurocognitive measures and functional decline in personal care. In addition, individuals with mild cognitive impairment (MCI) or individuals in the beginning stages of progressive deterioration do not experience substantial functional decline (though there may be very subtle decline) in personal care or basic ADLs. As such, traditional neurocognitive measures may lack sensitivity with regard to a decline in personal hygiene, grooming, and other aspects of self-care. Likewise, some studies have found that only 40% of the variance in functional decline is accounted for by cognitive decline, suggesting that these processes are overlapping, yet different (Mortimer, Ebbitt, Jun, & Finch, 1992).

There is some evidence that global measures of neurocognitive function are correlated with declines in basic ADLs. For example, moderate correlations between the Mini-Mental State Examination (MMSE) (Folstein, Folstein, & McHugh, 1975) and caregiver ratings of basic ADLs have been reported (Leckey & Beatty, 2002); a correlation also exists between basic ADLs and direct assessments of functional performance (Burns, Mortimer, & Merchak, 1994). However, the variance accounted for by the MMSE is reduced dramatically when sample populations are restricted to individuals with mild to moderate dementia (Leckey & Beatty, 2002). This is consistent with previous observations that a decline in personal care is somewhat resilient to the initial effects of progressive neurodegenerative disease. These findings also suggest that the MMSE, used in isolation, is not an adequate tool for the prediction of functional declines in basic ADLs.

Previous studies have found a relationship between the Mattis Dementia Rating Scale (DRS) (Mattis, 1988) and basic ADLs (Fitz & Teri, 1994). In a recent study, Fields et al. (2010) examined the predictive utility of the DRS relative to basic and instrumental ADLs in a sample of 2469 community-dwelling individuals with varying degrees of cognitive functioning. Functional activity was assessed via the Record of Independent Living (ROILS), which is an informant-based rating of basic and instrumental ADLs (Weintraub, 1986). The basic ADLs measured with this instrument include eating, toileting, dressing, and washing/grooming. The results of this study suggest that at least 50% of individuals with DRS scores below 120 may have some difficulty with washing/grooming, but require no more than verbal prompts for completion of these tasks. Of individuals with DRS scores below 45, 50% could no longer perform washing/grooming and dressing activities, and had difficulty with eating and toileting. This study also provides corresponding MMSE scores. Thus, an MMSE score of 23/30 roughly translates to a DRS score of 118, and an MMSE score of approximately 10/30 roughly translates to a DRS score of 45. This study is particularly important given that 40% of individuals with cognitive complaints live alone, and as such, there are no collateral informants who can provide additional information about function. The study also provides a promising step toward understanding the relationship between neurocognitive measures and personal care. However, the authors also acknowledge that the use of the ROILs may be limiting because of the restricted descriptors (i.e., simple phrases) on the instrument. These descriptors are open to interpretation and are less specific than those provided in other measures of function (e.g., Lawton & Brody, 1969).

Although cognitive and functional decline represent different processes and the rates of decline may differ between these processes, Mortimer and colleagues (1992) suggest that lower baseline scores on specific nonverbal neuropsychological measures of visuospatial function and visual memory predict faster rates of functional decline in activities of daily living. In this study, 65 patients with probable AD (initially mildly to moderately impaired) were followed for up to 4 years. Although lower scores on verbal neuropsychological tests at the time of entry were related to faster cognitive progression, lower scores on nonverbal neuropsychological tests (as well as other symptoms such as the presence of paranoid ideation, hallucinations, and activity disturbances) were related to faster functional decline. In this study, the measure of functional decline was a summation of scores on Lawton and Brody's (1969) Instrumental Activities of Daily Living Scale and Physical Self-Maintenance Scale. Other studies have reported similar findings. Perry and Hodges (2000) examined 24 patients with possible or probable AD using a neuropsychological test battery. Functional assessment was completed using a 25-item analogue scale that included items that assess instrumental activities of daily living and self-care. The Visual Object and Space Perception Test (Warrington & James, 1991) was related to a decline in self-care. In this study, self-care included basic ADLs such as bathing/showering, dressing unaided, eating meals unaided, retaining levels of concern over appearance, and shaving or applying cosmetics.

Additional research suggests that visuospatial decline is related to dependency among patients with progressive neurodegenerative disease. For example, Sarazin and colleagues (2005) found that copying a figure from a modified MMSE is predictive of severe dependency among patients with probable AD. It is thus reasonable to presume that this is also predictive of a decline in personal care. In accounting for these findings, Perry and Hodges (2000) suggest that "intact visuospatial function would clearly be a prerequisite to efficient tool and object use in a dynamic environment." Likewise, Sarazin and colleagues (2005) suggest that deficits in visuospatial constructive functions are related to changes on posterior temporoparietal and occipital association areas, and that "visuoconstructive abilities provoke a severe dependency outcome because the integrity of visuospatial and praxic functions, which both rely on parietal lobe function, is involved in daily activities." These findings suggest that nonverbal neuropsychological tests may be useful for referrals where personal care is questioned.

Although executive function is often linked to decline in IADLs (see, for instance, Cahn-Weiner et al., 2000), it seems reasonable that poor ability to initiate behavior, multitask, and concentrate would be related to poor performance of basic ADLs as well. It is interesting to note, however, that some studies have not found a relationship between executive function and some basic ADLs such as hygiene. For example, Nadler and colleagues (1993) found that the Initiation/Perseveration subscale of the DRS was related to a decline in the activities of daily living such as safety and cooking, but not hygiene. As discussed previously, it is plausible that the overlearned nature of basic ADLs does not require heavy utilization of executive function skills.

SELF-REPORT AND INFORMANT RATINGS OF BASIC ADLs

A variety of self-report and informant rating instruments exist for the evaluation of basic ADLs or personal care. A review of all of the instruments is beyond the scope of this chapter, and the reader is referred to a handbook for psychologists written by the American Bar Association (ABA) Commission on Law and Aging–American Psychological Association (APA) for more extensive information about rating scales (American Bar Association Commission on Law and Aging & American Psychological Association, 2008). The reader may also wish to consult McDowell's (2006) book entitled *Measuring Health: A Guide to Rating Scales and Questionnaires*, the extensive compendium of tests provided by Strauss, Sherman, and Spreen (2006), and the following link: http://www.chcr.brown.edu/pcoc/functi.htm. This website reviews several different measures, including IADLs and basic ADLs, that may be useful to the clinician.

One well-known instrument is the Barthel ADL Index (BI), which was developed to measure the level of disability in patients whose disease (i.e., neuromuscular disorders) interfered with limb movements (Mahoney & Barthel, 1965). However, the items of this index are considered basic ADLs, and thus it is useful for examining changes in independent function observed in progressive neurodegenerative disease. The BI's reliability and internal consistency have been well established, and it can be administered by a clinician or through self-report. However, self-report is least correlated with other evaluators such as nurse clinical observation or physical therapists. The BI was also found to be quick and reliable, and suitable for use by both experienced and less skilled clinicians (Collins et al., 1988). The BI correlates with clinical judgment, and results from the use of the BI were shown to predict mortality and influence discharge outcome (Wylie & White, 1964). Granger, Albrecht, and Hamilton (1979) reported a test–retest reliability of 0.89 with severely disabled adults; the interrater agreement exceeded 0.95. Construct validity and face validity have also been established between the BI and the Functional Independence Measure (Gosman-Hedstrom & Svensson, 2000).

Another instrument is the Katz ADL, which assesses basic ADLs such as toileting and eating. This measure was originally created as a survey instrument to track the course of chronic illness and the aging process, and has since been used as a complement to medical intakes (Hartigan, 2007; Katz, Ford, Moskowitz, Jackson, & Jaffe, 1963). Although the BI is not hierarchical in nature, the Katz ADL is a Guttman-type scale, which presents items in a hierarchy of difficulty based on the idea that recovery and regression (as it happens in the aging process) occur in a predictable order (Katz et al., 1963). For example, the ability to bathe independently would presumably be lost prior to loss of the ability to eat independently. Research that has not utilized the Katz ADL confirms the notion that loss of function begins with more complex activities and subsequently progresses to the least complex of activities. For example, in one study, bathing was the first ADL to pose difficulty, followed by mobility, toileting, dressing, transfer, and feeding (Jaggor, Arthur, Spiers, & Clarke, 2001). Little formal reliability and validity information exists for the Katz ADL compared to the BI, but the utility of its specificity and its predictive value are notable when compared to the judgments of a small sample of nurses (Tornquist, Lovgren, & Soderfeld, 1990). The Katz ADL requires a skilled observer, in contrast to the BI. Both of these scales have limited sensitivity to detect small changes over time, and it has been suggested that the use of either of these scales should be coupled with an assessment of IADLs (Rodgers, Holm, & Stone, 1997).

Another rating scale that exists for the evaluation of personal care is the Physical Self-Maintenance Scale (PSMS) that was developed by Lawton and Brody (1969) to address self-care or basic ADLs. This scale contains items that evaluate dressing, grooming, hygiene, and feeding, and is substantially different from Lawton and Brody's (1969) other scale that evaluates IADLs. This instrument is a Guttman scale containing six items of self-care, and was designed as a disability measure for use in planning and evaluating treatment in elderly people living in the community or in institutions. Similar to the Katz ADL, it is based on the theory that human behavior is ordered on a hierarchy of complexity. Within each category, a further hierarchy of complexity progresses from basic to complex activities. The PSMS includes both ADL and IADL items. Although the scale was developed decades ago, the interrater reliability between a variety of professions is more than adequate (Hokoishi et al., 2001). For example, interrater reliability was demonstrated among pairs of nurses who rated 36 patients ($r = 0.87$).

Clinicians may also choose to use the Adult Functional Adaptive Behavior Scale (AFABS; Spirrison & Pierce, 1992). The AFABS assesses both ADL and IADL functions along with those skills that allow the individual to adhere to societal norms for personal responsibility, which are referred to as "requisites for personal responsibility" (Spirrison, 1992). The AFABS was compared to the Vineland Adaptive Behavior Scale and the AAMD Adaptive Behavior Scale in a group of elderly patients with mental retardation (Kerby, Wentworth, & Cotton, 1989). Construct validity for the AFABS was supported through significant correlations with both the Vineland Adaptive Behavior Scale ($r = 0.72$) and the AAMD Adaptive Behavior Scale ($r = 0.85$). Scores on the AFABS were also found to predict the patient's level of residential placement, even to a greater extent than the other two measures, which is useful for this population, especially as the other measures take four to five times longer to administer than the AFABS (Kerby et al., 1989; Spirrison, 1992).

Although many measurements are available for clinical assessment of independence and self-care capacities, limited empirical support and testing leave much to be desired for choosing specific tests. Haywood and colleagues (2005) warn that instrument reliability and responsiveness are both neglected areas of instrument evaluation. In addition, dementia patients and hospitalized elders consistently overestimate their ability (Marson & Hebert, 2006), and ratings from caregivers typically result in low to moderate correlations with performance-based functional assessment (Angel & Frisco, 2001). Based upon the noted shortcoming of such instruments, rating scales should not be the only means of assessment used by clinicians. Likewise, the actual cognitive and judgment skills of the examinee should be taken into account (American Bar Association Commission on Law and Aging & American Psychological Association, 2008).

DIRECT OBSERVATION AND PERFORMANCE-BASED ASSESSMENTS

As discussed above, there are shortcomings in the use of neuropsychological instruments, self-reports, and informant ratings of an individual's ability to perform self-care independently. Direct observation of the performance of activities that are associated with personal hygiene such as grooming and dressing may provide the clearest evidence of the capacity to complete such activities independently. For a variety of reasons, direct observation of some functions (e.g., toileting) may not be practical for the neuropsychologist, and may seem inappropriate to the patient within the context of the evaluation. Relatedly, well-developed conceptual models and direct assessment are available for other domains of function (e.g., financial capacity), but are currently lacking with regard to personal care (Marson & Hebert, 2006). To this extent, research pertaining to reliable and valid direct assessment of personal care remains in its infancy.

Review of the patient's medical record may provide some evidence of the capacity for performing such functions, as other disciplines (physical therapy, occupational therapy, and nursing) may perform home safety evaluations. In addition, a scale for the direct assessment of some of these functions exists that is reliable and valid (Loewenstein et al., 1989). The Direct Assessment of Functional Status (DAFS) consists of multiple scales that require direct observation. One subscale evaluates dressing/grooming skills, where the patient is taken to a bathroom and asked to do the following: take the cap off a tube of toothpaste, put the toothpaste on a toothbrush, turn on the tap, brush teeth, dampen washcloth, put soap on washcloth, wash face, and turn off the tap. The patient is also asked to use a hairbrush, put on a coat, button a coat, zip, and tie shoelaces. Another subscale exists for feeding abilities; it requires the patient to sit at a table, show how he or she would cut a steak, take a bite, eat soup, and pour water into a glass and drink it. The reliability and validity of the use of this instrument are high, with coefficients >0.9 across many of the subscales. However, for a variety of reasons, direct observation of these function(s) is not practical during examination and reliance on the medical chart or the evaluations available from other disciplines may be necessary. An additional criticism of these assessments is their potentially limited ecological validity, given that this procedure is likely to be performed outside of the patient's everyday environment.

OTHER RELATED RESEARCH ON PERSONAL CARE AND INDEPENDENT LIVING SKILLS

When determining the degree of independence and level of self-care it is important to consider factors secondary to neurocognitive impairment, such as comorbid psychiatric conditions, environmental variables, and psychosocial factors. It is widely known that comorbid psychiatric disorders, predominantly depression and psychosis, occur secondary to dementia. For example, a recent estimate suggests that 27% of individuals with dementia have a depressive disorder as well (Castilla-Puentes & Habeych, 2010). Although the prevalence of depression is higher in individuals with dementia compared to controls, the relationships appear complex and research findings have varied widely. For example, depression has been linked to less severe dementia, but has also been associated with more severe cognitive deficits (Ownby, Harwood, Acevedo, Barker, & Duara, 2001;

Rovner, Broadhead, Spencer, Carson, & Folstein, 1989; Teri & Wagner, 1991). A recent study found that depression was most common among individuals with vascular dementia, with 44% of the sample meeting criteria for depression compared to only 18% of individuals with AD (Castilla-Puentes & Habeych, 2010).

Recent research has also examined the relationship among depression, dementia, and poor self-care. Katon and colleagues (2010) examined dementia prevalence and self-care in patients with diabetes and depression, and found that those individuals with dementia had a much more difficult time with self-care including poor diet, lack of medication adherence, and lack of other health-related behaviors, such as exercise (Katon et al., 2010). Another study that examined the quality of life in dementia patients focused on the development and comparison of two competing path models composed of quality of life variables including dementia, pain, behavioral disturbances, and ADLs. Results revealed that cognitive, emotional, and behavioral variables interact in complex ways with one another to predict patients' activities of daily living (Cipher & Clifford, 2004).

The cumulative effects of cognitive impairment and psychiatric complications have direct implications for self-care and independence. Because many studies are correlational rather than causal, it is difficult to determine the role of psychiatric problems in cognitive impairment and independent living skills. There is a complicated and bidirectional relationship between cognitive impairment and psychological impairment that is biological and environmental. For example, poor cognitive functioning may cause problems in activities of daily living. Awareness of these problems may lead to feelings of hopelessness and/or inadequacy that can lead to the development of depression. Upon examining a number of demographic and environmental characteristics associated with the quality of life in dementia patients, the best predictor of quality of life was a high level of independence in activities of daily living (Andersen, Wittrup-Jensen, Lolk, Andersen, & Kragh-Sorensen, 2004). There is also substantial evidence that depression can cause neurocognitive impairment as well as loss of independence. For example, in stroke patients with moderate to severe deficits, poststroke depression has been found to significantly impair activities of daily living such as eating, walking, dressing, and understanding spoken language. Remission of depression was found to improve activities of daily living (Chemerinski, Robinson, & Kosier, 2001). Therefore, self-care is impacted by both cognitive impairment and mood disorders and worse outcomes are expected when both conditions are present.

Although AD and depression are fundamentally quite different, there is some overlap in the pathophysiology of these two disorders. The diminishing neurotrophic factors and neuroinflammation observed in depression are also thought to be associated with the development of AD (Wuwongse, Chang, & Law, 2010). Similarly, the relationship between executive functioning and depression has been explored, and has been linked to loss of independence in those with dementia. Thomas and colleagues have proposed a new subtype of depression, "depression-executive dysfunction syndrome," that occurs later in life due to frontostriatal dysfunction and is characterized by a diminution of spontaneous activity, lack of drive and motivation, and inability to plan ahead. Thomas and colleagues examined various subpopulations of individuals with cognitive impairment including AD, vascular dementia, mild cognitive impairment (MCI), Lewy body dementia, and frontotemporal dementia (FTD). Those participants who were depressed had more impaired executive functioning, which was associated with impaired self-care and independent living. The depressed patients with impairment in executive functioning were more likely to have behavioral disorders, lack of motivation, problems with instrumental acts of daily life, increased risk of falls, and malnutrition (Thomas et al., 2009).

Psychosis is sometimes observed in various types of dementia such as AD and Parkinson's disease. Although some studies have found psychosis to be associated with more severe cognitive impairment, others have found only a nonsignificant trend between psychosis and severity of cognitive impairment (Bylsma et al., 1994; Jeste, Wragg, Salmon, Harris, & Thal, 1992). Still, the presence of psychosis should be carefully assessed, as it is directly related to elements of independence and self-care. In a Chinese study examining the relationship between noncognitive symptoms of dementia and functional impairment in AD, the presence of hallucinations was an independent predictor of activities of daily living and instrumental activities of daily living (Mok, Chu, Chung, Chan, & Hui, 2004). Oliveria and colleagues (2006) examined adverse events in a nursing home among participants with dementia with psychosis. Of these participants who suffered from dementia with psychosis, 90% had another cormorbid psychiatric disorder not otherwise specified by researchers. Among these nursing home patients who had AD with psychosis, the most common adverse outcomes occurring within a 2-year follow-up period included accidental injury, death, pain, infection, anorexia, and weight fluctuation (Oliveria et al., 2006). A limitation of this study is the lack of a control group of patients that had dementia without psychosis.

Another comorbid condition to be aware of when assessing an individual's level of independence is chronic pain. An estimated 50% of individuals with dementia who are living in the community suffer from chronic pain (Shega et al., 2007). Patients with dementia who have chronic pain are more likely to be depressed and may manifest discomfort due to pain through behaviors such as agitation, disruptive behavior, and social withdrawal. Chronic pain may also influence neurocognitive functioning and increase the likelihood of physical disability and impairment in ADLs (Shega et al., 2007; Snow et al., 2009). There is also evidence that persistent pain is poorly treated in nursing home residents (Won et al., 2004).

The literature on various neurocognitive conditions and independence highlights the importance of the individual's interpretation of his or her situation. In a study examining cognitive impairment in elderly participants with epilepsy, perceived cognitive impairment was a better predictor of poor psychosocial adjustment than objective cognitive impairment (Baker, Taylor, & Hermann, 2009). These participants had difficulty getting around familiar places, difficulty remembering names of familiar people, difficulty learning how to do something new, and were lethargic and sluggish. Similarly, in a sample of patients with multiple sclerosis (MS), perceived depression and fatigue were linked to level of disability and difficulty completing ADLs such as cooking, transportation, cleaning, and shopping, regardless of the degree of cognitive impairment (Johansson et al., 2007).

Another key issue is the living arrangement of the patient. Approximately 20–30% of individuals with dementia who live in the community live alone. Not only do dementia patients who live alone underestimate the severity of their neurocognitive deficits and minimize the impact of these deficits on ADLs, but a recent study found that knowledgeable informants and physicians also underestimate their deficits (Lehmann, Black, Shore, Kasper, & Rabins, 2010). Many neuropsychologists and other healthcare professionals rely heavily on informant reports in both interview format and standardized measures when determining an individual's level of independence. Therefore it is important to specifically assess the involvement of family members and other informants when gathering information and making decisions regarding patient care.

GUIDELINES AND SUGGESTIONS FOR EVALUATION OF PERSONAL CARE AND INDEPENDENCE

Assessing independence and personal care capacities can be challenging for neuropsychologists, especially when one considers the value placed on the ability to remain independent and care for one's self. The choice of assessment instruments or procedures may be overwhelming due to the lack of consensus among clinicians and the lack of empirical support for measures of independence and self-care (Haywood, Garratt, & Fitzpatrick, 2005). It is also challenging to assess these capacities given the amount of information a neuropsychologist must synthesize. From the paragraphs above, the examination of personal care must include data from a variety of sources including neurocognitive testing, self-report and collateral informants, and,wherever possible, direct assessment. The assessment of capacity for personal care will also involve chart review, and on many occasions, assistance from other disciplines that may be in a better position to assess directly personal care [e.g., physical therapy (PT) and occupational therapy (OT)].

To assist with the assessment process, a three-part framework was proposed by the American Bar Association and the American Psychological Association for the functional elements associated with independent living (American Bar Association Commission on Law and Aging & American Psychological Association, 2008). This framework consists of requiring an individual to exhibit an *understanding* of the requirements for living independently, a functional *application* of this understanding, and problem-solving abilities with an appreciation of the consequences of potential choices, also known as *judgment*. Although this framework was created for the evaluation of a multitude of functions associated with independent living, it can be readily applied to the specific aspects of self-care including grooming, dressing, and bathing. Approaching the assessment in this manner assists with the conceptualization and the evaluation of the ways in which cognitive factors, maladaptive behaviors, and physical deficits may interfere with independence and personal care capabilities. The following sections offer information about psychological and neuropsychological tools that can help a clinician complete such an assessment.

Understanding. The first task for the clinician within this framework is to assess a patient's understanding of the requirements for living independently and, in particular, self-care. During the clinical interview it is important to ask the patient about daily requirements of taking care of the home and self. Regardless of the individual's circumstances, it is vital to assess that he or she understands the significance of personal hygiene, cleanliness in the home, safety, health and diet, and the consequences of not being able to fulfill these obligations. In other words, does the individual have insight into the necessities of independent living and personal care? Interviewing a reliable informant can also provide crucial information regarding a patient's insight. This will allow the clinician to gauge the individual's insight into his or her own abilities or deficits and how they relate to independence and self-care capacities.

The clinician can begin forming hypotheses about a patient's functioning and capacity from the interview and then choose assessments that will appropriately test these hypotheses. Many factors must be considered when choosing these assessments. For example, the appropriateness of a self-report versus a "proxy"-based measure must be considered; both of these types of assessment have limitations, as previously discussed. Declining cognitive function or lack of insight may influence the validity of a self-report measure, while having a caregiver perform the ratings could also provide questionable information if, among other things, the caregiver does not spend much time with the patient.

Application. If the patient does indeed seem to demonstrate good understanding, the focus of assessment then becomes one of application (American Bar Association Commission on Law and Aging & American Psychological Association, 2008). For example, can the individual maintain personal hygiene and perform daily and weekly chores to maintain cleanliness in the home and to eat the right kinds of food to maintain health? Physical and cognitive impairments may limit the ability to perform these types of tasks, in which case an assessment of problem-solving abilities is important. For example, if the patient can no longer write checks to fulfill financial obligations due to a limitation in visual acuity, will the individual accept help from a trusted loved one to do so? In this case, it becomes important to assess the patient's ability to communicate with others as they will need to do so in order to give directions. It is also essential to assess the individual's ability to perform ADLs including toileting and mobility, for example, as difficulties with these could lead to overall loss of self-esteem and could exacerbate the effects of any other disability. The assessment of basic ADLs can be performed via the use of previously described instruments. Likewise, as discussed, performance of basic ADLs may be assessed via direct observation or through information obtained from the assessments completed by other disciplines (i.e., home safety evaluations performed by OT or PT).

Judgment. In some cases, an individual will demonstrate good understanding and application of the requirements needed for independent living and personal care, but will exercise poor judgment in carrying out these abilities. A psychological or cognitive disorder could be hindering an individual's ability to use good judgment in order to consistently fulfill obligations, avoid high-risk behavior, and respond appropriately in emergency situations. Indeed, a variety of conditions (e.g., stroke, depression, dementia) may contribute to poor judgment and ultimately self-neglect (Naik, Teal, Pavlik, Dyer, & McCullough, 2008). For these reasons, the evaluation of medical records for diagnoses that could hinder good judgment and consulting with the individual's physicians for any suspected diagnoses are imperative. In the case of an individual exhibiting cognitive deficits or poor insight, assessing the extent to which these deficits hinder the individual from carrying out necessary tasks to live independently is just as important as identifying the deficit itself. In fact, one of the main goals of performing a cognitive assessment, as it relates to assessing the capacities of independent living and personal care, is to find ways that the patient can use his or her strengths or make adjustments in the environment to overcome any observed cognitive deficits. Thus, a comprehensive evaluation of neurocognitive function is an important and integral part of the evaluation of capacity for personal care.

Within the neuropsychological report, the examiner may elect to highlight the degree to which the patient demonstrates understanding, application abilities, and judgment with regard to the elements associated with personal care. Synthesis of data from the neurocognitive examination, self-report and informants, and direct observation should provide the information needed to make concise statements about each of the three aspects (i.e., understanding, application, and judgment) previously described. Provision of these statements (with quantitative data included where appropriate) will enable the examiner or other healthcare professionals to track change over time.

CASE STUDY

The following abbreviated case study highlights the importance of the use of a variety of resources for the examination of a patient's ability to perform self-care, and how the model for assessment proposed by the American Bar Association Commission on Law and Aging & American Psychological Association (2008) may be utilized to assist with the determination of capacity within this domain. This case is not meant to be comprehensive. Rather, it is offered to address the specific question of capacity for self-care. It is acknowledged that other issues exist with regard to this case, such as performance of IADLs. However, the primary focus is on personal care.

Mr. JH is an 84-year-old right-handed white male with a history of reported memory decline. He was initially referred for a neuropsychological examination to assist with diagnostic clarity and to make recommendations concerning independent living. Six months prior to the evaluation he was placed in an assisted living facility following a broken left leg. At some point during hospitalization and placement, he was diagnosed with probable AD. However, no information regarding how the diagnosis was reached was evident from a review of the medical chart and a neuropsychological examination had not been completed. Mr. H recovered from his physical problems to the extent that there was no noted physical barrier to living independently, and he no longer required physical care. As a result, he expressed a desire to return to his home and live independently. However, his son, who already had guardianship and control of his finances, disagreed with this, given the diagnosis of AD. As a result of this disagreement, Mr. H retained an attorney for legal assistance. It is within the context of the patient's desire to return home that this evaluation was requested.

His medical history was remarkable for bypass surgery in 1980. He previously underwent three hernia repair surgeries, all of which occurred 15 years ago. There is no previous psychiatric history. At the time of this examination his medications included Namenda, Cardizem, Nexium, Lasix, aspirin, and Plavix. Magnetic resonance imaging (MRI) of the brain was unremarkable, as were clinical laboratory studies. An EEG was within normal limits. Mr. H completed the ninth grade. He previously served in the military. He was widowed in 2003. He has one son and four grandchildren.

Examination Findings: *Mr. H was transported to the examiner's office by his son, which is noteworthy given the legal tension between the two. Yet the relationship between Mr. H and his son remained amicable despite the disagreement about independent living. Lawton and Brody's (1969) Instrumental Activities of Daily Living (IADL) and Physical Self-Maintenance (PMS) scales were completed by his son. According to Mr. H's son, he required some assistance with traveling, shopping, preparing meals, housework, and taking medication. He also required assistance with the management of money. He also indicated that he does not think his father can make reasoned decisions. Regarding physical self-maintenance, there were no concerns with regard to personal care such as toileting, feeding, dressing, grooming, ambulation, or bathing (as indicated on the PMS). His son stated that memory problems have been evident for about 18 months, and that there is possibly a slow decline.*

Also with the patient's written consent, a telephone interview was conducted with a physical therapist who had worked closely with Mr. H during his hospitalization and placement within assisted living. This physical therapist recently performed a "home safety" direct assessment that consisted of an examination of this patient's ability to perform basic ADLs. Mr. H was capable of performing all of the basic ADLs independently. In contrast, the physical therapist indicated that there was concern about Mr. H's ability to perform IADLs, such as handling money, food preparation, and remembering to take medications. The physical therapist also stated that Mr. H had a tendency to repeat questions and, in general, appeared forgetful of some conversations. On some occasions, he required prompts and reminders to perform basic ADLS, though he was capable of completing them without additional prompts.

On examination, Mr. H was appropriately dressed. Grooming and hygiene were intact. He was alert and oriented to person, place, and time. He admitted to sadness associated with his current living arrangements. However, he denied suicidal or homicidal ideation. His mood and affect were mildly depressed. His thought processes were goal directed. He correctly named the current president and his predecessor. He was vaguely familiar with current events. His interpretation of a familiar proverb was appropriately abstract. He made errors on serial subtractions of 7s from 100. Immediate recall of three words was 3/3 as well as brief delayed recall.

During the clinical interview he denied the presence of memory disorder and he stated that he was capable of living by himself. In essence, he denied having any difficulties with ADLs including instrumental and basic. When asked direct questions about independent living, he was capable of a discussion about the importance of self-care (and associated steps) as well as IADLs. To this extent, he understood the importance of these activities. He was no longer driving and had no desire to do so.

Neuropsychological testing was completed over the course of two sessions. Mr. H was compliant with testing procedures. On some occasions he displayed difficulty understanding instructions. Repeated attempts to explain them were of little utility. He sometimes demonstrated that he understood the instructions but then later became confused on the task. This was particularly evident on tests that required high cognitive load or cognitive flexibility such as the Stroop Neuropsychological Screening Test. Test scores are detailed in Table 7.1.

On neuropsychological testing there is evidence of impairment across multiple cognitive domains (see Table 7.1). Overall, the profile is consistent with progressive cortical disease, including impairment on measures of fluency, spatial processing, new learning and memory, and executive functioning. Accelerated forgetting and poor recognition memory were also prominent features. Mr. H also completed an abbreviated version of the Geriatric Depression Scale. His score on this measure was 6/15, which falls within the depressed range. He endorsed feeling helpless, and having fears about what would happen to him.

Summary and Impressions. *This was an 84-year-old white male with a history of reported progressive cognitive decline. He was referred for a neuropsychological examination to assist with diagnostic clarity and to make recommendations regarding the capacity for independent living. Given the information obtained from chart review, clinical interview, and psychometric testing, the diagnostic impressions were as follows: (1) Probable dementia of the Alzheimer's type. (2) Depressive disorder NOS.*

All reversible causes of dementia were excluded and the most likely diagnosis was dementia of the Alzheimer's type, particularly given the salient impairment on memory measures. Within this domain, there was accelerated forgetting and impaired recognition memory. However, he was also impaired on measures of executive function, language, and spatial processing. Information provided by his son, as well as his physical therapist, was consistent with the findings from neuropsychological testing in that there is a history of forgetfulness. Likewise, Mr. H's son and his physical therapist reported a decline in IADLs. In contrast, there was no noted decline in Mr. H's ability to perform basic ADLs, though at times he required prompts to initiate the behaviors associated with self-care.

Table 7.1 NEUROPSYCHOLOGICAL TEST RESULTS

Test	Score	Percentile
General Function		
North American Adult Reading Test	85	16
Wechsler Adult Intelligence Scale-III (WAIS—III)		
Picture Completion	8	25
Digit Symbol Coding	2	<1
Similarities	7	16
Arithmetic	5	5
Matrix Reasoning	6	9
Digit Span	7	16
Information	7	16
Verbal IQ Estimate	80	9
Performance IQ Estimate	75	5
Full Scale IQ Estimate	76	5
Fine Motor Control		
Grooved Pegboard		
Dominant Hand	174″	<2
Nondominant Hand	159″	10
Language		
Dean-Kaplan Executive Function System (D-KEFS)	2	<1
Letter Fluency		
Semantic Fluency (Animals)	10	<1
Boston Naming Test (15 Items Short Form)	11/15	25
Spatial Processing		
Clock Drawing	14/20	
Rey-Osterrieth Complex Figure	13/36	<1
New Learning and Memory		
Hopkins Verbal Learning Test—Revised		
Trial 1	3/12	
Trial 2	6/12	
Trial 3	6/12	
Total Recall	15/36	5
20 Minute Delayed Recall	0/12	<1
Recognition	7, 3fp	<1
Wechsler Memory Scale—III		
Logical Memory I	4	2
Logical Memory II	7	16
Brief Visuospatial Memory Test—Revised		
Trial 1	2/12	10
Trial 2	2/12	1
Trial 3	2/12	<1
20 Minute Delayed Recall	0/12	<1
Recognition	4, 2fp	3–5
Test of Memory Malingering Trial 1	46/50	
Test of Memory Malingering Trial 2	49/50	

(Continued)

Table 7.1 NEUROPSYCHOLOGICAL TEST RESULTS (CONT'D)

Test	Score	Percentile
Attention and Executive Function		
Brief Test of Attention	12/20	25–74
Trailmaking Test		
Part A	168″	2
Part B	Discontinued	
Stroop Neuropsychological Screening Test	33	<1
Mood and Affect		
Geriatric Depression Scale—Short Form	6/15	
Basic ADLS and IADLS		
Instrumental ADLs (IADLS)	4/8	
Physical Self-Maintenance (PSMS)	6/6	

Understanding, Application, and Judgment: *During the clinical interview, Mr. H was capable of discussing the relevant aspects of IADLs and basic ADLs and thus he currently has* understanding *of the importance of these elements to independent living. With regard to the application of these skills, his son and physical therapist indicated concerns about money management. His son provided some instances of forgetfulness and possible poor use of funds. In contrast, Mr. H's son and physical therapist indicated no concerns with his ability to perform personal care. His physical therapist performed a direct assessment of this functional domain and Mr. H was readily capable of completing these tasks. To this extent, although there were concerns about his ability to perform IADLs, there was no evidence to support impaired performance of basic ADLs (*application*). Mr. H denied cognitive impairment and denied any functional decline, yet neurocognitive testing and reports from his son and physical therapist suggest that there is cognitive decline. Likewise, his physical therapist indicated that he sometimes required prompting to initiate basic ADLs, though he was readily capable of completing these activities without additional assistance. To this extent, Mr. H lacked full insight into his cognitive and functional decline, and may have diminished* judgment *when performing these functions.*

Recommendations: *The results from this examination indicated cognitive impairment, functional decline with regard to IADLs, and possibly some difficulty initiating personal care. There was also diminished insight with regard to his cognitive deficit and functional decline. A return to his home would require assistance and supervision to ensure his safety and to ensure that he is not taken advantage of. Supervision would be most important with regard to IADLs. In contrast, he would require only minimal prompting for performance of basic ADLs, as he readily demonstrated an understanding and application of these skills.*

Case Outcome: *The testing results, diagnostic impressions, and recommendations were shared with Mr. H. After providing feedback, Mr. H continued to deny cognitive or functional impairment. However, he was readily agreeable to hiring a personal assistant who could provide the necessary supervision within the home (he had the financial means to do so), if it would allow him to return. He indicated that he felt as if he were being held hostage in the assisted living facility, and he thought that the depressed mood would improve if he were to return to his home. Ultimately, with the assistance of his attorney, the courts decided that Mr. H could return to his home provided that he had supervision. Likewise, Mr. H and his son were able to come to an agreement about the hiring of a personal assistant, rather than having Mr. H's son serve as a primary caregiver. To this extent, their relationship also improved. The decision to allow Mr. H. to return to his home was based on the fact that he could complete basic ADLs independently including toileting, feeding, dressing, grooming, and bathing, and that he did not require any physical assistance. Thus, there was little risk for self-neglect or difficulty in self-care. In contrast, he required assistance with money management and other IADLs. The personal assistant was hired to ensure that IADLs were managed and that he was not taken advantage of. This was a good solution because Mr. H. did not want his son to manage his affairs. Likewise, it was anticipated that he would continue to decline cognitively (and well as his ability to perform self-care skills independently), and the personal assistant could assist with monitoring his future status.*

SUMMARY AND FUTURE DIRECTIONS

As reviewed above, there is no single technique or tool available for the evaluation of personal care. In general, the use of global and specific neurocognitive tests for the evaluation of personal care may not yield useful data, particularly given the fact that most individuals within the beginning phases of decline do not exhibit discernible personal care deficits. However, there is promising research (Fields et al., 2010) that provides some corresponding cutoff scores for the DRS and the MMSE that may be helpful in tracking patient decline within this modality. Likewise, some models suggest that a decline in nonverbal skills is more associated with functional decline (Perry & Hodges, 2000). Further investigation of these models, as they pertain to functional decline, will likely assist the examiner in reaching conclusions with regard to capacity for personal care and independence. For now, it is important to note that spatial deficits noted on the neuropsychological examination appear more predictive of decline in basic ADLs than verbal deficits.

A plethora of self-report and informant rating scales that are specific to functional decline in basic ADLs exist. The examiner should use caution when incorporating these instruments, as it is well known that patients often overestimate their ability to perform these activities and caregiver ratings provide only modest correlations with direct assessment techniques. In addition, the time required to complete these measures should be taken into account, as some instruments require lengthy instruction and investment from the clinician. Direct assessment techniques may provide useful information within the context of the evaluation of personal care, as these procedures require patients to perform the exact duties that are being evaluated (grooming, dressing, etc.). For a variety of reasons, direct assessment or observation may not be practical or appropriate during the neuropsychological evaluation. Likewise, the ecological validity of this type of assessment has been criticized, as the site or place of the evaluation may be out of the context in which the patient would normally perform these duties (i.e., not in the patient's home). From other disciplines, there is a trend toward providing reliable and valid instruments that screen for capacity for self-care, some of which are similar to direct assessment. For instance Naik et al. (2008) provide the methodological steps for validating a screening tool that provides an assessment of basic cognitive abilities, decisional capacity, and executive capacity. This three-step model uses case scenarios and requires patients to articulate how they would perform certain activities that are associated with safety and independent living. Although the individual elements of this concept are not necessarily novel, the validation of a device that incorporates all elements could eventually serve as a useful initial screener that could provide information about the need for more in-depth assessment.

Within the context of the evaluation, it is important to consider a multitude of factors that could influence functional decline. For example, sometimes the examiner must determine whether physical decline (rather than cognitive) accounts for the loss of ability to perform personal care; this determination is important for the diagnosis. Likewise, the functional decline may be static or progressive. Instead, a multitude of factors such as depression and psychosis may variably influence functional capacity, and improved capacity may be observed as depression and psychosis abate. To date there is little research that examines the extent to which physical, psychological, and cognitive deficits interact to produce a decline in personal care.

The use of the American Bar Association Commission on Law and Aging & American Psychological Association (2008) model consisting of *understanding, application*, and *judgment* may provide some utility with regard to the conceptualization of a patient's capacity for personal care. From the case study reviewed above, it was evident that the patient demonstrated an understanding of and the ability to apply knowledge to personal care requirements. However, he sometimes lacked judgment (i.e., forgetfulness and executive function deficits) in doing so and as such required prompts. Although this case study demonstrates the potential application of this model, to date there is limited research on how this proposed model may facilitate reaching decisions concerning supervision or placements for patients who may suffer from deficits in self-care.

References

American Bar Association Commission on Law and Aging & American Psychological Association. (2008). *Assessment of older adults with diminished capacity: A handbook for psychologists.* Washington, D.C.: Author.

Americans with Disabilities Act of 1990, Pub. L. No. 101–336, § 2, 104 Stat. 328 (1991).

Andersen, C. K., Wittrup-Jensen, K. U., Lolk, A., Andersen, K., & Kragh-Sorensen, P. (2004). Ability to perform activities of daily living is the main factor affecting quality of life in patients with dementia. *Health and Quality of Life Outcomes, 2*, 52.

Angel, R. J., & Frisco, M. L. (2001). Self-assessments of health and functional capacity among older adults. *Journal of Mental Health and Aging, 7*, 119–135.

Baker, G. A., Taylor, J., & Hermann, B. (2009). How can cognitive status predispose to psychological impairment? *Epilepsy & Behavior, 15*, S31–S35.

Baum, C., Edwards, D., Yonan, C., & Storandt, M. (1996). The relation of neuropsychological test performance to performance of functional tasks in dementia of the Alzheimer's type. *Archives of Clinical Neuropsychology, 11*, 69–75.

Burns, T., Mortimer, J. A., & Merchak, P. (1994). Cognitive performance test: A new approach to functional assessment in Alzheimer's disease. *Journal of Geriatric Psychiatry and Neurology, 6*, 46–54.

Bylsma, F. W., Folstein, M. F., Devanand, D. P., Richards, M., Bello, J., Albert, M., & Stern, Y. (1994). Delusions and patterns of cognitive impairment in Alzheimer's disease. *Neuropsychiatry Neuropsychology and Behavioral Neurology, 7*, 98–103.

Cahn-Weiner, D. A., Farias, S. T., Julian, L., Harvey, D. J., Kramer, J. H., Reed, B. R., & Chui, H. (2007). Cognitive and neuroimaging predictors of instrumental activities of daily living. *Journal of the International Neuropsychological Society, 13*, 747–757.

Cahn-Weiner, D. A., Malloy, P. F., Boyle, P. A., Marran, M. E., & Salloway, S. (2000). Prediction of functional status from neuropsychological tests in community-dwelling elderly individuals. *The Clinical Neuropsychologist, 14*, 187–195.

Castilla-Puentes, R. C., & Habeych, M. E. (2010). Subtypes of depression among patients with Alzheimer's disease and other dementias. *Alzheimers & Dementia, 6*, 63–69.

Cipher, D. J., & Clifford, P. A. (2004). Dementia, pain, depression, behavioral disturbances, and ADLs: Toward a comprehensive conceptualization of quality of life in long-term care. *International Journal of Geriatric Psychology, 19*, 741–748.

Chaytor, N., & Schmitter-Edgecombe, M. (2003). The ecological validity of neuropsychological tests: A review of the literature on everyday cognitive skills. *Neuropsychology Review, 13*, 181–197.

Chemerinski, E., Robinson, R. G., & Kosier, J. T. (2001). Improved recovery in activities of daily living associated with remission of poststroke depression. *Stroke, 32*, 113–117.

Collins, C., Wade, D., Davies, S., & Horne, V. (1988). The Barthel ADL Index: A reliability study. *International Disability Studies, 10*, 61–63.

Fields, J. A., Machulda, M., Aakre, J., Ivnik, R. J., Boeve, B. F., Knopman, D. S., Petersen, R. C., & Smith, G. E. (2010). Utility of the DRS for predicting problems in day-to-day functioning. *The Clinical Neuropsychologist, 24*, 1167–1180.

Fitz, A. G., & Teri, L. (1994). Depression, cognition, and functional ability in patietns with Alzheimer's disease. *Journal of the American Geriatrics Society, 42*, 186–191.

Folstein, M., Folestein, S., & McHugh, P. (1975). Mini-mental state: A practical guide for grading the cognitive state of the patient for the physician. *Journal of Psychiatry Research, 12*, 189–198.

Galasko, D., Bennett, D. A., Sano, M., Marson, D., Kaye, J., & Edland, S. D. (2006). ADCS prevention instrument project: Assessment of Instrumental Activities of Daily Living for community-dwelling elderly individuals in dementia prevention clinical trials. *Alzheimers Disease and Associated Disorders, 20*, S152–S169.

Goode, K. T., Haley, W. E., Roth, D. L., & Ford, G. R. (1998). Predicting longitudinal change in caregiver physical and mental health: A stress process model. *Health Psychology, 17*, 190–198.

Gosman-Hedstrom, G., & Svensson, E. (2000). Parallel reliability of the Functional Independence Measure and the Barthel ADL Index. *Disability and Rehabilitation, 22*, 702–715.

Granger C. V., Albrecht G. L., & Hamilton B. B. (1979). Outcome of comprehensive medical rehabilitation; measurement by PULSES Profile and the Barthel Index. *Archives of Physical Medicine and Rehabilitation, 60*, 145–154.

Hartigan, I. (2007). A comparative review of the Katz ADL and the Barthel Index in assessing the activities of daily living in older people. *International Journal of Older People Nursing, 2*, 204–212.

Haywood, K. L., Garratt, A. M., & Fitzpatrick, R. (2005). Older people specific health status and quality of life: A structured review of self-assessed instruments. *Journal of Evaluation in Clinical Practice, 11*, 315–327.

Hokoishi, K., Ikeda, M., Maki, N., Torikawa, S., Nomura, M., Fujimoto, N., Fukuhara, R., Komori, K., & Tanabe, H. (2001). Scale and the Instrumental Activities of Daily Living Scale in a variety of health professional representatives. *Aging & Mental Health, 5*, 38–40.

Jaggor, C., Arthur, A. J., Spiers, N. A., & Clarke, M. (2001). Patterns of onset of disability in activities of daily living with age. *Journal of the American Geriatrics Society, 49*, 404–409.

Jeste, D. V., Wragg, R. E., Salmon, D. P., Harris, M. J., & Thal, L. J. (1992). Cognitive deficits of patients with Alzheimer's disease with and without delusions. *American Journal of Psychiatry, 149*, 184–189.

Johansson, S., Ytterberg, C., Claesson, I. M., Lindberg, J., Hillert, J., Andersson, M., & von Koch, L. (2007). High concurrent presence of disability in multiple sclerosis. Associations with perceived health. *Journal of Neurology, 254*, 767–773.

Jorm, A. (1986). Controlled and automatic information processing in senile dementia: A review. *Psychological Medicine, 16*, 17–88.

Katz, S., Ford, A. B., Moskowitz, R. W., Jackson, B. A., & Jaffe, M. W. (1963). Studies of illness in the aged. The Index of ADL: A standardized measure of biological and psychosocial function. *Journal of the American Medical Association, 185*, 914–919.

Katon, W. J., Lin, E. H. B., Williams, L.H., Ciechanowski, P., Heckbert, S. R., Ludman, E., Rutter, C., Crane, P. K., Oliver, M., & Von Korff, M. (2010). Comorbid depression is associated with an increased risk of dementia diagnosis in patients with diabetes: A prospective cohort study. *Journal of General Internal Medicine, 25*, 423–429.

Kerby, D. S., Wentworth, R., & Cotton, P. C. (1989). Measuring adaptive behavior in elderly developmentally disabled clients. *Journal of Applied Gerontology, 8*, 261–267.

Lawton, M. P., & Brody, M. P. (1969). Assessment of older people: Self-maintaining and Instrumental Activities of Daily Living. *Gerontologist, 9*, 179–186.

Leckey, G. S., & Beatty, W. W. (2002). Predicting functional performance by patients with Alzheimer's disease using the problems in everyday living (PEDL) test: A preliminary study. *Journal of the International Neuropsychological Society, 8*, 48–57.

Lehmann, S. W., Black, B. S., Shore, A., Kasper, J., & Rabins, P. V. (2010). Living alone with dementia: Lack of awareness adds to functional and cognitive vulnerabilities. *International Psychogeriatrics, 22*, 778–784.

Loewenstein, D. A., Amigo, E., Duara, R., Guterman, A., Hurwitz, D., Berkowitz, N., & Eisdorfer, C. (1989). A new scale for the assessment of functional status in Alzheimer's disease and related disorders. *Journal of Gerontology: Psychological Sciences, 44,* 114–121.

Loewenstein, D. A., & Mogosky, B. J. (1999). The functional assessment of the older adult patient. In P. A. Lichtenberg (Ed.), *Handbook of assessment in clinical gerontology* (pp. 529–554). New York: Wiley.

Mahoney, F., & Barthel, D. (1965). Functional evaluation: The Barthel Index. *Maryland State Medical Journal, 12,* 61–65.

Marson, D., & Hebert, K. R. (2006). Functional assessment. In D. K. Attix & K. A. Welsh-Bohmer (Eds.), *Geriatric neuropsychology* (pp. 158–197). New York: Guilford Press.

Mattis, S. (1988). *Dementia Rating Scale.* Odessa, FL: Psychological Assessment Resources.

McDowell, I. (2006). *Measuring health: A guide to rating scales and questionnaires, Third Edition.* New York: Oxford University Press.

Mok, W. Y. W., Chu, L. W., Chung, C. P., Chan, N. Y., & Hui, S. L. (2004). The relationship between non-cognitive symptoms and functional impairment in Alzheimer's disease. *International Journal of Geriatric Psychiatry, 19,* 1040–1046.

Mortimer, J. A., Ebbitt, B., Jun, S. P., & Finch, M. D. (1992). Predictors of cognitive and functional progression in patients with probable Alzheimer's disease. *Neurology, 42,* 1689–1696.

Nadler, J. D., Richardson, E. D., Malloy, P. F., Marran, M. E., & Hostetler-Brinson, M. E. (1993). The ability of the Dementia Rating Scale to predict everyday functioning. *Archives of Clinical Neuropsychology, 8,* 449–460.

Naik, A. D., Teal, C. R., Pavlik, V. N., Dyer, C. B., & McCullough, L. B. (2008). Conceptual challenges and practical approaches to screening capacity for self-care and protection in vulnerable older adults. *Journal of the American Gerontological Society, 56,* S266–S270.

N.C. Gen. Stats ch. 35AN.C. Gen. Stats ch. 35A (2001), § 111.

Oliveria, S. A., Liperoti, R., L'Italien, G., Pugner, K., Safferman, A., Carson, W., & Lapane, K. (2006). Adverse events among nursing home residents with Alzheimer's disease and psychosis. *Pharmacoepidemiology and Drug Safety, 15,* 763–774.

Olmstead V. L. C. (98–536) 527 U.S. 581 (1999) 138 F.3d 893.

Ownby, R. L., Harwood, D. G., Acevedo, A., Barker, W., & Duara, R. (2001). Factor structure of the Cornell Scale for Depression in Dementia for Anglo and Hispanic patients with dementia. *American Journal of Geriatric Psychiatry, 9,* 217–224.

Patterson, M. B., Mack, J. L., Neundorfer, M. M., Martin, R. J., Smyth, K. A., & Whitehouse, P. J. (1992). Assessment of functional ability in Alzheimer disease: A review and a preliminary report on the Cleveland scale for activities of daily living. *Alzheimer Disease and Associated Disorders, 6,* 145–163.

Perry, R. J., & Hodges, J. R. (2000). Relationship between functional and neuropsychological performance in early Alzheimer's disease. *Alzheimer Disease and Associated Disorders, 14,* 1–10.

Ranhoff, A. H., & Laake, K. (1993). The Barthel ADL Index: Scoring by the physician from patient interview is not reliable. *Age and Ageing, 22,* 171–174.

Rodgers, J. C., Holm, M. B., & Stone, R. G. (1997). Evaluation of daily living tasks: The home care advantage. *American Journal of Occupational Therapy, 51,* 410–422.

Rovner, B. W., Broadhead, J., Spencer, M., Carson, K., & Folstein, M. F. (1989). Depression and Alzheimer's disease. *American Journal of Psychiatry, 146*, 350–353.

Sarazin, M., Stern, Y., Berr, C., Riba, A., Albert, A., Brandt, J., & Dubois, B. (2005). Neuropsychological predictors of dependency in patients with Alzheimer's disease. *Neurology, 64*, 1027–1031.

Schinka, J. A. (2010). Use of informants to identify mild cognitive impairment in older adults. *Current Psychiatry Reports, 12*, 4–12.

Shega, J., Emanuel, L., Vargish, L., Levine, S. K., Bursch, H., Herr, K., & Weiner, D. K. (2007). Pain in persons with dementia: Complex, common, and challenging. *Journal of Pain, 8*, 373–378.

Snow, A. L., Chandler, J. F., Kunik, M. E., Davila, J. A., Balasubramanyam, V., Steele, A. B., & Morgan, R. O. (2009). Self-reported pain in persons with dementia predicts subsequent decreased psychosocial functioning. *American Journal of Geriatric Psychiatry, 17*, 873–880.

Spirrison, C. L., & Pierce, P. S. (1992). Psychometric characteristics of the Adult Functional and Adaptive Behavior Scale (AFABS). *The Gerontologist, 32*, 234–239.

Strauss, E., Sherman, E. M. S., & Spreen, O. (2006). *A compendium of neuropsychological tests, third edition*. New York: Oxford University Press.

Teri, L., & Wagner, A. W. (1991). Assessment of depression in patients with Alzheimer's disease-concordance among informants. *Psychology and Aging, 6*, 280–285.

Thomas, P., Thomas, C. H., Billon, R., Peix, R., Faugeron, P., & Clement, J. P. (2009). Depression and frontal dysfunction: Risks for the elderly? *Encephale-Revue de Psychiatrie Clinique Biologique et Therapeutique, 35*, 361–369.

Tornquist, K., Lovgren, M., & Soderfeld, B. (1990). Sensitivity, specificity, and predictive value in Katz's and Barthel's ADL indices applied on patients in long term nursing care. *Scandinavian Journal of Caring Sciences, 4*, 99–105.

U.N. General Assembly, Convention on the Rights of Persons with Disabilities. G.A. res. U.N. Doc A/RES/61/106 (2006).

U.N. General Assembly, Universal Declaration of Human Rights. G.A. res. 217A (III), U.N. Doc A/810 at 71 (1948).

Uniform Guardianship and Protective Proceedings Act § 102(5) (1997).

Warrington, E. K., & James, M. (1991). *The Visual Object and Space Perception Battery*. Bury St. Edmunds, UK: Thames Valley Test Company.

Weintraub, S. (1986). The Record of Independent Living: An informant-completed measure of activities of daily living and behavior in elderly patients with cognitive impairment. *American Journal of Alzheimer Care and Related Disorders, 7*, 35–39.

Wolinsky, S. L., Callahan, C., Fitzgerald, J., & Johnson, R. (1993). Changes in functional status and the risks of subsequent nursing home placement and death. *Journal of Gerontology: Social Sciences, 48*, S93–S101.

Won, A. B., Lapane, K. L., Vallow, S., Schein, J., Morris, J. N., & Lipsitz, L. A. (2004). Persistent nonmalignant pain and analgesic prescribing patterns in elderly nursing home residents. *Journal of the American Geriatrics Society, 52*, 867–874.

Wuwongse, S., Chang, R. C. C., & Law, A. C. K. (2010). The putative neurodegenerative links between depression and Alzheimer's disease. *Progress in Neurobiology, 91*, 362–375.

Wylie, C. M., & White, B. K. (1964). A measure of disability. *Archives of Environment Health, 8*, 834–839.

8

Adult Guardianship

GEORGE J. DEMAKIS

INTRODUCTION

An Associated Press (Bayles & McCartney, 1987) series about guardianship in the United States found that a Vermont woman learned that she had a guardian only when told by her nursing home that she could no longer spend money without the permission of her guardian-daughter. A Florida woman learned that she had a guardian only when she was turned away at the polling booth, whereas a court in Montana had no record of what happened to the $131,000 estate of a 92-year-old man found ill and alone in his cabin after a couple—described as friends—had been assigned guardians. The cases demonstrated the failings of our guardianship system, as well as the continuing challenges facing the judicial system's responsibility to adjudicate whether an adult is competent and, if not competent, to subsequently determine and monitor guardianship. A host of legal and psychological issues are raised: How should incompetency be determined and are current statutory definitions acceptable? What is the role of psychological experts in aiding the court in such determinations? If psychologists are used, what sort of data should they provide to the court? Who should represent the respondent (i.e., the person alleged to be incompetent) and should they testify at their incompetency hearing? In terms of guardianship, who makes the best guardian and how should psychological (and other) data inform such choices? Should the courts monitor guardians and, if so, how should they do this?

In this chapter I address these and other questions relevant for the psychologist working with guardianship issues. As described in detail below, guardianship is determined only after the court has adjudicated an individual incompetent. Competency or capacity issues are, in fact, the focus of this volume and there are chapters on testamentary, financial, healthcare, driving, and personal care capacity. In my view, clinical psychologists are uniquely suited to assist the court with both competency and guardianship issues because of their broad training in psychopathology, psychological assessment, family systems and dynamics, as well as psychological treatment. Clinical neuropsychologists bring particular expertise to cases in which cognitive difficulties, most likely due to neurological dysfunction or disease, are present. In any case, guardianship issues may be more challenging and complex than competency. For example, in contested cases, there is typically significant family conflict and the family system is likely to be at its most chaotic and vulnerable. Interviewing the various family members, seeking compromises where appropriate, and working with the family and court to craft a workable guardianship plan require considerable clinical skill and sensitivity. As will be discussed later in this chapter, state statutes tend to be much less detailed about guardianship than competency; the relative lack of legal or statutory guidance on this issue is challenging for the clinician. In comparison, competency is typically well specified in state statute. Finally, unlike most competency evaluations, guardianship may be continually monitored and evaluated by the court to ensure that the ward is being properly cared for. In some states, the guardian submits a yearly report of the ward's status and updates on the estate (if that is part of the guardianship plan). Guardianship may also change due to the death or incapacity of a guardian or failure to perform adequately in that role. Although competency issues may be revisited (see below), these are probably less likely than guardianship changes or reevaluations, particularly in wards with dementia.

Adult competency and guardianship cases are not only about older adults, as some guardianship cases involve young- or middle-aged adults with mental illness or mental retardation. Nonetheless, elders are overrepresented in these cases (Demakis, 2010). With the graying of the United States' population and the increase in dementia, state courts are likely to see an increase in probate issues, elder abuse, and competency/guardianship issues (van Duizend, 2008). It thus behooves psychologists to be educated about such issues, particularly if they work with older adults, their families, or in the family law arena. Much work has been done in this area since Hafemeister and Sales' (1982) early article that detailed the roles and responsibilities (and statutory limitations) of psychologists in guardianship laws across the United States. Relatively little research or advocacy, however, has been explicitly from a psychological perspective; rather, it has come from an array of legal, gerontological, social services, and advocacy group perspectives. Where possible, I detail this work, but also seek to integrate relevant psychological research and theorizing.

Guardianship[1] is a formal legal relationship between the guardian and ward by which the court gives the guardian the duty and power to make decisions for a ward who has been adjudicated incompetent. Ideally, the relationship is to protect the ward who, by virtue of medical, neurological, psychological, or other condition, is no longer able to manage safely and independently his or her affairs. Typically, guardianship may be of the person (i.e., with responsibilities for medical,

1. In some states (e.g., California), this is referred to as conservatorship. For ease of communication, I refer to this relationship as guardianship throughout, unless otherwise noted.

living, and related decisions), of the estate (i.e., with responsibilities for financial and estate decisions), or, more commonly, a plenary or general guardianship that includes both of these. This latter type of guardianship may be viewed as a "one-size-fits-all" approach. A limited or partial guardianship is when guardianship is only of the person or estate (or other specific domain of functioning that the individual is incapable of). These guardianships are tailored to the respondents' unique retained capacities as well as areas for which they have been adjudicated incompetent. Furthermore, because guardianship is so restrictive and the ward relinquishes autonomy and decision making, it is typically considered a measure of "last resort." There are other less restrictive ways of assisting adults with decisional impairments: a representative payee to receive federal benefits such as Social Security, assignment of an individual to have power of attorney for financial and/or healthcare decision making, healthcare advanced directives, joint-ownership of cash, properties, and assets with a trusted family member or friend, or establishment of a trust managed by an individual or institution. These are beyond the scope of this chapter (see Quinn, 2005, pp. 105–131 for a review). In any case, competency and guardianship proceedings represent a significant tension between, on the one hand, respecting the autonomy and independence of individuals (even to make poor decisions) and the need to protect the most vulnerable and easily manipulated members of our society.

HISTORY AND DEVELOPMENT OF GUARDIANSHIP IN THE UNITED STATES

Guardianships issues received relatively little legal and media attention until a series of newspaper reports illustrated the abuses, lack of legal protections, and poor oversight over the guardianship process (see Quinn, 2005, pp. 161–163). The Associated Press report was prominent and included an examination of more than 2200 randomly selected court files in every state. Examples of findings included the following: in 44% of the cases the proposed ward was not represented by an attorney, about 34% of the files contained no medical evidence, 49% of the proposed wards were not at their incompetency hearing, and 25% of the files contained no evidence that the hearing had even been held. Similarly, others have found that in about 90% of the cases reviewed in Florida there was no data on the behavioral information necessary to establish incompetency per Florida statute (Peters, Schmidt, & Miller, 1985). And, once guardianship was assigned, financial reviews of the guardians' work were "almost nonexistent." In Ohio and Washington state, Bulcroft et al. (1991) found that the proposed elderly ward was not at his or her own hearing 97% of the time and that guardianship was contested either formally or informally only 11% of the time. Though more recent research and newspaper articles continue to illustrate similar problems in various states (see, e.g., Uekert & Dibble, 2008), the 1980s and 1990s was a time in which there was a growing awareness of the need to change fundamentally how competency hearings are conducted and how guardianship is determined and monitored.

A variety of legal and elder-advocacy groups have helped to initiate such changes. Two prominent efforts were the Wingspread and Wingspan national guardianship conferences held in 1988 and 2001, respectively. The sponsors of these conferences were, among others, the National Academy of Elder Law Attorneys, the National College of Probate Judges, the America Bar Association, and the National Guardianship Association. Although the recommendations of these conferences are too numerous to list here, a few will illustrate how thinking about guardianship has changed. The Wingspan Conference recommended that: the respondent has a right to appear in court and to be heard; the court should fashion appropriate limited guardianship orders (vs. plenary or complete guardianship); there should be mandatory annual reports of the person and annual financial accountings; and professional guardians (i.e., not family members) should be licensed, certified, or registered (Wingspan, 2002). Some of these same recommendations were also made by the National Conference of Commissioners on Uniform State Laws in their model act titled "Uniform Guardianship and Protective Proceedings Act" (UGPP, 1997). Six states and the Virgin Islands had adopted this act as of October 2010. This latter group also developed a model act titled "Uniform Adult Guardianship and Protective Proceedings Jurisdiction Act" in 2007 that addressed a variety of legal issues in guardianship such as interstate transfer of guardianship. This has been adopted by 20 states. Because guardianship varies by state and U.S. society is so mobile, this act assists in resolving what can sometimes be complex jurisdictional issues. Furthermore, because of the limited data in guardianship in general, there have also been frequent calls for collecting additional and more systematic data on guardianship (e.g., a joint resolution by the Conference of Chief Justices and Conference of State Court Administrators as cited in Uekert, 2010). Overall, there have been consistent calls to collect additional data on the adult guardianship process and, more importantly, to safeguard respondents and to ensure that competency and guardianship decisions are done in ways that protect the rights of the proposed ward.

Partly as a result of the above recommendations, many states have made significant statutory reforms to their adult guardianship procedures. Moye, Wood, Edelstein, Wood, Bower, Harrison, and Armesto (2007) noted that from 1988 to 2006, 28 states enacted such changes. Quinn (2005, pp. 31–21) summarized changes in state laws as occurring in the following four areas: enhancing procedural due process safeguards for the proposed ward; moving toward a functional determination of incapacity (i.e., how the person actually functions) versus relying on medical labels or diagnoses; emphasizing the least restrictive alternative, including limited guardianships, versus plenary guardianships; and strengthened guardianship accountability. How successful have such reforms been? Keith and Wacker (1994) comprehensively evaluated guardianship cases in three states—Colorado, Iowa, and Missouri—before and after adult guardianship legislation was passed. They found some, but clearly not consistent, improvements. Regarding full versus limited guardianship, they found essentially no differences for Iowa and Missouri across time, but in Colorado, there was an increase in the use of limited guardianships. Before the legislation changes in this state, only 4% of the cases were awarded limited guardianship; this increased to 15% after the legislation was enacted. In terms of a statement from a health professional about the proposed ward's medical status (and presumed competency), Missouri remained the same prelegislation and postlegislation, but this increased in both Iowa and Colorado. For instance, before the legislation, there was medical evidence in 59% of the Iowa cases, but this increased to 73% after legislation. Moye, Wood, Edelstein, Armesto, Bower, Harrison, and Wood (2007) selected three states (Colorado, Massachusetts, and Pennsylvania) that had different degrees of statutory reform to their adult guardianship statutes and examined older adult guardianship case files. Colorado enacted significant changes in 2000 based substantially on the Uniform Guardian Protective Proceeding Act, Pennsylvania made some progressive changes in 1992, and Massachusetts' adult guardianship statute has seen little change over the past 30 years. Colorado's cases were, for the most part, significantly different than these states. For instance, proposed wards in that state were more likely to attend their own hearing and their case files were more likely to contain evidence of their functional abilities and cognitive or psychiatric symptoms. In Colorado, evaluations were also more likely be completed by professionals other than a physician. Although the above two studies point to potential value of reform, these findings are limited by relatively small samples in select jurisdictions and, in the latter study, because prereform and postreform data were not reported and preexisting differences between these states cannot be ruled out. In any case, these are the best data we currently have on the effect of guardianship statute reform and, unfortunately, what is happening more broadly across the nation is poorly understood.

THE GUARDIANSHIP DETERMINATION PROCESS

Assignment of a guardian or conservator is at the "back end" of what can be a lengthy competency determination process. Only after an adult is adjudicated incompetent is a guardian assigned. Although states vary in legal statutes and terminology as well as the legal process guiding competency and guardianship (see Mayhew, 2005; Karp & Wood, 2006, p. 52), there are usually four main procedures that are dealt with sequentially (see Melton, Petrila, Poythress, & Slobogin, 1997, pp. 338–345).

Petition: An adult is presumed to be legally competent. The petition is a formal mechanism brought before the court that seeks to challenge this and have the person adjudicated incompetent. The petition spells out the reasons for this and may, for instance, address issues such as why the individual's presumed disability is affecting financial management, cognitive abilities, and/or the ability to care for oneself. Based on the allegations, the petitioner may seek a general or plenary guardian for both the person and estate or a guardian for either the person or the estate. Some states have petitions available on-line to expedite the process. Once a petition is filed, the alleged incompetent person or proposed ward, now typically known as the respondent, is notified about this as are other family members, friends, and possibly healthcare providers. In emergency cases in which, for instance, the proposed ward is in imminent physical danger, or where his or her assets are being drained a temporary or emergency guardian may be assigned until the formal process below may be initiated. These are typically time-limited procedures.

Hearing: Prior to the hearing at which competency and guardianship are determined, the court seeks information (in addition to that in the petition) about the proposed ward, his and her current circumstance, and the proposed guardianship plan. This will typically include interviews with the proposed ward, family members, healthcare providers, as well as other interested parties. Review of relevant records is also common. The person conducting such fact-finding varies by jurisdiction but may be a court investigator, or the attorney or the guardian *ad litem* (GAL) assigned to the proposed ward. Once this information is collected the hearing officer, either a judge or clerk, holds a hearing or hearings on the matter. During the hearing, the respondent may be represented by a privately retained or a court-appointed attorney or GAL depending on the jurisdiction. There is some confusion about the role these individuals are supposed to take and most state laws are silent on this issue. Two primary models that govern the GAL or court-appointed attorney are the best interest and the zealous advocacy models (see Saxon, 2005, for a review). In the first, they represent the best interest of the respondent and are charged with determining, representing, and protecting his or her best interest based on the attorney's judgment. Notably, such a determination may be at odds with the expressed wishes of the respondent; as such, it is sometimes considered a responsible advocate model. In such cases, the respondent may also retain an attorney to represent his or her preferred desires. The other model—zealous advocacy—requires that the attorney represent the respondent as he or she would any client in a pending legal proceeding and to advise the respondent on a chosen course of action. They zealously advocate for and, if necessary, negotiate for the course of action chosen by their client. These two models represent fundamentally different ways of viewing the guardianship process as one tends to be viewed as more therapeutic and the other as more adversarial (see Kapp, 2002, for a review of this issue).

The actual hearing may include testimony from the respondent, petitioner, witnesses, as well as experts appointed by the court to assist in competency and guardianship determination. The type of professional and the type of expected evaluation vary jurisdictionally. It appears that in most states psychologists can now statutorily serve as evaluators; this is a welcome change since Hafemeister and Sales' (1982) early work that demonstrated a statutory preference for physicians versus psychologists for this type of work. Drogin and Barrett (2010) describe the requirements of who conducts the evaluation and the issues he or she is supposed to evaluate in three different states—New York, Vermont, and Kentucky. New York's guardianship statute is particularly detailed and asks the evaluator to address, among other issues, whether the proposed ward can attend the hearing, resources available to provide for the ward without a guardian, how the proposed ward is functioning with respect of activities of daily living, the prognosis of any mental disabilities and/or substance abuse, and what would be the least restrictive form of intervention. The evaluator is tasked with deciding if the proposed guardian, including if nominated by the proposed ward, is appropriate. Although jurisdictions vary, an important recent development has been the recommendation that the respondent be present at the hearing—even in the recent past, this was unfortunately rarely the case (see below).

Adjudication: As a result of the hearing or hearings, the judge or clerk determines competency and, if the respondent is adjudicated incompetent, a guardian is appointed. Each state has a statute defining competency: in North Carolina an incompetent adult is one who "lacks sufficient capacity to manage the adult's own affairs or to make or communicate important decisions concerning the adult's person, family, or property" [North Carolina General Statutes 35A—1101 (7)]. In Nevada, incompetency is defined as an adult person who is "unable, without assistance, properly to manage and take care of himself or herself or his or her property, or both" (Nevada Revised Statutes 159.019). Nevada statute also includes a provision for "limited capacity," which is an adult who "is able to make independently some but not all of the decisions necessary for the person's own care and the management of the person's property" (Nevada Revised Statutes 159.022). Via testimony, possibly including a competency evaluation, the hearing officer reviews the respondent's medical condition, psychiatric status, cognitive functioning, activities of daily living, and safety/harm issues to guide decision making (see recommendations from the American Bar Association—American Psychological Association, 2006). If allowed by the jurisdiction, the hearing officer may find that the respondent has some specific retained competencies—perhaps in medical, self-care, and living decisions, but not financial decisions. In such cases, partial or limited guardianships can be imposed and they are increasingly recommended (e.g., UPPGA, 1997). The hearing officer also decides who will serve as guardian. This is most frequently a family member or perhaps a professional guardian hired by the family, but, in the majority of states a public agency may serve in this role if there is no family or the family is unwilling or unable to serve in this capacity. In most states, this agency is a social services or mental health agency, but may also be the county government, an independent state office, or the courts (Teaster, Wood, Lawrence, & Schmidt, 2007).

Guardianship monitoring and succession: Once a guardian is assigned, the court may seek continuing information on guardianship, typically via status updates and financial reporting. Though this is recommended, there is huge variability across jurisdictions in whether this is done and how this is implemented. Historically, oversight by the court has been lax (see, e.g., Peters et al., 1985) and this has been a frequent issue of continuing concern. Court oversight, however, has been changing and there have been calls for increasing resources for courts to perform this role (Uekert, 2010). For instance, Karp and Wood (2007) in an American Association of Retired Persons survey found that 74% of guardians reported that they were required to file a personal status report, up from 68% in a similar 1991 survey. In 1991, only five state statutes required a guardianship plan on the future care of the ward; this increased to 10 states by 2005. In addition to such monitoring, states have provisions for successor guardianship, when a guardian dies, becomes incompetent themselves, or no longer wishes to serve in this capacity.

An additional issue is that competency restoration is possible, assuming the ward has meaningfully improved. Restoration may be feasible for a mentally ill ward who is able to comply successfully with a treatment regimen and attain psychiatric stability. Another example is an individual who is in the acute phases of traumatic brain injury when adjudicated incompetent, but eventually demonstrates significant recovery. Restoration is obviously less likely in individuals with dementia.

WHAT WE KNOW ABOUT GUARDIANSHIP IN THE UNITED STATES

In this section, I describe some of the basics about what we know about guardians and their wards. As competency adjudication and guardianship determination are done at the state level, there are unfortunately few reliable national statistics in this area. There are several national surveys, but these tend to be limited by modest return rates that, in some cases, rely on estimations from some states rather than actual data about, for instance, the number of guardianship filings and caseloads (Uekert, 2010). For instance, in a survey of state court administrators conducted by the American Bar Association Commission on Law and Aging (Wood, 2006), it was found that only 34% of states or territories that responded actually reported guardianship cases of the person or estate to the state court administrative office. Despite this, this survey clearly demonstrated that there were multiple locales throughout the county that did maintain notable data collection practices. Although some of it is described below, some states do not collect such data systematically and, if they do, it does not appear to be widely disseminated or publically available. Nevertheless, with the little published research in the area, as well as information from national surveys, the information below provides a reasonable overview of basic guardianship issues.

How many individuals in the United States have guardians? Because nationwide records are not kept and state record keeping tends to be poor, this is a difficult question to answer accurately and estimates vary. In a comprehensive study using the 1995 National Health Interview Supplement on Disability that asked about the presence of a legal guardian, Reynolds (2002) found a prevalence of 0.3%. Assuming that this percentage is still the same today, extrapolating based on today's United States population (approximately 300 million), the number of adults with a legal guardian is approximately one million. Although valuable because these findings and related ones described below were collected on a nationally representative sample, they are somewhat limited because they are based on self-report data. With our aging society, this number is likely to increase. For instance, in an internet survey conducted by Uekert (2010) with those working in the guardianship field (e.g., judges, state court administrators), 37% responded that their guardianship filings have increased and 43% responded that they have seen an increase in caseloads.

What are the characteristics of those who are ultimately assigned a guardian? Using a nationally representative sample, Reynolds (2002) found that increasing age was associated with having a guardian. Compared to those without a guardian, those who had a guardian tended to be older, less educated, poorer, to live without a spouse, and, not surprisingly, to have more sensory impairments, more impairments in daily living, and to be suffering from alcohol or substance abuse. Reynolds and Wilber (1997) compared individuals with public conservators in Los Angeles County California to a nationally representative sample. Their findings were quite similar to those above, but they also found that older conservatees (70+) were, among other things, significantly more likely to have dementia (54% vs. 37%), to have diabetes (20% vs. 13%), and to be childless (73% vs. 15%). It is important to note that these findings were obtained on those with public conservators from the Department of Mental Health and that findings are likely to differ for those with family or privately hired conservators. When Moye, Wood, Edelstein, Armesto et al. (2007) examined guardianship practices in three states (Colorado, Massachusetts, and Pennsylvania), the most common diagnosis for respondents was dementia (59%), followed by mood disorder (14%) and other neurological disorders such as Parkinson's disease (11%). These individuals were also described as having a range of other cognitive (e.g., confusion, memory) and functional (e.g., health and money management) deficits. Using a relatively small Veteran's Affairs geropsychiatry sample ($n = 39$) in Texas, Burruss, Kunik, Molinari, Orengo, and Rezabek (2000) found that for patients for whom guardianship was recommended, the guardianship process (presumably including adjudication of incompetency) was actually completed for only 33% of patients. Those assigned a guardian were more depressed and had a greater number of medical conditions; there were no differences in, among other variables, marital status, living arrangement, presence of dementia, or medications. Although this study is limited as it is a small convenience sample, this appears to be the only one that has reported actual psychological test findings (however limited) on those ultimately adjudicated incompetent and assigned a guardian. To my knowledge only one study (Keith & Wacker, 1994) has examined the causes or critical incidents leading to guardianship. Though these findings are not about wards per se, they illustrate the types of issues these individuals face. The three primary reasons leading to guardianship, accounting for over 75% of cases, were a physical emergency (45%), incapacity and dependency (25%), and altered personal relationships (7%).

Little research has been done about guardianship in younger or middle-aged adults with developmental disabilities or severe mental illness. A study by Millar and Renzaglia (2002) is an exception, as they studied guardianship court files for developmentally delayed adults aged 17 to 28 in Michigan for whom a final guardianship decision had been made. They found that 100% of guardianship requests were granted and that those with mental retardation accounted for almost 90% of their sample. There was predictable variability in the type of guardianship assigned. Respondents with mild mental retardation were more likely to be appointed partial guardianship (either of the person or estate) whereas those with severe or profound retardation were more likely to be appointed plenary guardianship.

Who are the petitioners and guardians? Not surprisingly, family members are the majority of both petitions and guardians. In Millar and Renzaglia's (2002) Michigan study of developmentally delayed young adults, 75% of the petitioners were family members and approximately 90% were assigned guardianship. In the study by Moye, Wood, Edelstein, Armesto et al. (2007) of court practices in three states with elderly respondents, the petitioner tended to be a family member or friend. In Massachusetts, 81% of the petitioners were family or friends and, in Colorado, 56% were family or friends. Agencies petitioned in 34% of the cases in Pennsylvania, but in only 8% of the cases in Massachusetts. Dudley and Goins (2003) found that family members were petitioners in 75% of guardianship cases for elderly respondents in West Virginia and Pennsylvania. In terms of actual guardianship, Keith and Wacker's (1994) study of court records in three states—Iowa, Colorado, and Missouri—found that 79% of the guardians were family members and 51% were involved in caring for the proposed ward before guardianship assignment. Only 5% of guardians were the Department of Human Services or a county attorney/public administrator. In 82% of the cases reviewed, the petitioner was assigned guardianship; when they were not, it tended to be in cases in which a government agency or representative petitioned, but a family member was assigned guardianship. Studies of court records in Florida (Peters, Schmidt, & Miller, 1985) and Ohio and Washington (Bulcroft, Kielkopf, & Tripp, 1991) found that approximately 70% of guardians (primarily of the elderly) are family members.

What do guardians actually do and what is their experience of guardianship? Answering these questions is difficult, as guardians' experiences vary tremendously based on the needs, abilities, and expectations of the ward, as well as where the ward is placed (e.g., in their home vs. an assisted living facility). Moreover, their experiences vary depending on the type of guardianship—plenary or partial. Nonetheless, three studies are illustrative. In a 2001 Virginia study of 191 wards served by public guardians (see Quinn, 2005, pp. 101–103), guardians spent an average of 12 hours per case before being appointed and, once appointed, most individuals in guardianship were seen several times per month. These public guardians provided an average of 4.5 hours of service to each ward per month and they spent their time in the following ways (ranked from most to least time): financial assistance, medical/physical health, caregiver support, and home/physical environmental needs. In a small qualitative sample of conservators and conservatees in California, Wilber, Reiser, and Harter (2001) found that both public and private conservators considered their role to be decision makers and supervisors/managers. Moreover, family members were more likely to describe their primary role as providing direct care and support such as bathing, unless there were sufficient funds to pay for a caretaker. In a quantitative study noted above, Keith and Wacker (1994) used multiple regression analyses to predict role strain for guardians in men and women. Not surprisingly, for both genders, the "demandingness" of the ward, the need for instruction on how to care for the ward, hours per week spent on guardianship, and interference on personal health were all positively associated with role strain. Interestingly, a positive relationship with the ward was associated with less strain in women, but not men, whereas for men only, the perceived importance of the role was related to role strain. These authors also created a typology of guardian types based on their written descriptions of the most difficult aspects of their roles and how they managed guardianship. In this exploratory study they described the following guardian types with percentages: the tough (15%), the sympathetic (35%), the sad (25%), and the challenged (25%). Among other findings, for instance, they found the tough guardian had been guardian for the shortest period of time, whereas the sad guardian had served for the longest period of time. Not surprisingly, the tough guardian reported higher role strain than the other types and was more likely to disagree about the need for a guardian, disagree with their selection as guardian, and to have experienced a change in family relationships as a result of the guardianship. These findings about the stresses of guardianship echo findings from the broader caregiving burden literature that show, for instance, those who care for an older adult with dementia have higher rates of depression and are at risk for physical health problems (Schulz, O'Brien, Bookwala, & Fleissner, 1995; Vitaliano, Zhang, & Scanlon, 2003).

MAKING RECOMMENDATIONS ABOUT GUARDIANSHIP

In this next section, I detail issues that are relevant when the court has asked for the psychologist's assistance in actually determining who the guardian should be. This is, of course, assuming that the person has already been adjudicated incompetent by the court. Typically, the family member who has petitioned the court is seeking guardianship, but this is not always the case and the petitioner may have another family member or a governmental agency in mind to serve as guardian. Either way, the proposed guardian may not be acceptable to certain family members. Particularly in cases with large estates, there may be considerable conflict about who will serve as guardian. Much like a child custody hearing, the psychologist provides a recommendation to the court about which family member is best suited to serve as guardian. Some of these cases are highly contentious with chaotic, high-conflict families. Or, in some cases, the determination is between a family member (whether petitioner or not) and a government agency. In other cases, a government agency may both petition and seek guardianship; in these cases, because the nature and quality of the guardianship are known, there is relatively little to evaluate or examine. The information below is designed to be most useful in cases in which guardianship is contested.

Unfortunately, state guardianship statutes provide little in the way of assistance in providing guidelines or criteria for determining standards or criteria for guardianship assignment. However, the recommendation from the Wingspan Conference is that "The court consider the best interest of the person with diminished capacity in selecting the guardian." Similarly, the Uniform Guardianship and Protective Proceedings Act (UGPPA, 1997) states: "A guardian at all times shall act in the ward's best interest and exercise reasonable care, diligence, and prudence." Best interest in not defined in either of these recommendations.

However, it has been articulated by some states in regards to child custody cases, in which some of the decision-making dynamics are similar. For instance, in Minnesota judges are provided a variety of factors to consider and evaluate including, among a total of 13, the intimacy of the relationship between each parent and the child, the interaction and interrelationship between each parent and the child, as well as the capacity and disposition of the parties to give the child love, affection, and guidance (Minnesota Statutes 518.17). Again, though one might argue that these criteria themselves are subjective, they at least direct the judge to thoroughly and carefully review the child's particular circumstance (again, only a few factors are listed above). In the absence of clear standards for adult guardianship in some states, including the fairly vague best interest standard, it appears as if evaluators and judges have some latitude in their guardianship recommendations and determinations, respectively. In the determination of the best interest of the respondent, factors related to the proposed guardian—such as resources and plans—and the fit or match between these and the respondent's needs is key. Below I describe relevant issues to guide such recommendations to the court.

The respondent or proposed ward: Even though the respondent may be decisionally impaired and have self-care difficulties, he or she may still have a preference, perhaps well-articulated, about who they would like to serve as guardian. If so, the evaluator should seek to obtain as much information on this preference as possible including why the respondent desires one individual and not the other (assuming that it is a family conflict). Learning of the respondent's perception of what the relationship will be like, how their life will change (oftentimes it won't substantially if the proposed guardian is already assuming care for them), and how selecting one family member will affect other relationships can all be important in thinking about guardianship. Obtaining information on difficulties and challenges in the relationship can also be helpful.

There are two caveats to the above: In some cases, the respondent will be so impaired, typically due to dementia or mental retardation but possibly also psychiatric illness, that they may not be able to articulate who they desire to serve as guardian. More likely, however, they will not be able to provide a sufficient rationale for their choice. More pernicious, however, is cases in which there may be an attempt to unduly influence or control the proposed ward's wishes. In such cases, the respondent may be manipulated by the proposed guardian to select them as the guardian, perhaps for emotional, but most likely for financial reasons. Relatively little research has been done on this issue, but Quinn (2005, p. 193) reports a finding from San Francisco that in one study of guardianship in 2000, 35% of individuals with diminished capacity were at risk for undue influence; how undue influence was defined was not specified in this source. Shulman, Cohen, Kirsh, Hull, and Champine (2007) have detailed some of the indicators of undue influence in cases of testamentary (i.e., will-making) capacity, but these dynamics may be relevant in a guardianship situation as well. They state that some of the indicators of undue influence (adapted for guardianship issues) are as follows: there is a confidential relationship between the proposed guardian and ward that allows the former to control or influence the latter; the proposed guardian uses the relationship to secure a change in what the proposed ward would have wanted; there is undue benefit to the proposed guardian; and, obviously, the proposed ward is vulnerable to being influenced as a result of neurological or mental disorder or because of specific emotional circumstance. Quinn (2002) described some the interpersonal dynamics of undue influence and found that common factors include an abuser who isolates the ward, engenders feelings of dependence, isolation, and powerlessness, and seeks to keep the ward unaware or uninformed. In one of the few research studies on this topic, Spar, Hankin, and Stodden (1995) surveyed U.S. probate judges on their opinion and perceptions of undue influence. Interestingly, approximately half disagreed with the statement that susceptibility to undue influence requires mental illness and the majority agreed with the statement that age alone does not increase undue influence. In other words, these judges believed that undue influence may occur at any age and that even individuals without diagnosed psychological or neurological disorder may be vulnerable. In any case, determination of what the proposed ward desires in such cases is obviously difficult, and the examiner should, at minimum, seek to evaluate the proposed ward separately from the proposed guardian in cases in which such concerns exist. Collateral information is also often useful in such cases. Although beyond the scope of this article, Quinn (2002) details some of the methods health-care professionals can use to counter undue influence.

The proposed guardian(s): The proposed guardian or guardians should be carefully and thoroughly examined for their knowledge of the respondent, as well as their actual abilities, plans, and resources to serve as guardian (see Table 8.1 for sample questions). A key consideration is the extent to which they have either made concrete plans or arrangements for this role, which may be substantial. In one case I evaluated, a father petitioned to become guardian for his adult son with mental retardation with whom he had not lived for many years. When queried about how he would manage this transition (if assigned guardian, it would have been in less than 1 month), it was clear he had made no plans about their living situation, his son's daily caretaking needs, or schooling. Needless to say, this was problematic. Another key consideration is the prospective guardian's understandings of the role of guardian and the associated duties and responsibilities. Some will have done research and may have asked questions of the court or the respondents' GAL and be relatively knowledgeable by the time of the evaluation, but others will have relatively little knowledge. I am less concerned about their formal or legal knowledge about what guardianship is (though this is eventually important), but more concerned if they have not considered how this new role (to the extent that they understand it) will impact them, their family, and the respondent. A final consideration refers to the fitness of the proposed guardian: those with cognitive impairments, severe or poorly controlled psychiatric issues, and/or medical issues may not be able to best serve as guardian. In one case on which I worked, a woman with poorly controlled bipolar disorder and an active substance abuse disorder sought to serve as guardian for her elderly mother. Though the petitioner was adamant that she could serve in this role and tentative plans were being arranged for her to do so, 1 week before the hearing she impulsively

Table 8.1 Suggested Questions for Prospective Guardianship

Are you interested in becoming a guardian for the respondent? Why?
If so, what is you plan in regard to living arrangements?
What is your plan in regards to his or her care?
What assistance (if any) from family, friends, or others will you have?
What arrangements would you make in regard to visitation with other family members?
In case something happens to you (illness or other emergency), what would be your backup plan?
What would you take into consideration when making medical decisions on behalf of the respondent?
How would you deal with end of life issues in regard to involving the respondent?
Are you aware of any burial plans? If not, what would you take into consideration to make the burial arrangements?
Do you have any medical problems or mental illness? Are you receiving treatment? Please describe.
What plans would you put into place if you are not able to serve as guardian?
Do you have a criminal record? If so, please describe.

Adapted with permission from a questionnaire by T. Luong, MSW, Guardianship Social Worker.

withdrew and angrily confronted the respondents' GAL about a host of issues. She was not assigned guardian. Other problematic issues include a proposed guardian with poor knowledge of or unrealistic expectations about the proposed ward's capacities and medical or psychiatric condition, lack of knowledge concerning caretaking roles and responsibilities, limited time and/or resources, and an inability or unwillingness to work with other family members or treatment providers.

Collateral informants: Guardianship recommendation is particularly difficult in high-conflict and chaotic families in which members are divided about who should serve as guardian. These conflicts can be quite contentious with frequent unfounded allegations and sometimes shifting family allegiances. In such cases, obtaining objective and reliable information about guardianship issues can be quite difficult. A home visit, although time intensive, can provide a wealth of information about the proposed ward's current living situation and how well he or she is managing at least some activities of daily living, as well as the proposed guardian's ability to manage or care for the proposed ward (if he or she already has assumed some of such responsibilities). Objective information from objective collaterals can also be very useful and might include a long-time family physician who knows the family well, neighbors, or uninvolved and unaligned family members. Probably the most informative collateral I interviewed was the principal of the respondent's school (he was just turning 18 and attending a small, private school for students with special needs). He was able to speak to the strengths and weaknesses of each of the parents who were divorced and who were each seeking guardianship and, more broadly, the family dynamics. Though extraordinary helpful, having such objective and well-informed collaterals is, in my experience, a rarity.

The recommendations: Based on the information collected from the respondent, proposed guardians, and collaterals the psychologist seeks to determine which guardian would be in the best interest of the respondent. This may, or may not, be a family member. It is important to consider that it is a recommendation to the court, and just that—the court decides the ultimate legal issues of competency and guardianship assignment. Although it is beyond the scope of this chapter to address this issue in detail, much has been written about the ultimate legal issue and whether psychologists should express opinions on it or not (e.g., Melton, Petrila, Poythress, & Slobogin, 1997, pp. 16–18, 539–546; Slobogin, 1989). In addition, if the proposed ward has some retained abilities, this should be communicated to the judge or legal decision maker to allow for a limited guardianship. For instance, an 18-year-old man I evaluated suffered a moderate to severe traumatic brain injury and eventually received a large monetary settlement for which he did not have the capacity to manage independently. I recommended a guardian of the estate only and that he retain other rights; the judge agreed. Carving out such retained capacities in a guardianship recommendation is, in fact, consistent with current recommendations to support the ward's autonomy and independence (e.g., see UGPPA, 1997; Wingspan, 2002).

ILLUSTRATIVE CASE STUDIES

I describe two cases below that highlight the role of the psychologist in competency and guardianship cases. In each of these cases my evaluation (termed Multidisciplinary Evaluation in North Carolina) was used by the court to assist with the initial competency decision and then guardianship issues. As can be seen, in the first case the court followed my recommendation, but the final chapter on this case has yet to written, whereas the court disagreed with my initial recommendation in the second case. I did provide another alternative, though, that the court followed and the outcome, at least to the degree that it can be expected, was favorable. Identifying details have been altered where appropriate and I have provided only a relatively brief overview of each case as they were both quite complex and lengthy.

The respondent with severe-persistent mental illness: *A 56-year-old African-American woman had multiple prior psychiatric hospitalizations, essentially throughout her adult life, and had been diagnosed primarily with schizophrenia. She had been poorly compliant with her medication, homeless for periods of time, and had been evicted from the various homes and assisted living facilities where she had resided, primarily because of hostility, defiance, and persecutory delusions. She had been previously adjudicated incompetent 1 year prior to my evaluation, during an acute psychiatric exacerbation, and her brother was assigned general or plenary guardianship. He was also the representative payee of her*

Social Security Disability check; he had been assigned this role prior to the guardianship hearing. After she had been psychiatrically stabilized, she was released to a local hotel where she was living fairly independently, but her brother still had full control over her finances as well as healthcare (she was receiving depot antipsychotic medication). He ensured that she attended all healthcare appointments. On a daily basis, she was able to prepare simple meals, keep herself and her room reasonably neat, and use public transportation appropriately. As a result of increasing psychiatric stability, she petitioned the court for competency restoration as she believed that she could manage her affairs independently and that she did not need her brother's oversight. On psychological evaluation she presented as hostile, irritable, with marked, but fairly vague, persecutory delusions involving, for instance, the courts and her GAL, as well as the Mafia. Insight and judgment were quite poor as she stated that if adjudicated incompetent she would stop taking her medications. She had a vague and poorly developed plan on how she would leave the area and go to the beach. On formal testing, she did not demonstrate any cognitive or functional deficits, but psychological assessment was invalid as she did not respond to a sufficient number of items on a self-report measure (even after encouragement, she refused to respond). Overall, though she did appear to be managing her activities of daily living reasonably well at the time of the evaluation and was psychiatrically stable, this appeared to be primarily due to her brother's supervision and monitoring. Though I was primarily concerned because I did not have a good sense of what she could do on her own, I was also concerned that if adjudicated competent at this time she would decompensate psychiatrically. I shared this with the court in my written report and recommended a limited guardianship in which she would be provided with increasing rights and responsibilities. For example, at the time of my evaluation, she was provided with only a small monthly sum of money from her check from her brother; I recommended that she be provided the entire sum at the beginning of the month to evaluate how well she could manage the money independently. I also recommended that she be increasingly responsible for doctor's appointments and other mental health treatment to evaluate how well she could manage her healthcare independently. These two recommendations sought to limit the existing plenary guardianship and provide opportunities for her to demonstrate her ability to manage her affairs independently. The court agreed with these and asked to re-evaluate the situation in 6 months. I recommended that if she could manage these issues, and others, she should be adjudicated competent.

The respondent with dementia and a conflicted family: *This 83-year-old fragile white man was hospitalized in a skilled nursing facility and had previously been diagnosed with dementia and depression, as well as multiple health problems such as hypertension, hypothyroidism, and gastrointestinal difficulties. He was prescribed multiple medications including anticholinesterase inhibitors as well as antidepressants. Furthermore, he was described as a "total care patient" according to a physical therapy evaluation and it was stated that he needed assistance with multiple activities of daily living such as bathing, grooming, ambulation, and car transfers. In this context, there was significant family strife between the wife and multiple siblings who were at odds about his care. One side of the family, comprised of the wife and one of the children, was allied against the other children. The former side believed that he was competent and that he should return home, whereas the other side of the family disagreed and believed that he was incompetent and in need of 24-hour care. Their disagreements were long-standing and, at times hostile; in one situation, the family members got into a physical altercation in front of the respondent at the nursing facility. My evaluation of the respondent was limited because he was so compromised cognitively, but I relied heavily on medical records as well as interviews with healthcare providers to arrive at my recommendation that he was not competent. In terms of guardianship issues, I interviewed several of the family members and it was clear that there was still substantial disagreement about care and placement issues, as well as some overt hostility. Because of this I recommended that a public guardian be appointed. In making this recommendation, I also provided the court with another option, which was to have one side of the family serve as Guardian of the Estate (the child who was already managing some of these responsibilities) and the other to serve as Guardian of the Person. Moreover, if this was to be done, I recommended several specific issues such as each side informing the other about decisions about his care or estate, that the side of the family assigned Guardian of the Estate be allowed reasonable visitation, and that each side of the family refrain from making hostile or disparaging remarks about the other in the ward's presence. The court chose to follow this latter recommendation, believing that it would be prudent to try a family solution prior to assigning a public guardian. A follow-up status hearing was set for 3 months after the initial hearing; the social worker who had been assigned to this case reported that this agreement was working well and that there were no difficulties.*

CONCLUSIONS

Competency and guardianship go hand-in-hand. Once a respondent or proposed ward is adjudicated incompetent, the court assigns guardianship. Not surprisingly, guardianship determination can be a difficult task, particularly in respondents with complex healthcare needs and conflicted and chaotic families. Courts sometime look to psychologists to assist and to provide recommendation with these decisions. Clinical psychologists, by virtue of their training and experience in areas such as psychopathology, neuropsychology, family dynamics and systems, psychological treatments, as well as forensic issues, are uniquely suited to provide guidance to the court. Such guidance may include, for instance, who should serve as guardian, how the guardianship order should be crafted (e.g., limited vs. plenary), and care recommendations (e.g., the guardian should provide a particular type of treatment). Unfortunately, at present, there is relatively little empirical research to guide such recommendations. The current research is primarily descriptive about the legal process and guardianship orders, who petitions and is ultimately assigned guardianship, and how assigned guardians experience their work. There have been consistent calls for more research in the area, particularly by advocacy groups.

Moving forward, there are two broad areas that could benefit from additional research. First, considerably more work needs to be done on what makes guardianship successful and viable over time. Family structure and dynamics, available social support and other resources, as well as the psychological characteristics of guardians would seem important to evaluate. Clearly the ward and his or her disabilities need to also be addressed as these are likely to affect guardians. Work on what maintains the guardianship relationship over time is particularly needed; in my review of the literature, I could not find any longitudinal work on how the guardianship relationship changes (or remains the same) over time. This would seem to be especially important in younger individuals with developmental disabilities or severe mental illness. In such cases, a related issue is how the ward deals with and transitions to a new guardian (if that even occurs). A second area of needed research is in the legal arena. Even though much of the current research is on legal processes and issues, because these tend to be state specific, it remain unclear how accurate this work portrays wider guardianship issues. Research on more jurisdictions would be welcomed. What does not appear to have been studied, however, is how legal decision makers reason about, conceptualize, and ultimately arrive at their decisions about guardianship. Such work has been done with judges in the criminal realm and it has been broadly useful in better understanding their preferences about mental health findings and testimony (e.g., see Redding, Floyd, & Hawk, 2001). In any case, a better understanding of how legal decision makers use psychological evidence or testimony about guardianship issues is needed. In particular, an understanding of how they weigh various pieces of evidence (e.g., preferences of the proposed ward vs. preferences of the proposed guardian) and consider issues such as the long-term viability of the guardianship relationship, family dynamics, and psychological well-being of the proposed ward is important. Overall, because guardianship statutes vary by state and there is enormous variability in what is done locally, these remain difficult issues to research on a large scale. Yet the needs of our society—with a likely increase in competency and guardianship hearings—demand that we improve our understanding of this process to better serve some of society's most vulnerable members.

References

American Bar Association Commission on Law and Aging—American Psychological Association (2006). *Judicial determination of capacity of older adults in guardianship proceedings*. Washington, D.C.: American Bar Association & American Psychological Association.

Bayles, F., & McCartney, S. (1987). *Guardians of the elderly: An ailing system*. Associated Press.

Bulcroft, K., Kielkopf, M. R., & Tripp, K. (1991). Elderly wards and their legal guardians: Analysis of county probate records in Ohio and Washington. *The Gerontologist, 31*, 156–164.

Burruss, J. W., Kunik, M. E., Molinari, V., Orengo, C. A., & Rezabek, P. (2000). Guardianship applications for elderly patients: Why do they fail? *Psychiatric Services, 51*, 522–524.

Demakis, G. J. (2010). *Promises and pitfalls of the Multidisciplinary Evaluation.* Presentation to the North Carolina Guardianship Association. Asheville, North Carolina.

Drogin, E. Y., & Barrett, C. L. (2010). *Evaluation for guardianship.* New York: Oxford University Press.

Dudley, K. C., & Goins, R. T. (2003). Guardianship capacity evaluations of older adults: Comparing current practice to legal standards in two states. *Journal of Aging & Social Policy, 15*, 97–115.

Hafemeister, T., & Sales, B. D. (1982). Responsibilities of psychologists under guardianship and conservatorship laws. *Professional Psychology, 13*, 354–371.

Kapp, M. B. (2002). Reforming guardianship reform: Reflecting on disagreements, deficits, and responsibilities. *Stetson Law Review, 31*, 1047–1055.

Karp, N., & Wood, E. (2007). *Guardianship monitoring: A national survey of court practices.* Washington, D.C.: American Association of Retired Persons Public Policy Institute.

Keith, P. M., & Wacker, R. R. (1994). *Older wards and their guardians.* Westport, CA: Praeger.

Mayhew, M. (2005). Survey of state guardianship laws: Statutory provisions and clinical evaluations. *Bifocal, 27*, 1–19.

Melton, G. B., Petrila, J., Poythress, N. G., & Slobogin, C. (1997). *Psychological evaluations for the courts: A handbook for mental health professional and lawyers* (2nd ed.). New York: Guilford.

Millar, D. S., & Renzaglia, A. (2002). Factors affecting guardianship practices for young adults with disabilities. *Exceptional Children, 68*, 465–484.

Minnesota Statutes Annual 518.17.

Moye, J., Wood, S., Edelstein, B., Armesto, J. C., Bower, E. H., Harrison, J. A., & Wood, E. (2007). Clinical evidence in guardianship of older adults is inadequate: Findings from a tri-state study. *The Gerontologist, 47*, 604–612.

Moye, J., Wood, E., Edelstein, B., Wood, S., Bower, E. H., Harrison, J. A., & Armesto, J. C. (2007). Statutory reform is associated with improved court practice: Results of a tri-state comparison. *Behavioral Sciences and the Law, 25*, 425–436.

National Conference of Commissioners on Uniform State Laws (1997). Uniform Guardianship and Protective Proceedings Act. Retrieved October 23, 2010 from http://www.law.upenn.edu/bll/archives/ulc/fnact99/1990s/ugppa97.htmm.

Nevada Revised Statutes 159.019 & 159.022.

North Carolina General Statutes 35A—1101 (7).

Peters, R., Schmidt, W. C., & Miller, K. S. (1985). Guardianship of the elderly in Tallahassee, Florida. *The Gerontologist, 25*, 532–538.

Quinn, M. J. (2002). Undue influence and elder abuse: Recognition and intervention strategies. *Geriatric Nursing, 23*, 11–16.

Quinn, M. J. (2005). *Guardianship of adults: Achieving justice, autonomy, and safety.* New York: Springer.

Redding, R. E., Floyd, M. Y., & Hawk, G. L. (2001). What judges and lawyers think about the testimony of mental health experts: A survey of the courts and bar. *Behavioral Sciences and the Law, 19*, 583–594.

Reynolds, S. L. (2002). Guardianship primarvera: A first look at factors associated with having a legal guardian using a nationally representative sample of community-dwelling adults. *Aging & Mental Health, 6*, 109–120.

Reynolds, S. L., & Wilber, K. H. (1997). Protecting persons with severe cognitive and mental disorders: An analysis of public conservatorship in Los Angeles County, California. *Aging & Mental Health, 1*, 87–97.

Saxon, J. L. (2005). The role and responsibilities of court-appointed lawyers in guardianship proceedings. *Administration of Justice*, No. 2005/06.

Schulz, R., O'Brien, A. T., Bookwala, J., & Fleissner, K. (1995). Psychiatric and physical morbidity effects of dementia caregiving: Prevalence, correlates, and causes. *Gerontologist, 35*, 771–791.

Shulman, D. I., Cohen, C. A., Dirsh, F. C., Hull, I. M., & Champine, P. R. (2007). Assessment of testamentary capacity and vulnerability to undue influence. *American Journal of Psychiatry, 164*, 722–727.

Slobogin, C. (1989). The "ultimate issue" issue. *Behavioral Sciences and the Law, 7*, 259–266.

Spar, J. F., Hankin, M., & Stodden, A. B. (1995). Assessing mental capacity and susceptibility to undue influence. *Behavioral Sciences and the Law, 13*, 394–403.

Teaster, P. B., Wood, E. F., Lawrence, S. A., & Schmidt, W. C. (2007). Wards of the state: A national study of public guardianship. *Stetson Law Review, 37*, 193–241.

Uekert, B. K. (2010). Adult guardianship court data and issues results from an online survey. Williamsburg, VA: National Center for State Courts.

Uekert, B. K., & Dibble, T. (2008). Guardianship of the elderly: Past performance and future promises. *The Court Manager, 23*, 9–15.

Uniform Guardianship and Protective Proceedings. (1997). National Conference of Commissioners of Uniform State Laws. Chicago, IL.

Van Duizend, R. (2008). The implications of an aging population for the state courts. *Future Trends in State Courts*, 1–5.

Vitaliano, P. D., Zhang, J., & Scanlan, J. M. (2003). Is caregiving hazardous to one's physical health? A meta-analysis. *Psychological Bulletin, 129*, 946–972.

Wilber, K., Reisser, T., & Harter, K. (2001). New perspectives on conservatorship: The views of older adults conservatees and their conservators. *Aging, Neuropsychology, and Cognition, 8*, 225–240.

Wingspan—The Second National Guardianship Conference (2002). Wingspan—The second national guardianship conference recommendations. *Stetson Law Review, 31*, 596–609.

Wood, E. F. (2006). State-level adult guardianship data: An exploratory survey. Washington, D.C.: American Bar Association on Law and Aging For the National Center on Elder Abuse.

PART THREE

Applications

9

Assessment of Civil Capacities: An Evaluative Framework and Practical Recommendations

STACEY WOOD AND MERYL O'BRYAN

A probate attorney calls a neuropsychologist with a potential referral of a 75-year-old client, Candice, who suffered a left hemisphere middle cerebral artery (MCA) stroke approximately 8 months previously. According to her attorney, Candice evidenced difficulty speaking and writing after the stroke. The attorney was retained by the adult children of the client because of their concerns regarding their mother's capacity to manage finances and to engage in estate planning. The attorney reported that he handled Candice's original estate planning when her husband had been living and that she has recently changed attorneys and initiated changes to her durable powers of attorney and estate plans. Candice's original plans made it clear that she wanted her adult children to serve as her health care proxies and that her estate should be divided equally between her two adult children. However, more recent estate planning appears to favor her partner of 2 years, Robert. Upon completion of the new documents, Robert plans to move with Candice out of state. The attorney wants to know if the client "has capacity" to change her documents. This chapter will describe an overview of the procedures that a neuropsychologist may apply to a range of similar referrals in the area of civil capacities. It will begin with the presentation of a framework developed by the American Bar Association/American Psychological Association (ABA/APA) working group on capacity issues and will then provide more specific guidance regarding assessment tools. A case study will also be provided to illustrate issues in capacity assessment.

NEUROPSYCHOLOGISTS AND CAPACITY ASSESSMENTS

Neuropsychologists bring a number of critical skills to questions related to decisional capacity. Because they have extensive training in standardized assessment, neuropsychologists can bring objective data to the bench as evidence, which is important because research in the area has revealed the generally poor quality of clinical assessment data (Markson, Kern, Annas, & Glantz, 1994; Marson, McInturff, Hawkins, Bartolucci, & Harrell, 1997; Moye et al., 2007; Rutman & Silberfeld, 1992). Neuropsychologists, especially those who work in rehabilitation, are also familiar with the importance and nature of functional assessments. Probate code has evolved toward emphasizing the importance of the description of specific capacities versus a global statement regarding incompetence (Moberg & Kniele, 2006). Neuropsychologists already conceptualize cognition in terms of domains and can use this approach to help the courts craft a more nuanced order that recognizes strengths as well as weaknesses. The role of the psychologist as consultant rather than as treating clinician is also already familiar to many neuropsychologists. Neuropsychologists are required to explain complex medical disorders to patients and families, and these skills are necessary when working with attorneys and judges. Taken together, neuropsychologists bring a number of strengths to the assessment of civil capacities.

However, there are some key differences between a standard clinical assessment and an assessment of civil capacity (Melton, Petrila, Poythress, & Slobogin, 2007; Moye, 1999). These types of referrals have a more extensive pre-assessment phase to determine the nature of the referral and to clarify ethical obligations up front (i.e., privilege and confidentiality). Psychologists must know relevant legal standards, and because these standards often are functional in nature, a functional assessment must be part of the assessment. Clinicians must be aware of admissibility standards in their jurisdiction and design a test battery that meets them. Finally, unlike a clinical evaluation, a forensic evaluation requires the clinician to voice a clear opinion regarding the client's ability to make a decision, either contemporaneously or retrospectively (Spar & Garb, 1992). These key differences have been incorporated into a conceptual framework that can be applied to diverse referrals in this area.

A FRAMEWORK FOR THE EVALUATION OF CIVIL CAPACITIES

In 2003, under the auspices of the interdisciplinary task force on facilitating ABA/APA relations, a working group was formed comprised of psychologists and attorneys. The working group has produced a series of three handbooks to provide guidance in capacity issues for attorneys, judges, and psychologists [American Bar Association Commission on Law and Aging & American Psychological Association, 2005; American Bar Association/American Psychological Association Assessment of Capacity in Older Adults Project Working Group, 2008; American Bar Association (ABA), American Psychological Association (APA), & National College of Probate Judges (NCPJ), 2006]. One product of this collaborative venture has been the development of a conceptual framework for capacity assessments. Because of the nature of capacity referrals, which can address a wide range of behaviors from capacity to drive, marry, vote, manage finances, make a will, give a gift, make medical decisions, or consent to research, a one-size-fits-all battery is not appropriate. The conceptual framework helps clinicians design more specific batteries and ensures that they have gathered the information necessary to formulate an opinion.

Theoretical conceptualizations of clinical assessments of capacity draw heavily from the seminal work of Thomas Grisso (Grisso, 1986, 2003). The Grisso model includes a causal component (medical diagnosis), a functional component (including cognition and functional skills), a contextual component (complexity of decision making), an interactive component (person-fit component), and a judgmental and dispositional component (the clinician must render a judgment that may have a dispositional impact on the client). The ABA/APA framework begins with this model and expands it by specifying the nine components of clinical capacity assessment of older adults: Legal Standard, Functional Elements, Diagnosis, Cognitive Underpinnings, Psychiatric or Emotional Factors, Values, Risk Considerations, Steps to Enhance Capacity, and Clinical Judgment of Capacity. An introduction to the model is included below, but for a more thorough treatment of the model and its application, the reader is referred to the *ABA/APA Assessment of Older Adults with Diminished Capacity: A Handbook for Psychologists*, which is available at http://www.apa.org/pi/aging/programs/assessment/index.aspx. In addition to these nine components, there are several other methods available for performing functional assessments that are described elsewhere (e.g., Allen et al., 2003; Fitten, Lusky, & Hamann, 1990; Fitten & Waite, 1990; Schmand, Gowenberg, Smit, & Jonker, 1999; Vellinga, Smit, van Leeuwen, van Tilburg, & Jonker, 2004).

Legal standard. Legal standard refer to the legal question, relevant legal statutes, and case law necessary for completing an assessment. Legal definitions of capacity vary from state to state, so it is important to become familiar with the specific language that is used in the relevant jurisdiction and how these standards and language have been interpreted in legal decisions. Legal standards also vary by type of capacity. For example, in a capacity assessment it will be necessary to answer a specific legal question, such as "Does this individual have the capacity to manage his or her finances?" Because the clinical assessment will be used to determine the legal rights of the alleged incapacitated person to make financial decisions, the clinician must be familiar with the specific legal standards in his or her state. The first consideration is that of the legal setting in which the examinee is evaluated. For example, many capacity assessments are done to assist in conservatorship/guardianship matters that are handled in probate courts. Cases of elder abuse and neglect may be handled in criminal courts that follow criminal law and legal standards. Some questions of capacity, such as the capacity to make medical decisions and participate in research, are typically handled outside of the judicial context. To determine the specific legal standards in a particular jurisdiction, there are a number of resources available. For example, the referring attorney can usually provide the information, as well as clarify any legal questions. In California, reference books such as the *California Department of Mental Health Laws and Regulations* (2010) provide much of the needed information. Many states (including California) have probate (conservatorship)-related codes posted on-line as well (e.g., see http://law.onecle.com/california/probate/811.html). Probate courts are usually open to the public and allow for observations of some matters. Once familiar with the legal standards, the neuropsychologist then discusses with the referral source the legal standard in his or her jurisdiction. Some states have forms that must be completed as part of a capacity assessment that specifically ask about different cognitive domains, and may be required to be submitted with a report. For example, California requires a "Capacity Declaration" form to be submitted when petitioning for guardianship hearings. The clinician should discuss with the referral source exactly what is required for the evaluation and write-up (ABA/APA, 2008).

Functional assessment. One of the key distinctions between a traditional neuropsychological assessment and an assessment of decisional capacity is the added emphasis on functional assessment. A common referral question relates to the potential need for a guardianship over person and estate (or conservatorships, in some jurisdictions). Many states (e.g., Alabama, Colorado, Hawaii, Minnesota, and Montana) have adopted laws similar to the model law from the Uniform Guardianship and Protective Proceedings Act (UGPPA, 1997) regarding guardianship proceedings. The UGPPA emphasizes the need for domain-specific recommendations versus an all-or-none determination of capacity. The Act defines an incapacitated person as "an individual that lacks the ability to meet essential requirements for physical health, safety, or self-care, even with appropriate technological assistance" (UGPPA, 1997, pp. 45–102). Note that the Act combines cognitive and functional elements, and as such, clinicians completing these assessments need to be able to explicitly discuss how the client is performing at a functional level. To be able to address the functional question, most commonly, clinicians will use their typical neuropsychological battery and add a section for the "functional" domain in question. It is difficult to overstate the importance of collecting valid functional data to augment the traditional neuropsychological battery. Below is an example of a functional assessment of money management using the Independent Living Scales with a woman who received a large inheritance.

Ms. Gray performed in the ***low range*** *on a test designed to assess financial knowledge and skills (standard score = 21). She had difficulty on items referring to dates that she would pay taxes, knowing how much a loaf of bread might cost, reading a bill, and writing two checks. Although she was able to write a check, she was not able to subtract the balance of money from a beginning balance, including the two checks. She had difficulty on any task that required her do more than very simple math. For example, she was able to count out coins but was not able to do addition or subtraction problems for more than a few dollars. Her performance did not improve when given a calculator, as she was unsure of the basic processes. It is possible that she has limited experience with a calculator. Her performance on this measure is consistent with the skill set that she needs in her current circumstances: earning and spending a few dollars at a time. She was not able to describe health insurance or medical insurance, explain how co-pays work, or provide a rationale* *for how someone can keep from being cheated out of money or why it is important to pay bills.*

In summary, her performance on this task is consistent with her self-report as a primarily dependent adult on her parents, who was also homeless, without an income, and without concomitant need to manage finances. She is anxious and confused regarding math. When asked about the importance of receiving independent advice regarding her upcoming inheritance, she seemed confused, and when the examiner stated, for example, "It is important for you to find someone who you pay hourly that has no interest in the outcome of the decisions regarding financial management. That type of person could be truly independent." She responded with a suggestion that she could have a friend of hers, who is a street performer in Los Angeles, help manage her finances because that person had an accounting background. It was very difficult for her to understand management of money that was more than about five dollars. In summary, she is financially naive with poor knowledge, skills, and judgment in financial matters.

Diagnosis. A diagnosis, obtained by history or documented by neuropsychological testing, is a critical part of the model as it establishes a "causal" component. That is, a medical reason exists as to why the alleged incapacitated person may be at risk for cognitive and functional impairment. A diagnosis further allows the neuropsychologist to inform the court if the cognitive impairment is likely to stay the same, get worse, or improve. A clinician may sometimes be asked to make a retrospective determination of capacity. In these cases, a clinician may voice an opinion regarding a client's level of functioning in the past and must use his or her knowledge of the course of the dementia process to support that opinion. However, it is important to note that a diagnosis in itself is not sufficient for the presumption of incapacity. Thus, although a neuropsychologist should provide a diagnosis, it is equally important to provide a rationale for how that particular diagnosis impacts cognition and functional behavior so that the neuropsychologist can connect the dots for the courts (ABA/APA, 2008).

Cognitive underpinnings. A thorough understanding of the client's cognitive functioning obtained through neuropsychological testing allows the clinician to describe the strengths and weaknesses of the client's decisional abilities. However, these test results must be employed with some understanding of the cognitive underpinnings of the capacity in question. Other chapters in this volume specifically review those topics (driving, financial, and testamentary). It is important to note that neuropsychological constructs do not perfectly map to the legal constructs. For example, the ability to make medical decisions requires four subabilities including understanding (i.e., comprehension of relevant information), appreciation (i.e., the ability to integrate relevant information with the current situation), reasoning (i.e., the ability to give rational explanations for decision), and expressing a choice (i.e., the ability to communicate a choice) (Moye, Karel, Azar, & Gurrera, 2004). In the assessment of medical consent capacity, tasks of verbal memory, comprehension, abstract reasoning, confrontational naming, and executive functioning have been linked to these four elements (ABA/APA, 2008;

Marson, Chatterjee, Ingram, & Harrell, 1996). However, the relationships between individual neuropsychological tasks and the legal constructs underlying medical consent capacity show considerable variance (ranging from about 10% in expressing a choice to 78% of understanding) (Gurrera, Moye, Karel, Azar, & Armesto, 2006; Wood, 2007). Based on a series of studies in patients with mild cognitive impairment (MCI) and moderate dementia, the following neuropsychological domains have been linked to financial capacity: arithmetic abilities, as well as executive functioning and memory.(Marson, Earnst, Jamil, Bartolucci, & Harrell, 2000; Marson & Hebert, 2008; Marson, McInturff, Hawkins, Bartolucci, & Harrell, 1997; Marson et al., 2000). In summary, when crafting a neuropsychological battery for a capacity evaluation, understanding the cognitive basis of the task in combination with a thorough cognitive assessment and some knowledge of the client's history makes it possible to comment on possible cognitive impairment.

Psychiatric and emotional factors. When psychiatric or emotional disturbances are severe, it may limit judgment and, as such, diminish capacity (Grisso, 2003). In addition to severe depression and psychosis, neuropsychologists are likely to confront complex neuropsychiatric disorders in which the interaction of psychiatric symptoms, such as delusions, and even mild cognitive impairment may result in very poor judgment (Grisso & Appelbaum, 1995). These symptoms can also help to build an effective undue influence case. Undue influence refers to a dynamic between two individuals in which the stronger person exploits or "bends" the will of the weaker, typically resulting in financial gain. Undue influence may take place in the absence of frank cognitive impairment and factors such as depression, dependence, and grief increase the susceptibility to undue influence (ABA/APA, 2008). An assessment approach should include an assessment of psychiatric and emotional factors that may impact decisional capacity, functional abilities, and susceptibility to undue influence. Below is an example of the role emotional and psychiatric factors may play in an evaluation of undue influence:

Ms. Chase had a well-documented history of paranoia that included a fear that others were out to get her, spying on her, gossiping about her, that strangers were looking at her in a negative way, and that someone was harassing her. This condition specifically impacted her ability to make good decisions regarding her safety. These beliefs were so salient that they drove Ms. Chase to hire two private investigators, both of whom reported that there was no current threat and that Ms. Chase was suffering from paranoid beliefs. They reported to her that there was no evidence of a threat. However, Ms. Chase was not reassured and hired a third "private investigator," Mr. Con. Mr. Con immediately took advantage of her paranoia by planting a false "wire," increasing her fears and ensuring his employment. From that point on, he and his father fabricated increasingly unrealistic scenarios to fuel the fire of her paranoia and then stepped in to "protect" her from these fabrications. Ms. Chase's mental impairment impacted her ability to protect herself from this scam. Her inability to accurately assess risks impaired her judgment regarding the need for 24 hour protection. It was only after a fourth private investigator, Mr. Mays, investigated Mr. Cons' credentials and motives that Ms. Chase learned that she was being scammed. In summary, the suspects took advantage of the victim at a time when her paranoia was at its peak and when she was unable to accurately assess her safety and their intent.

Values and preferences. Capacity evaluations require an assessment of an individual's values and preferences. Many factors may inform an individual's values including their culture, sexual orientation, religion, ethnicity, and gender (ABA/APA, 2008). In many cases, there is a mismatch between the clients' preferences and that of the clinician, and as such, the clinician needs to be aware of their values (Karel, Moye, Bank, & Azar, 2007). For example, a client may have issues with hoarding in his or her home. In these cases the emphasis should be on the ability to manage personal safety in that environment versus evaluating the home environment in relation to the clinician's personal standards. In addition to asking the clients about their choices and preferences for care, determining how clients have made decisions in the past can be of use to examine consistency of preferences. For example, in cases of disputed testamentary capacity, it can be useful to look at how the individual's values guided previous dispositions and see if there has been a shift.

Risk of harm and level of supervision needed. Clinicians must perform their assessment with an understanding of the decision context and setting of the alleged incapacitated person. A balance must be struck between protection of the person and his or her assets and respecting autonomy (Sabatino & Basinger, 2000). Capacity opinions on two individuals with identical standardized test scores may be quite different based on the complexity of the decision-making context and support available to each individual.

Enhance capacity. It is prudent for a clinician to perform an assessment that optimizes functioning (e.g., quiet, hearing aids present, frequent breaks, cultural issues). If the clinician identifies factors that may be improved (e.g., medication, new glasses) these should be noted in the report along with the recommendation to consider retesting after the accommodations have been made if improvements are noted. Below is an example of a set of recommendations for enhancing capacity:

Mrs. Chavez evidenced significant expressive aphasia, so it is recommended that she seek speech therapy in an outpatient rehabilitation setting. It is also noted that Mrs. Chavez appeared to be anxious and depressed throughout the interview, and she scored in the depressed range on formal testing of mood. It is recommended that a consultation be done for treatment of her psychological distress, and that after treatment, capacity should be retested. Lastly, Mrs. Chavez needed glasses for part of the evaluation, but she was only able to locate a broken pair that she apparently bought at a drug store some time ago. A referral to an optometrist is recommended.

Clinical judgment of capacity. Some commentators (Melton, Petrila, Poythress, & Slobogin, 2007) suggest that it is inappropriate for a clinician to ever answer what is fundamentally a legal question, whereas others argue that proffering an opinion is appropriate and useful as long as the clinician can adequately justify his or her conclusions based on sound psychological practice (Goldstein, 2006). In our opinion, it is appropriate to offer a clear clinical opinion for the courts to consider in capacity cases. At the end of the report in a clearly marked section, the clinical opinion regarding the capacity in question should be noted. One should seek to clearly make the link between specific data points and the opinion. There are also cases in which it may not be possible to reach an opinion about capacity. In these cases, there may be mixed evidence regarding capacity and it is necessary to clearly state the specific reasons for that opinion and list evidence that may be helpful to clarify it.

In summary, the model developed in the ABA/APA Handbook (2008) provides a useful framework for conceptualizing the assessment and assembling a test battery that will allow clinicians to address all of the steps in the model.

PRACTICAL ISSUES IN THE CIVIL CAPACITY EVALUATION

Working with referral sources. A large part of the orientation to the capacity assessment depends on the setting in which the psychologist works and his or her role. The context of the case will determine who the client is and the capacity in question. For example, in rehabilitation settings and medical settings, the referral source for a medical capacity evaluation will likely be a physician or other treatment team member. For the purposes of this chapter, we will focus on working with referral sources in guardianship-type cases. A referral involving a petition for guardianship (conservatorship in some jurisdictions) requiring a capacity evaluation can arise from a number of sources. It may be brought by an agency, such as adult protective services, concerned family members or family members in conflict, a probate attorney, or the court seeking an independent expert. When working on a case that is initially brought by family members, it is critical to ascertain who the client is and who will have access to the report. Also, it can be helpful to recommend to a family that is considering guardianship that they speak with an experienced probate attorney about the legal process, including a discussion of alternatives to the guardianship procedure. The evaluation will be critical evidence as part of a guardianship hearing, but it will be most effective if used by an attorney.

Probate attorneys and the courts provide the bulk of referrals in the area of capacity assessments. It can be helpful to plan an initial phone consultation to gain an understanding of the nature of the case, timeframe, the legal standards involved, the quality of evidence available (usually past medical records), and billing information. The psychologist's role should be clarified, including who will see the report. It is necessary to work with the referring attorney to establish a procedure for the evaluation. For example, the attorney may want a verbal description of the client's capacity prior to the generation of a written report. The attorney may have a hearing date in the near future and may need a particular piece of information prior to that time. The attorney will also have some history and potentially other evaluations, so the psychologist should ask about these and access them prior to drafting the opinion to ensure that all the relevant information has been included. It is unusual to be asked to testify in an uncontested guardianship (conservatorship) proceeding, so typically the report and local forms will suffice. However, on occasion it may be necessary to testify, and at that point, the psychologist will need to work with the referring attorney to assist with trial preparation.

A third type of referral source may be the courts themselves. As the assigned expert in these cases, the psychologist will receive a court order from a local probate judge laying out the essentials in terms of timeline, who the alleged incapacitated person is, the fees, and other critical players. Depending upon the jurisdictions, a court investigator or other court representative for the alleged incapacitated person may also be involved in the case. Typically, these referrals will begin after the psychologist has been established in a practice area, and it may also be necessary to be placed on a county panel of experts. It is important to clarify to whom the report will be submitted and the date it is required. As stated above, the psychologist should clarify his or her role with the referral source and explicitly identify others who will see the report so that the limits of confidentiality can be presented accurately to the client.

Interviewing. Similar to all types of assessments, the clinical interview is a critical tool in differential diagnosis and expert decision making. Usually, the interview will be longer and include supplemental questions focused on the capacity in question (e.g., finances, daily living). In addition, collateral interviewing becomes especially important as one seeks to ascertain the client's true level of functioning and his or her level of insight into his or her abilities and weaknesses. Because of the nature of capacity assessments, it is not atypical for clients to present themselves in the most favorable light. The clinical interview can be an opportunity to develop a rich set of observations that will help support the capacity findings and provide a context for the test data. For example, asking the client about salient current events, such as sports or recent natural disasters, may help to track his or her functional memory and may provide a compelling example for the lawyers and judge reading the report. Although there are limited data regarding the effectiveness of neuropsychological data in courts, the literature suggests that clinical observations are more persuasive than data presented only as numbers, at least to juries in sexually violent predator cases (Lieberman, Kraus, & Kryger, 2007). These observations should be included in the written report, as it is not typical to testify in capacity cases. Some examples are included in the sample report at the end of the chapter.

Collateral interviews are important in capacity assessments. Whether the family is "on the same page" or hardly speaking, it is recommended that a collateral interview be conducted with each significant family member and invested party, not just the individuals that retained the psychologist. To facilitate this, it can be useful to create a list of a few standard questions that will be asked of all involved, such as "What changes have you noticed in your mother's memory over the past year?" and "What do you think the best case scenario is for her situation?" A good rule of thumb in writing forensic reports is to always seek out third party confirmation for all data that are collected. For example, a family member may mention that their father has made several poor investments resulting in losses. It is not only acceptable to ask for financial statements, but prudent in order to corroborate these statements. One of the most valuable aspects of the collateral interviews is ascertaining the clients' insight into their limitations and assessing their judgment. When discrepancies emerge between the clients' report and the other data, it is possible to begin to understand their particular vulnerabilities in context.

PSYCHOLOGICAL TESTING

Building a capacity battery. Because of the diversity of capacity questions (e.g., testamentary, financial, independent living, medical decision making, sexual consent), there is no one battery that will be appropriate for all capacity referrals. Neuropsychologists thus may use a variety of tests to assess cognition based upon their particular context and the particulars of the case. In general, a complete assessment of cognition including attention, language, memory, visuoperceptual abilities, speed of processing, executive functioning, judgment and reasoning, and motor functioning is useful. Just as in clinical cases, a neuropsychologist uses these tests to determine strengths and weaknesses, differential diagnosis, and prognosis.

There has been some progress in terms of identifying the underlying cognitive mechanisms of decisional capacity, especially for the domains of medical and financial decision making. The relationship between cognitive functions and medical consent abilities has been one of the better studied areas in the decisional capacity literature in dementia patients (ABA/APA, 2008; Gurrera, Moye, Karel, Azar, & Armesto, 2006; Palmer & Salva, 2007). In terms of assessment tools, tasks of verbal memory, comprehension, abstract reasoning, confrontational naming, and executive functioning have been linked to medical consent abilities among dementia patients (ABA/APA, 2008; Marson, Chatterjee, Ingram, & Harrell, 1996). However, it should be noted that the relationships between individual neuropsychological tasks and medical decision making are moderate at best (Gurrera et al., 2006; Wood, 2007). This means that neuropsychological testing can provide the information regarding diagnosis and prognosis, and that additional testing with a functional measure of medical decision making is necessary.

Financial capacity is perhaps the decisional capacity with the highest "cognitive load." A conceptual framework developed by Marson and Hebert (2008) suggests that financial capacity is comprised of three types of knowledge, including declarative knowledge, skills (e.g., checkbook balancing), and judgment. Based on a series of studies in patients with mild cognitive impairment (MCI) and moderate dementia, the following neuropsychological measures have been linked to financial capacity: arithmetic abilities, executive functioning, and memory. Decline in arithmetic skills has been linked to impairments in financial capacity even in early stages of Alzheimer's disease and suggests that financial capacity may be impacted earlier than other types of decisional capacities (Griffith et al., 2003; Marson et al., 2000; Martin et al., 2008). In a preliminary study of a population of older adults that had been documented victims of financial exploitation and subsequently deemed to lack financial capacity, numeric skills and executive functioning were found to be consistently impaired (Wood et al., 2010). Neuropsychological measures help to ascertain an individual's cognitive functioning and risk, but to assess all three core areas of knowledge, skills, and judgment, it is recommended that neuropsychologists include a measure of financial capacity [e.g., Independent Living Scale (ILS), Financial Condition Index (FCI)] and interview questions that relate to the individual's situation.

In summary, psychologists should build a cognitive battery that provides the ability to determine the diagnosis and prognosis for each examinee. It may be necessary to augment the testing battery with tests that tap into arithmetic abilities (WRAT-IV) and to include a strong assessment of executive functioning. Tests that tap into judgment such as the Kaplan Practical Problem Solving task or the reasoning items from the Neurobehavioral Cognitive Status Examination (COGNSTAT) can be useful measures of judgment.

Functional assessment. In general, a neuropsychologist augments his or her test battery with a functional tool in the domain of interest to obtain a more proximal measure of a specific decisional domain. Three of the most common referral questions include the capacity to manage the person, to manage the estate, and to make medical decisions. An assessment of functional elements may include a home visit, an explicit assessment of Activities of Daily Living (ADL), and Instrumental Activities of Daily Living (IADL), the use of functional test instruments to assess medical decision-making capacity and financial capacity, or some combination of the above (e.g., Hopemont, Independent Living Scales, Financial Capacity Instrument) (Griffith et al., 2003; Loeb, 1996; Marson et al., 2000; Staats & Edelstein, 1995). In addition to the instruments that provide hypothetical situations, it is helpful to ask questions regarding the specific incidents in question. For example, if the client seems to be making poor medical decisions, questions designed to assess his or her knowledge of the current medical situation will be critical. In cases of financial decision making, specific questions regarding the client's financial situation (based on collateral information) will allow the clinician to ascertain his or her practical day-to-day knowledge.

Generating an opinion. After describing the client's neuropsychological profile and diagnosis, the report should state a clear opinion regarding the findings. The opinion should clearly state the legal questions (i.e., financial capacity) rather than make a plenary statement regarding decisional capacity in general. The opinion should integrate the findings from the neuropsychological assessment and functional assessment.

REPORT WRITING EXAMPLE

In the next section, a sample report is presented with comments as a teaching case to help clinicians understand how to apply the model and concepts described above into a coherent assessment and clear opinion. The report is structured similarly to clinical neuropsychology reports, but includes expanded collateral interviews, sections on independent living skills and financial skills, and formal functional assessments. The original case came from private practice, but it has been modified for confidentiality purposes and to provide a clear example of common issues in capacity evaluations. It is an example of a client who was at one point high functioning and a successful businesswoman, but now her capacity to manage person and estate was questioned by family members. The family members were in disagreement regarding the best course of action, and this case was referred by the probate attorney representing the interests of her niece L.S. Ultimately, the client was deemed to lack capacity by the courts to manage her person and estate. Notes in italics have been added to highlight relevant details.

Name: Jones, Jane
Date of Birth: 9/1/19
Age: 89 years
Gender: Female
Handedness: Right
Highest Grade Completed: Some College
Date of Evaluation: 07/21/2009

Reason for Referral

I performed a comprehensive geriatric neuropsychological evaluation of Jane Jones in order to assess Mrs. Jones's ability to manage her finances, manage her person, and make medical decisions.

This section should lay out the referral source as well as legal questions of interest.

Sources of Information

1. *Clinical interview and neuropsychological testing with Mrs. Jane Jones.*
2. *Collateral interview with Mr. F. (brother), Ms. Lisa F. (niece). 7/12/09.*
3. *Collateral interview with Ms. J.S. (niece). 7/12/09.*
4. *Collateral interview with Dr. P.K. 7/12/09.*
5. *Medical Records Hospital A: 5/29/09–6/08/09.*
6. *Medical Records Hospital B: 6/08/09–present.*

Collateral interviews are completed with all interested parties and documented.

Background Information

Mrs. Jones is an 89-year-old female currently residing in a postacute care facility status post a fall on May 29, 2009. According to available records, Mrs. Jones was found by her apartment manager and by her cousin, Frank R., and his daughter, Ms. J.S., on May 30, 2009 in a distressed state in her condominium. Per Ms. J.S.'s report, Mrs. Jones was lying on the floor covered in feces and urine and wearing only a thin sweater. Per Ms. J.S., the home was in disarray with piles of mail covering most kitchen surfaces, no bed linen, urine and feces on the bed, a soiled bathroom, and no food in the home. Mr. R. and Ms. J.S. brought her to the emergency room at Hospital A where she was admitted for observation, testing, and follow-up. Following an initial observation and treatment, she was transferred to a Postacute Care facility on June 8, 2009.

This section lays out the history of the problem and addresses the issue "why is a conservatorship necessary right now?"

Family and Social History

Mrs. Jones was able to recall some aspects of her autobiographical past. She reported that she was born in New Jersey as one of three siblings. Mrs. Jones reported that her elder sister was deceased. Her younger brother S.F., with whom she maintains a close relationship, lives in a nearby California city. She graduated from high school and moved to California as a young adult. She married and worked with her husband at their sound stage, C. Studios.

Medical History

Current diagnoses included altered mental status, functional decline, hypertension, hyperglycemia, hypothyroidism, osteoarthritis, cataracts, and coronary artery bypass surgery (CABG). The family medical history is positive for Alzheimer's disease (mother) and cancer (unspecified).

Mrs. Jones was hospitalized on 5/29/09. Records from that hospitalization were obtained. According to these records, a neurological evaluation was done. It is noted that on 6/01/09 by Dr. C.M. that "Mrs. Jones is oriented to self only, but not place or time." It was reported that Mrs. Jones would not cooperate with a full mental status examination. Mrs. Jones' mental status was described as waxing and waning, and she was diagnosed with a moderately severe encephalopathy related to multiple factors including a urinary tract infection, dehydration, and hypothyroidism. Stroke was ruled out.

Neuroimaging

A computed tomography (CT) scan of the brain done on 5/29/09 demonstrated mild diffuse atrophy, but was otherwise within normal limits. Magnetic resonance imaging (MRI) done on 6/02/09 revealed moderate diffuse atrophy and mild periventricular small vessel changes.

Current Medications

Based on a review of the Postacute Home medical charts on 7/19/09, Mrs. Jones is currently taking the following:

1. *Baby Aspirin for hypertension.*
2. *Colace 100 mg for constipation.*
3. *Lexipro 10 mg for depression.*

4. Nexium 40 mg for gastroesophageal reflux disease (GERD).
5. Synthroid 0.1 mg for hypothyroidism.
6. Lisinopril 2.5 mg for high blood pressure.
7. Ritalin 2.5 mg for mood.

Previous Psychiatric History

This was noncontributory.

Independent Living Skills

Mrs. Jones is currently residing at a postacute care center in Los Angeles. Per her report, she was independent in all activities of daily living, although she noted that she used a taxi service for transportation. She also reported that she was independent in all ADLs at the care center including walking, toileting, grooming, and eating. However, her report is at odds with the description of her level of functioning at home by family members. For example, it appeared that Mrs. Jones' usually reasonable housekeeping had declined, and her home was described as significantly unkempt. Also, she appeared to be ordering her meals for some time and was not cooking much. Her medication compliance was poor, and it is stated in her medical records that she had not been taking her prescription for thyroid (Synthroid) for an unknown length of time, resulting in hypothyroidism. According to the nursing staff at the care home, Mrs. Jones is dependent across ADL domains with the exception of feeding. They reported that Mrs. Jones has difficulty maintaining posture in a chair at the present time. It was also reported that she got out of bed and tried to walk the previous day, but fell. Overall, Mrs. Jones has poor insight into her functional abilities and will need assistance as she transitions back to her home.

This section highlights the discrepancy between the client's self-report and the level of functioning reported by staff and collaterals.

Financial Knowledge

Mrs. Jones was a mixed historian regarding her finances. She reported accurately that she receives approximately $2,000 per month from Social Security. She also knew that she owned her condominium "free and clear." She did not know the current market value of her condominium. When asked if she had any other investments or accounts, she reported that she didn't know. She thought her bank was Bank of America. She was unable to estimate her estate. Given Mrs. Jones' history as a shrewd and very successful businesswoman, these findings likely represent a decline in her functional abilities.

Note the specific examples of her basic life skills and financial knowledge in these sections.

Behavioral Observations

Mrs. Jones was in her bed when the examiner arrived. Her brother S.F. and niece Lisa F. arrived for a visit approximately 30 minutes into the interview and were present for about 30 minutes to assist with Mrs. Jones' social and medical background information. The entire interview and testing lasted approximately 3.5 hours.

Interpersonally, Mrs. Jones was friendly, but repeatedly would halt and ask, "What is this all about?" and needed to be reminded of the purpose of the interview. She presented as a charming woman who would use catch phrases such as "baby" rather than people's names. Her speech was normal in tone and prosody, although difficulties in finding words were noted. Her thought processes were at times tangential, but she was easily redirected. There was no evidence of perceptual disturbances.

Mrs. Jones's evidenced memory difficulties throughout the evaluation. She was not oriented to time, place, or situation. She stated the year as 2006, the season as winter, and the date as "March sometime." She reintroduced the examiner to her brother and niece when they returned to the room at the end of the assessment, forgetting they had been present earlier in the interview. She had difficulty recalling some aspects of her autobiographical past. A delirium screen assessing agitation, sleep/wake disturbances, perceptual disturbances, and variability in cognitive status indicated her delirium had resolved. Mrs. Jones appeared to be motivated to do her best. It is believed that these results provide a reasonable assessment of her current level of cognitive functioning.

Tests Administered

1. *Folstein Mini-Mental State Examination (MMSE)*
3. *Clock Drawing*
4. *Logical Memory I & II from the Wechsler Memory Scales–Revised.*
5. *Boston Naming Test*
6. *Digit Span*
7. *Trail-Making Test, Part A and B*
8. *FAS Word Fluency Test*
9. *Independent Living Scale (ILS) (Money Management Subtest select questions)*
10. *Geriatric Depression Scale*
11. *Delirium Scale*

This test battery contains all the aspects of a typical capacity battery with verbal memory, calculation, and executive functioning represented, among other domains. Although the MMSE has limited clinical utility in terms of diagnosis and capacity opinions, it is familiar to some attorneys and the courts and can be useful. In a higher functioning client, the CVLT-II may be added to evaluate verbal memory, as can additional executive functioning measures such as the Wisconsin Card Sort. Whereas the ILS has some calculation problems, the WRAT-IV arithmetic is a good addition for a less impaired individual. Finally, a grooved pegboard or another measure of motor activity may be helpful with laterality issues.

Table 9.1 Test Results*

Domain	Test	Score	Percentile	Interpretation
Mental Status	MMSE	19/30	<1	Severely impaired
Attention				
	Digit Span	12/16	90th	Superior
Language				
	Boston Naming Test	42	<10th	Moderately impaired
	FAS Fluency	16	<10th	Moderately impaired
Memory				
	MMSE recall	0/3		Impaired
	Orientation to time	0/5		Impaired
	Logical Memory I	9/75	2nd %	Moderately impaired
	Logical Memory II	0	<1	Severely impaired
Visual-Spatial				
	MMSE figure			Within normal limits
	Clock			Impaired
Executive Functioning				
	Trail-Making Test A	>3 minutes	< 1	Severely impaired
	Trail-Making Test B	>3 minutes	< 1	Severely impaired
Financial Skills	Money Management from ILS		SS = 20	Low range
Mood	GDS	3/15		Not depressed

* Using a table can help others read the report and make quick "apples to apples" comparisons between domains; it can also cut down on text for busy judges to read.

Test Results

Using a table (Table 9.1) can help others read the report and make quick "apples to apples" comparisons between domains; it can also cut down on text for busy judges to read.

Money Management

Mrs. Jones was administered the Managing Money subscale of the Independent Living Scale. She performed in the low range, indicating impaired performance. Mrs. Jones had difficulty writing a check and reading a "bill." She was able to do a simple calculation (make change from a $5.00) but did not attempt more complex items. Mrs. Jones presented as an individual with good baseline knowledge of financial matters. For example, she knew what Social Security was for, when taxes were due, and the general purpose of a will. However, her financial skills have declined, and she can no longer perform the steps necessary to manage her finances. These results likely represent a decline in her functional abilities related to financial management.

This section describes the functional assessment of independent living and financial management using the Independent Living Scales. This test allows for a standardized administration and some practical skills assessment such as bill paying.

SUMMARY/IMPRESSION

Neuropsychological Findings

The results of the neuropsychological test battery revealed that Mrs. Jones presents with significant neurocognitive deficits, greater than would be expected by age alone. Her neurocognitive profile appears consistent with a dementia syndrome as defined by the American Psychiatric Association's Diagnostic and Statistical Manual of Mental Disorders, 4th Edition, Text Revision (DSM-TR) (2000). Mrs. Jones retains some abilities (e.g., relatively intact attention, simple visual-spatial skills), but demonstrated significantly impaired performance across the domains of memory, language, executive functioning, and complex visual-spatial abilities. She reported that she was not depressed. A delirium screen assessing agitation, sleep/wake disturbances, perceptual disturbances, and variability in cognitive status indicated her delirium had resolved. When these findings are considered in light of her medical history, neuroimaging, and collateral data, they suggest a pattern consistent with a diagnosis of a progressive dementia process. Mrs. Jones has been reported to have evidenced a functional decline over at least the past 1 to 2 years, suggesting a progressive disorder. In addition, the MRI scan indicated moderate diffuse atrophy with no evidence of an acute event (stroke/traumatic brain injury), consistent with a progressive dementia process. Her clinical presentation, with intact social skills and adequate attention with very poor learning, word finding difficulties, impaired short-term and remote memory, and poor insight, is consistent with an diagnosis of Alzheimer's disease. Mrs. Jones is also at some increased risk given her family history of Alzheimer's disease.

This section describes cognitive impairment, differential diagnosis, and prognosis, similar to any other neuropsychological evaluation.

Conservatorship of the Person

In my clinical opinion, with a reasonable degree of certainty, a conservatorship of the person is necessary for Mrs. Jones. Mrs. Jones lacks adequate appreciation of her overall healthcare needs, general care requirements, and medical needs. For example, she tried to walk independently recently and fell. Despite adequate financial resources, Mrs. Jones does not appear to be able to hire and direct staff, secondary to poor memory and executive functioning resulting from a dementia syndrome. Mrs. Jones lacks insight into her functional limitations. As such, Mrs. Jones would benefit from assistance in this domain.

Conservatorship of the Estate

In my clinical opinion, with a reasonable degree of certainty, a conservatorship of the estate is necessary for Mrs. Jones. Financially, Mrs. Jones has evidenced a significant decline in her skills. By all accounts, Mrs. Jones was a successful businesswoman who had good financial skills. Her financial skills have declined as documented by her low score on the money management subtest. In addition, her memory is extremely poor, so that any financial decision requiring the ability to retrieve information from memory (i.e., "Did I already pay that bill?") will be at risk. In summary, because of impaired cognitive functioning and poor financial skills secondary to a dementia process, Mrs. Jones would benefit from assistance with the management of her estate.

These two sections address the legal issues from the referral. It is important to note that a clear opinion is expressed that integrates the cognitive assessment with her functional presentation. These two sections are often all that is carefully read by some interested parties, and as such, there must be enough information to support the opinion, not simply state it. In this case, the court determined that Mrs. Jones lacked capacity and a conservatorship was initiated for her person and estate.

Some psychologists are not comfortable with voicing an ultimate opinion, and if so, the evaluation should be described as a clinical finding rather than being used as a legal finding. In the courtroom, evidence will be collected from a number of parties, all of whom will typically voice a clear opinion. As such, we believe that the neuropsychologist should be willing to state an opinion, understanding that it will be only one source of data that the judge will use.

CONCLUSIONS

Neuropsychologists bring a number of critical skills to the area of civil capacity assessments. Standardized tools allow for presentation of objective data to the court. At the same time, cognitive information needs to be interpreted in light of the clients' functional abilities. Working with the ABA/APA model (ABA/APA, 2008) for the assessment of capacity can be helpful to ensure that a thorough weighing of all relevant factors is completed prior to expressing an opinion.

Test batteries will vary depending on the legal standard in question and the patient population, but, typically, they should include, at minimum, a thorough assessment of verbal memory, literacy, calculation, and executive functioning. A typical capacity evaluation will include an assessment of functional abilities and integrate the information to develop an opinion. Because courtroom testimony is rarely sought in capacity cases, reports need to be significantly detailed, written in a manner that will be accessible to attorneys, and contain a clearly stated opinion.

References

Allen, R. S., DeLaine, S. R., Chaplin, W. F., Marson, D. C., Bourgeois, M., Dijkstra, K., et al. (2003). Advance care planning in nursing homes: Correlates of capacity and possession of advance directives. *The Gerontologist, 43*, 309–317.

American Bar Association/American Psychological Association Assessment of Capacity in Older Adults Project Working Group. (2008). *Assessment of older adults with diminished capacity: A handbook for psychologists.* Washington, D.C.: American Bar Association and American Psychological Association.

American Bar Association (ABA), American Psychological Association (APA), & National College of Probate Judges (NCPJ). (2006). *Judicial determination of capacity of older adults in guardianship proceedings.* Washington, D.C.: American Bar Association and American Psychological Association.

American Bar Association Commission on Law, Aging & American Psychological Association. (2005). *Assessment of older adults with diminished capacity: A handbook for lawyers.* Washington, D.C.: American Bar Association and American Psychological Association.

American Psychiatric Association. (2000). *Diagnostic and statistical manual of mental disorders* (Revised 4th ed). Washington, D.C.: American Psychiatric Association.

California Department of Mental Health. (2010). *California Department of Mental Health Laws and Regulations.* San Francisco, CA: Barclays Official California Code of Regulations.

Fitten, L. J., Lusky, R., & Hamann, C. (1990). Assessing treatment decision-making capacity in elderly nursing home residents. *Journal of the American Geriatrics Society, 38*, 1097–1104.

Fitten, L. J., & Waite, M. S. (1990). Impact of medical hospitalization on treatment decision making capacity in the elderly. *Archives of Internal Medicine, 150*, 1717–1721.

Goldstein, A. M. (2006). *Forensic psychology: Emerging topics and expanding roles.* Hoboken, NJ: John Wiley & Sons.

Griffith, H. R., Belue, K., Sicola, A., Krzywanski, S., Zamrini, E., Harrell, L, & Marson, D. (2003). Impaired financial abilities in mild cognitive impairment: A direct assessment approach. *Neurology, 60*, 449–457.

Grisso, T. (1986). *Evaluating competencies.* New York: Plenum.

Grisso, T. (2003). *Evaluating competencies: Forensic assessments and instruments,* 2nd ed. New York: Kluwer Academic.

Grisso, T., & Appelbaum, P. S. (1995). Comparison of standards for assessing patients' capacities to make treatment decisions. *American Journal of Psychiatry, 152*, 1033–1037.

Gurrera, R. J., Moye, J., Karel, M. J., Azar, A. R., & Armesto, J. C. (2006). Cognitive performance predicts treatment decisional abilities in mild to moderate dementia. *Neurology, 66*, 1367–1372.

Karel, M. J., Moye, J., Bank, A., & Azar, A. R. (2007). Three methods of assessing values for advance care planning comparing persons with and without dementia. *Journal of Aging and Health, 19*, 123–151.

Liberman, J. D, Krauss, D. A., & Kryger, M. (2007). Determining dangerousness in sexually violent predator evaluations: Cognitive-experiential self-theory and jury judgments of expert testimony. *Behavioral Sciences and the Law, 25,* 507–526.

Loeb, P. A. (1996). *Independent living scales.* San Antonio, TX: Psychological Corp.

Markson, L. J., Kern, D. C., Annas, G. J., & Glantz, L. H. (1994). Physician assessment of patient competence. *Journal of the American Geriatrics Society, 42*, 1074–1080.

Marson, D. C., Chatterjee, A., Ingram, K. K., & Harrell, L. E. (1996). Toward a neurologic model of competency: Cognitive predictors of capacity to consent in Alzheimer's disease using three different legal standards. *Neurology, 46*, 666–672.

Marson, D. C., Earnst, K. S., Jamil, F., Bartolucci, A., & Harrell, L. E. (2000). Consistency of physicians' legal standard and personal judgments of competency in patients with Alzheimer's disease. *Journal of the American Geriatrics Society, 48*, 911–918.

Marson, D. C., & Hebert, T. (2008). Financial capacity. In B. L. Cutler (Ed.), *Encyclopedia of psychology and the law* (Vol. 1, pp. 313–316). Thousand Oaks, CA: Sage.

Marson, D. C., McInturff, B., Hawkins, L., Bartolucci, A., & Harrell, L. E. (1997). Consistency of physician judgments of capacity to consent in mild Alzheimer's disease. *The American Geriatrics Society, 45*, 453–457.

Marson, D. C., Sawrie, S., McInturff, B., Snyder, S., Chatterjee, A., Stalvey, T., Boothe, A., & Harrell, L. (2000). Assessing financial capacity in patients with Alzheimer's disease: A conceptual model and prototype instrument. *Archives of Neurology, 57*, 877–884.

Martin, R., Griffith, R., Belue, K., Harrell, L., Zamrini, E., Anderson, B., Bartolucci, A., & Marson, D. (2008). Declining financial capacity in patients with mild Alzheimer's disease: A one-year longitudinal study. *American Journal of Geriatric Psychiatry, 16*, 209–219.

Melton, G. B., Petrila, J., Poythress, N. G., & Slobogin, C. (2007). *Psychological evaluations for the courts; A handbook for mental health professionals and lawyers.* New York: Guilford.

Moberg, P. J., & Kniele, K. (2006). Evaluation of competency: Ethical considerations for neuropsychologists. *Applied Neuropsychology, 13,* 101–114.

Moye, J. (1999) Assessment of competency and decision making capacity. In P. A. Lichtenberg (Ed.), *Handbook of assessment in clinical gerontology* (pp. 488–528). New York: John Wiley.

Moye, J., Karel, M. J., Azar, A. R., & Gurrera, R. J. (2004). Capacity to consent to treatment: Empirical comparison of three instruments in older adults with and without dementia. *Gerontologist, 44,* 166–175.

Moye, J., Wood, E., Edelstein, B., Wood, S., Bower, E. H., Harrison, J. A., et al. (2007). Statutory reform is associated with improved court practice: Results of a tri-state study. *Behavioral Sciences and the Law, 25*, 425–436.

Palmer, B. W., & Salva, G. N. (2007). The association of specific neuropsychological deficits with capacity to consent to research or treatment. *Journal of the International Neuropsychological Society, 13,* 1047–1059.

Rutman, D., & Silberfeld, M. (1992). A preliminary report on the discrepancy between clinical and test evaluations of competency. *Canadian Journal of Psychiatry, 37*, 634–639.

Sabatino, C. P., & Basinger, S. L. (2000). Competency: Reforming our legal fictions. *Journal of Mental Health & Aging, 6*, 116–144.

Schmand, B., Gouwenberg, B., Smit, J. H., & Jonker, C. (1999). Assessment of mental competency in community-swelling elderly. *Alzheimer Disease and Associated Disorders, 13*, 80–87.

Spar, J. E., & Garb, A. S. (1992). Assessing competency to make a will. *American Journal of Psychiatry, 149*, 169–174.

Staats, N., & Edelstein, B. (1995). *Cognitive changes associated with the declining competency of older adults.* Paper presented at the Gerontological Society of America, Los Angeles.

Uniform Guardianship and Protective Proceedings Act § 102(5) (1997). Retrieved on January 26, 2011 from http://www.law.upenn.edu/bll/ulc/fnact99/1990s/ugppa97.htm.

Vellinga, A., Smit, J. H., van Leeuwen, E., van Tilburg, W., & Jonker, C. (2004). Competence to consent to treatment of geriatric patients: Judgments of physicians, family members and the vignette method. *International Journal of Geriatric Psychiatry, 19*, 645.

Wood, S. (2007). Assessment of decisional capacity from a neuropsychological perspective. In M. Smyers & S. Qualls (Eds.), *Aging and decision-making capacity: Clinical family, and legal issues. Wiley Clinical Gerontology Series.* New York: John Wiley.

Wood, S., Rakela, B., Navarro, A., Fujikawa, K., Bernatz, S., Wilber, K., & Schneider, D. (2010). *Neuropsychological data as clinical evidence at the Los Angeles County Elder Abuse Forensic Center.* Part of the National Institute of Justice (NIJ) sponsored panel entitled "Memory, Capacity and Reliability Issues in Elder Abuse Prosecution and Research," presented at the American Psychology and Law Society Conference, March 20, 2010, Vancouver, CA.

10

Civil Capacity Instruments: Research Trends and Recommendations for Future Research

KAREN A. SULLIVAN

Almost 10 years ago, Edelstein and colleagues wrote that a major challenge for those developing tests of civil decision-making capacity was in knowing what to measure (Edelstein, Nygren, Northrop, Staats, & Pool, 1993, p. 182). The same challenge faces those wishing to evaluate such instruments, since such evaluations need to be based on an agreement about what these tests should measure. Although general definitions of decision-making capacity exist, defining what is an evolving construct and therefore identifying an appropriate methodology to assess it remain a challenge. It has been suggested that the only gold standard against which the criterion validity of capacity tests might be determined is the court decision (Hotopf, 2005), but this position is disputed by others (Mullaly et al., 2007).

The debate about how best to assess capacity is a long-standing and controversial one. Glass's early 1997 review of the literature on assessing mental competence concluded that despite a continuing lack of agreement about how to assess capacity, progress had been made as indicated by an apparent "evolution in thought" and a willingness "to view patients on an individual basis" taking account of their "beliefs, values and preferences established over a lifetime" (Glass, 1997, p. 33). At about the same time and prompted by Appelbaum and Grisso's early work on the MacArthur Treatment Competence Study, Kapp and Mossman (1996) wrote about the dangers of constructing a "capacimeter." They warned that the "continuing search for the elusive 'holy grail' test of capacity [should] proceed with great caution (if at all)" (p. 73). More recently, Moye and Marson (2009) writing about capacity assessment in older adults echoed both the optimism and caution evident in these statements. They argued that the accumulated body of knowledge about capacity assessment "provides a first pass at many of the key questions related to capacity assessment, but additional studies that replicate, extend and improve on this research are urgently needed" (p. 88). This position is endorsed in this chapter.

The on-the-ground experiences of clinical neuropsychologists who assess capacity are documented in the literature. Accounts of the clinical realities of capacity assessment in terms of time, cost, and in some cases, urgency, as well as the diversity of referral questions presented as capacity assessments are appearing (see Mullaly et al., 2007). The need to consider these practical aspects of capacity assessment with the evidence regarding optimal assessment practices is clearly important. The question of the place of capacity assessments in the work mix of a hospital-based clinical neuropsychologist has been raised vis-à-vis traditional diagnostic services. These issues cannot be ignored as they have the potential to impact both test selection and assessment approach and ultimately the standard of services offered. There is some evidence to suggest that such factors not only *could* but very probably *are* influencing the capacity assessment practices of neuropsychologists. For example, in the recent review by Pinsker, Pachana, Wilson, Tilse, and Byrne (2010) of financial capacity assessment instruments, the accessibility or availability of selected test instruments was noted as a factor in their utility, alongside traditional test selection criteria such as test reliability and validity. Thus, it is important to develop the empirical literature around capacity assessment, while at the same time addressing issues of the application of this research in professional practice settings. If adjustments in clinical practice need to be made on the basis of the best available evidence, appropriate solutions may be explored. Until that time, it is important to keep understanding of these issues advancing but separate so that the science is not hampered by the current limits on clinical practice.

In terms of the best available tests for assessing a specific type of decision-making capacity, the other chapters in this volume provide valuable guidance. Specific tests of capacity are not the focus of this chapter. The focus is on the broader issues of capacity assessment. This subject matter is approached in a number of ways, including an analysis of trends in the capacity assessment literature. Indeed, the question that drives this chapter is partly reflected by Glass's (1997, p. 10) comments about capacity assessment that, although we have come a long way, "there are no criteria or methodologies for determining competence in a medical context that are well accepted by all disciplines." A view of capacity assessments that considers the methods used by other professionals provides a broader perspective on these issues. This chapter also discusses clinical algorithms that describe an approach to capacity assessments used by medical professionals, some of which explicitly identify the point at which a neuropsychological assessment is indicated.

A key purpose of this chapter is to stimulate the ongoing efforts of clinicians and researchers to develop a richer evidence base for capacity evaluation, and this chapter thus concludes with practical recommendations. These are somewhat challenging; they suggest that additional research effort aimed at developing new tests may not be the best way forward and that optimizing the evidence base for existing measures may be a better use of resources. Implicit in this view is that neuropsychologists are facing a challenge to contribute to the research and debate around the issue of appropriate instrumentation and practice in relation to capacity assessments; if this is not done our place in this process will be determined for us. Moreover, it is timely that we extend our vision to develop and test a model of practice in this area.

Although the broader ethical issues associated with assessment of capacity are only touched on in this chapter, it is important to read this chapter keeping in mind the purpose of capacity assessments. This purpose is well described by Glass (1997), who suggests that capacity assessments have "dual ends, empowerment and protection, empowerment of those capable of making informed choices and protection of those who are unable to do so" (p. 32). Though this purpose is the fundamental reason why capacity assessments are conducted, there may be other uses to which such assessments could be put, depending on how they are conducted. It has been suggested that when such assessments occur in the context of a detailed neuropsychological assessment, they may be able to identify the reasons why capacity is impaired, if there are cognitive reasons for this impairment (Sullivan, 2004). Appropriate remediation strategies might then be developed on the basis of information about the client's cognitive strengths and weaknesses (Sullivan, 2004).

Furthermore, it has been argued that the timing of the assessment, whether it is to demonstrate current capacity in anticipation of future challenges as might occur in the assessment of testamentary capacity or it is to determine current capacity in an urgent medical situation, is also a factor that influences assessment practices (Sullivan, 2004). Thus, although the fundamental purpose of capacity assessments has not changed, the situations in which such questions arise have altered, as have important contextual factors. Early on, these situations predominantly involved questions about capacity to consent to treatment and research participation. At this time, the patient's capacity to make other decisions, such as about wills may also come into question. There is now greater variation in the critical parameters that may influence capacity assessment, including the urgency of the decision, and, indeed, the type of decision that has implications for the availability of specific tests. This change brings with it the opportunity to reconsider the purpose of a neuropsychological capacity assessment. Although at its core it must still address the fundamental issue of protection and empowerment, other important purposes might also be served by a comprehensive neuropsychological assessment of capacity.

TRENDS IN THE LITERATURE

Almost 10 years ago it was predicted that capacity assessment would be a growth area of neuropsychology (Sullivan, 2004). This prediction is one that continues to be echoed (Moye & Marson, 2007). The research in this area, including new test developments, has been steadily growing and changing in its emphasis. Some of the major trends in the literature are described in the following section.

Changing Terminology

Various terms are used in the literature to describe tests of decision-making capacity. In the area of testamentary capacity, for example, these terms include the word test. This term does not refer to a test as a neuropsychologist might understand it, but rather to the legal test that might apply. Shulman and colleagues refer to task-specific criteria for testamentary capacity, and Jacoby and Steer (2007, p. 155) have a list of the tests for testamentary capacity, both of which are in fact derived from legal judgments. Other terms that are used in the capacity literature include the following: "performance-based measures" (Leifker, Patterson, Bowie, Mausbach, & Harvey, 2010; Pinsker et al., 2010), "direct performance measures" (Baird, Solcz, Gale-Ross, & Blake, 2009), "direct assessment" (Lowenstein et al., 1989), "purpose-built tests" (Sullivan, 2004), and "direct assessment" methods (Griffith et al., 2003). Apart from neuropsychological tests, or tests in the legal sense of the word, the term that appears to be gaining the most traction in the literature to describe a method of assessing capacity is performance-based measures. In this chapter this term is used to denote those measures (including tests and interviews) that assess the ability to perform tasks that are thought to be more directly related to capacity than more indirect measures such as neuropsychological tests.

Debate about the Qualifications and Skills Necessary for Those Who Conduct Capacity Assessments

Professional debate continues as to who should conduct capacity assessments. Although this question may seem somewhat trivial, as it may not matter whether a physician or a neuropsychologist assesses capacity as long as the assessment is valid and reliable, it serves to highlight some important issues. At one level, it may be argued that this debate is consolidating in some areas, as indicated by the emergence of consensus statements and joint interprofessional guidelines (e.g., American Bar Assocation Commission on Law and Aging & American Psychological Association, 2005; Maeck & Stoppe, 2008). However, the issues that underline some of the debate are not fully resolved. For example, the recent European Dementia Consensus Network (EDCON) statement on the assessment of competence contains the following recommendation: "the assessment of competence requires special skills and should be performed by persons who can use currently available methods in an optimal manner" (Maeck & Stoppe, 2008, p. 10). Though emphasizing important general principles of assessment and test selection, the EDCON recommendations tolerate a diversity of practice. There is no definition of the special skills required to conduct such assessments, no specification of the minimum level of qualifications necessary to conduct such assessments, and no definition of "currently available methods."

Although absent in documents such as the EDCON statement, the statements of other entities provide recommendations about the skill set required to conduct capacity assessment. In some cases, the setting of standards in relation to appropriate assessment skills, knowledge, or training has been left to the test publishers. For example, the Independent Living Scales (ILS) (Loeb, 1996), which has subscales to assess both financial and health-related decision-making ability, is restricted to professionals from psychology or allied health areas. Individuals who interpret the ILS "ideally will have completed a master's level program, or the equivalent, that included individual standardized assessment; persons qualified to interpret the ILS may include psychiatrists, social workers, nurses, occupational therapists, and individuals in psychology or a related field" (p. 3). There may be other circumstances in which the test publisher defines the user qualifications or standard of training necessary to use a test in the absence of a professional consensus.

A different aspect of this issue is highlighted by Dunn and colleagues' (2006) review of instruments for assessing clinical research and treatment decision making. They reviewed 23 of these instruments for use among older adults, 15 of which assessed decisional capacity for treatment. This review found that only a handful of tests contained training materials. Thus, even if access to the test is not determined by the publisher's standards or supported by their training resources and documentation, independently produced tests *could* provide such support to users. A test with training materials is usually regarded as more likely to support standardized use and improve administration and scoring consistency and accuracy. Developing support and training materials for those capacity tests that do not already have them, and considering the quality and appropriateness of those materials for tests that already do, is an important focus for future research.

At another level, the question of who should conduct capacity assessments raises a related ethical issue about whether capacity assessments should be conducted by an independent party or the treating team. As in other spheres of clinical neuropsychology, these roles conflict and need to be considered separately. Most recently this issue was raised, albeit indirectly, in a letter to the editor by three psychiatrists (Querques, Kontos, & Freudenreich, 2010). Writing on the topic of who can evaluate capacity, and whether such assessments should be performed only by psychiatrists, Querques and colleagues offered a counter position, arguing that "Any physician can evaluate a [person's] decision-making capacity, and the physician most familiar with a patient is often best positioned to do so" (p. 1614). Whether this assumption is borne out in the empirical literature is unclear, but from an ethical standpoint we must consider the possibility that dual relationships may hamper, rather than facilitate, capacity assessments. Unless and until the evidence suggests otherwise, it may be wise to invoke established ethical and practice standards and avoid capacity assessments performed solely by the treating health professional.

A Broader Realm of Factors to Assess

Although Glass's comments highlighted the importance of assessing a range of aspects of functioning in a client whose capacity is in question, the need to include factors other than the interpersonal has been recently articulated. This idea may be implicit in the comment by Querques et al. (2010) above if this comment is read as suggesting that such assessments are facilitated by a thorough knowledge of the client, including his or her values and beliefs, as well as other contextual factors. However, such an aim can be achieved without risking the complications that can arise from dual relationships. With adequate history taking and efforts to corroborate data a full picture of the client can be gained. This general assessment principle—the need to corroborate data where possible—is one that is familiar to neuropsychologists. It is also indicated specifically in the capacity literature. Newberry and Pachet (2008) and others (e.g., O'Connor, Hall, & Donnelly, 2009; Pinsker et al., 2010) have highlighted the importance of assessing for the presence of undue influence. This group of authors make the point that decision-making capacity occurs in a social context, thus it behooves psychologists to assess a range of other factors such as psychological, social,and environmental influences on capacity, as well as the cognitive functions that underlie complex decision making.

Guidelines for Assessing Capacity in the Context of Specific Pathologies

Another trend in the literature is the emergence of practice statements and guidelines for assessing capacity for individuals with specific pathologies. For example, Johnson-Greene (2010) has written about capacity assessment in traumatic brain injury. Others have written about capacity assessment with the following client groups: older adults (Moye & Marson, 2009), persons with mild cognitive impairment and dementia (e.g., Okonkwo, Wadley, Griffith, Ball, & Marson, 2006), adults with intellectual disability (Willner, Bailey, Parry, & Dymond, 2010), people with psychiatric conditions, especially those likely to involve involuntary treatment (Etchells et al., 1997), and individuals with terminal illness (Meyers Sorger, Rosenfeld, Pessin, Kosinski Timm, & Cimino, 2007). The recent emergence of these articles provides valuable guidance specific to a particular client or work setting and highlights issues that are relevant to specific disorders, such as the likely course of cognitive change. More broadly, however, the emergence of these articles suggests a question about whether tests and assessment methods for specific disorders/diseases or age groups are needed or whether models of assessment that generalize across settings and pathologies can be developed. Rather than generating new and separate tests for each group, it may be possible to consolidate this effort to develop methodologies that are sensitive to the core principles of capacity assessment. Nevertheless, examining the performance of existing tests in diverse populations is an important consideration for future research.

What Do Neuropsychologists Do When They Assess Capacity?

Given that there are numerous approaches to assessing capacity, and numerous observations in the literature about which of these methods is most commonly used for this purpose, it is of interest to consider the data on this issue. There are a handful of studies that provide information on this issue, including some archival analyses and case reviews. This literature includes practice surveys of psychiatrists, for example, that seek to determine if those professionals know the elements of decision-making assessment as articulated by Grisso and Appelbaum (Hill, Mather, & James, 2006). However, such studies of professional knowledge do not address how capacity decisions are made nor do they specify the accuracy of such assessments. Although such studies might indicate whether there are professional development and training needs for capacity assessment, it is important that research that describes this practice move beyond the task of documenting whether professionals know what to do (or what they say they do) and move to assessing both what and how they actually perform capacity assessments, and how that practice relates to established external validity criteria.

The data most directly relevant to this chapter are from a recent practice survey of neuropsychologists. An emailed survey completed by 52 Australian neuropsychologists showed that most neuropsychologists use a combination of formal testing and targeted interviewing when assessing capacity (Mullaly et al., 2007). Standard neuropsychological tests, such as the Wechsler scales, were used by over 75% of this sample in capacity evaluations. Other methods of seeking information that were always used by at least half of these survey respondents were, in order from highest to least frequently endorsed, history-taking interview (92%), standardized tests (83%), information from files (79%), and semi-structured interview (71%). Over half of this sample reported that they never gathered information for their assessment from a questionnaire to family/carer (59%). The use of functional assessment as indicated by percentage endorsement was almost evenly split across the response options with between 10% and 25% of the sample indicating that this method was either always, often, sometimes, rarely, or never used. Thus, there appears to be a high degree of variability in the use of functional measures by neuropsychologists. Use of other methods of assessments was also reported, but this survey did not present data that would enable specific identification of neuropsychologists' use of performance-based tests.

Whether the capacity assessment approach that was most commonly used in this sample (i.e., the use of standard neuropsychological tests in combination with targeted interviewing) is optimal for capacity assessment is debated by Mullaly and colleagues (2007). The risk of this approach, they warn, is that it may introduce "further complexity and additional sources of uncertainty when conflicting information emerges" (p. 179). As noted elsewhere in this chapter, there may be different views about the purposes of a neuropsychological assessment of capacity, depending on the referral question or type of capacity being assessed. Nevertheless, although the point made by Mullaly and colleagues is an important one, it needs to be considered in context. That is, the general issue of how information from multiple sources should be weighted and interpreted is of concern in any neuropsychological assessment, not just capacity assessments. Thus, the broader clinical decision-making literature on identifying an appropriate methodology for investigating this issue empirically may provide guidance as to how such studies should proceed when the question of how to combine information from multiple sources in a capacity assessment arises.

Other issues highlighted in this survey include the issue of obtaining consent to assess decision-making capacity. When a specific capacity is in question it is possible that the capacity to consent to an assessment of that specific capacity is also impaired. Thus, akin to assessing capacity to consent to treatment or research specifically, the capacity to consent to an assessment of capacity is raised by this study. Less than 40% of respondents always "made their clients aware of the nature of the assessment" (Mullaly et al., 2007, p. 181), and when they did so, in most cases, consent was obtained verbally as opposed to in writing.

Professional confidence about contributing to capacity determinations was also assessed in this survey. Fifty-two percent of those people surveyed agreed with the statement "Assessing decision-making capacity is more difficult than other aspects of neuropsychological practice" (Mullaly et al., 2007, p. 182), and a slightly higher number (62%) agreed that "Once the assessment is completed, I usually feel confident about my conclusions." These data are important for several reasons. First, they highlight judgment confidence in capacity assessments, and this factor can be included in studies of capacity assessment accuracy as it has been in other areas of clinical decision-making research. Second, if this area of clinical practice is perceived to be a more complex area than other areas of practice, it suggests the need for further training. Third, if these data are seen as providing a general indicator of the level of professional confidence in capacity assessments, the level of confidence in these judgments appears to be relatively low. Although it would be ideal to have data on the level of confidence about the conclusions from capacity and noncapacity assessments to provide some context for these figures, these data may provide an explanation for why, with a few notable exceptions, neuropsychologists have been slow to develop practice models in this area.

The Question of External Validity: What Is an Appropriate Criterion?

The comments at the beginning of this chapter suggest that it may be difficult to reach agreement about an appropriate gold standard against which new tests of capacity might be compared. Mullaly et al. (2007) correctly observe that the outcome against which such comparisons are made requires careful consideration. They suggest that comparison of neuropsychologists' decision-making capacity recommendations against legal decisions may not be ideal given the differences between capacity assessments and legal determination of competence. Instead, they argue that a better standard is the ability of the patient to carry out decisions, and they suggest that this approach is preferred over outcomes that include the decision-making process itself. These observations are important, but they too need to be supported by the evidence. A prospective study that examines a patient's ability to carry out decisions is likely to be difficult in terms of feasibility and replicability. Furthermore, if the neuropsychologist's assessment of cognitive abilities reveals that an individual has intact decision-making capacity, and that outcome is compared with the results of an assessment from a functional test (e.g., counting money), this comparison, like the comparison between neuropsychological test scores and legal decisions, is arguably a comparison of related but different outcomes. A retrospective study of outcomes versus clinical decisions would be more cost-effective than a prospective study of the type just described; however, it too would provide limited insights into how such decisions were reached and therefore how they might be replicated or optimized. The issue of how to identify an appropriate external validity criterion is one that is discussed again later in this chapter where we will see that various standards are used. We will also see that the standard that is most often used is physicians' clinical judgment.

Algorithmic Approaches to Capacity Assessment

Several algorithms for structuring the clinical interview, and more broadly, the process for assessing decision-making capacity, have been published (e.g., Gibson & Ferrini, 2010; Jones & Holden, 2004; Michels et al., 2010; Miller & Marin, 2000). These algorithms appear as decision trees or flow charts whereby a set of actions or further questions are indicated dependent on the outcome of the preceding step, and the questions that flow from one outcome differ from the questions or actions that would be suggested by a different outcome at that step. Although an algorithm might include a set of questions, it may also recommend a method of generating an answer to such questions, such as when to refer to others for assistance.

The algorithm for assessing decision-making capacity described by Jones and Holden (2004) includes five key questions. First: Does the history and physical examination confirm that the patient can communicate a choice? Second: Does the person demonstrate an understanding of the necessary elements for this choice to be an informed one? Third: Can the person assign personal values to the risks or benefits of the choice? Fourth: Can the person manipulate information rationally and logically? Fifth: Is there stability in the choice expressed over time? In elaborating on the details forming the basis for each of these steps, Jones and Holden (2004) comment that some steps, such as steps one and two, may be impacted by disruption in short-term memory, or deficits in attention span, but no advice is given as to how to determine the presence of such deficits, and no advice is offered as to how to combine information gathered in response to these questions.

The family physician algorithm for assessing capacity to consent to treatment presented by Michels and colleagues covers an extended process (Michels et al., 2010). In this algorithm, decision-making capacity is assessed by the family physician and referral to a neuropsychologist is suggested if there is uncertainty about the conclusion or if an urgent decision is required and there is no advanced directive or surrogate decision maker (Michels et al., 2010). In driving capacity, Michels and colleagues (2010) advocate physician assessment of cognition using the Trail Making Test (Part B) and the clock drawing test; referral to a neuropsychologist is recommended to clarify the causes of cognitive impairment (if there are any) rather than to determine capacity per se. Thus, in fitness to drive assessments the use of selected cognitive tests by the assessing physician is a recommended part of the initial capacity assessment process rather than immediate referral to a neuropsychologist. These ideas are echoed by Hotopf, who writes that although "all registered medical practitioners should be able to assess capacity" (Hotopf, 2005, p. 583), a second opinion is recommended if "the decision has significant consequences" or if there are difficulties in identifying the cause of the impairments that are contributing to the incapacity (Hotopf, 2005).

The algorithm described by Gibson and Ferrini (2010) is particularly designed to assist with decision-making capacity assessments of individuals in long-term care because the formal assessments that can be provided by geriatric neuropsychology are "not available in all settings or at the time when decisions need to be made" (p. 25) and that such assessments may not be "justified" or "suited" to the types of questions that may arise in long-term care (e.g., "Does the person have the capacity to make a decision about engaging in an intimate relationship with another patient?"). Instead Gibson and Ferrini suggest that "formal geriatric neuropsychology may be more suited to 'legal' issues such as testamentary capacity" (Gibson & Ferrini, 2010, p. 25).

These three algorithms for assessing capacity have been primarily provided as a guide for medical practitioners and are helpful because they articulate a process that can be followed and they make the recommended steps explicit. These algorithms identify various roles for clinical neuropsychologists in this process. Jones and Holden's model does not formally identify a role for neuropsychologists; Michel and colleagues' algorithm identifies a role that is specific to capacity assessments, but they also recommend involving neuropsychologists in capacity assessments for more traditional "diagnostic" services; and Gibson and Ferrini see an important role for neuropsychological assessment in selected capacity assessments. It is important to consider the extent to which such recommendations align with the ways in which neuropsychologists contribute to such assessments, or indeed, the degree to which such recommendations match the evidence on best assessment practice. In Australia and elsewhere, it appears that some neuropsychologists in medical settings agree that their role is in complex cases only (e.g., Bradshaw, Pangnadasa-Fox, & McGregor, 2010). Similar views have been developed by other professional groups. Psychiatrists, for example, point out that capacity assessment does not require referral to a specialist as "any physician can evaluate capacity . . . [and they do so] . . . all the time without even realizing it" (Querques et al., 2010, p. 1614). Developing an understanding of the factors that determine when specialist input is warranted and when it is not is important. Clearly, capacity does not need to be tested for every decision or every time a decision is made. However, in some of this literature, constraints on practice appear to dominate the discussion on how to proceed. As a description of practice, these algorithms may be useful, but as a model of evidence-based best practice they are limited in what they communicate. Moye and Marson (2007) have already articulated the need to identify markers or indicators or triggers that might be helpful in suggesting when a formal capacity assessment is needed, but more research on this issue is needed.

Existing algorithms have yet to identify a role for clinical neuropsychologists in the remediation of causes of the lack of capacity, if these are remediable, or in the education of other health professionals about such assessments, even though such roles are discussed by neuropsychologists (Zombor, Mullaly, & Morriss, 2010). These algorithms also do not proscribe an initial neuropsychological examination prior to other examinations, even though this suggestion has been made in the driving capacity literature where individuals who fail a neuropsychological screen are sent for further examinations, such as an on-road driving test (Johansson & Lundberg, 2008). This possibility suggests a variation in the timing of neuropsychological assessment compared to the suggested points at which such assessments might occur in capacity assessment algorithms. However, the properties of tests that are used as early screens versus later in the diagnostic process vary considerably (e.g., sensitivity and specificity), as do the base rates related to capacity. This variability is currently difficult to factor into decisions about instruments, partly because of a lack of research in this area and partly because of the failure of some studies to include data on relevant clinical parameters such as sensitivity and specificity.

Clinical Interviews and Early Indicators of the Need to Assess Decision-Making Capacity

Clinical interviews are the most common method of assessing some types of decision-making capacity, such as financial decision making. This assessment method is also critiqued because some cognitive disorders may be difficult to detect solely on the basis of a casual office or bedside interview (Wood, 2007). The American Bar Association and the American Psychological Association warn that use of such methods may be particularly problematic if certain indicators are present, such as changes in communication or memory (American Bar Assocation Commission on Law and Aging & American Psychological Association, 2005).

Although important, this caveat may not be sufficient, for example, in cases of subtle cognitive decline in which such indicators are not yet manifest. It is possible that cognitive changes have occurred but they have not yet been reported or expressed as a history of changes in communication or memory. In situations that involve undue influence, where assessors may be particularly reliant on a history from other parties, the risk of missing such indicators may be even greater. The limitations of informant self-discrepancies in reports of functional skills or knowledge that may be related to financial capacity have recently been documented (Okonkwo et al., 2008). Assessments that rely on a clinical interview only, including ones that assess through question and answer responses to questions such as those articulated by Jones and Holden, may miss the detail that could be provided by a comprehensive neuropsychological assessment.

The attempt to identify the indicators that could be used as a guide to when to refer a patient for a neuropsychological assessment is an advance over the general guidelines that are provided elsewhere (e.g., refer for a neuropsychological assessment in "complex cases," or "when a second opinion would be helpful"); however, as argued above, this approach also has limitations. It should be possible to put the candidate variables to an empirical test to determine if and to what extent each of these variables is a significant predictor of incapacity.

Views on the Use of Neuropsychological Tests in Capacity Assessment

Mullaly and colleagues' (2007) neuropsychological capacity assessment practice survey highlighted divergent views about the role of neuropsychological tests in capacity assessments. The themes in the current discussion are also evident in earlier commentary on this issue. In 1997, Glass wrote that tests of intelligence, memory, mental status, and neuropsychological examinations were "commonly used to determine competency" (p. 15). This observation was followed by the comment that such tests are "insufficient" (p. 15) or "completely inappropriate" (p. 15) for the purposes of evaluating competency because they do not assess the specific task or factors relevant to a decision that needs to be made. As noted above, similar comments are evident in the literature today, albeit sometimes with further specification of situations that might constitute an exception to this rule (e.g., Gibson & Ferrini, 2010).

An opposite position has also been expressed (Pinsker et al., 2010; Sullivan, 2004), and indeed neuropsychological assessment has been described as playing a "critical" role in capacity assessments (Wood, 2007, p. 191). This tension about when and how neuropsychologists might be involved in capacity assessments provides an opportunity to develop this role, or indeed multiple roles, that, in Australia at least, has grown to include the education of other professionals about capacity assessments (Zombor et al., 2010).

Neuropsychological assessment commonly involves a clinical interview and standardized tests of cognitive and affective state. It may involve collateral information gathering, including interviews with family or other stakeholders (Michels et al., 2010). The cognitive functions assessed may include intellectual functioning, attention, memory, language, and executive functions. Neuropsychological tests measure purported correlates of capacity, rather than decision-making capacity per se (Pinsker et al., 2010). A challenge for neuropsychologists is to build on the existing, but limited, evidence base validating the relationships between neuropsychological measures and real-world decision-making abilities, since the findings from such studies have not always been positive or consistent. Nevertheless, the inclusion of both functional and neuropsychological measures in capacity decisions has been recommended (Pinsker et al., 2010; Sullivan, 2004).

Advice on Choosing Standard Neuropsychological Tests for Use in Capacity Assessments

There are several ways to approach the question of which cognitive domains or abilities should be assessed and, therefore, which neuropsychological tests may be most useful in capacity assessments. The comments on this issue offered here are, by necessity, relatively general and are followed up in detail elsewhere in this volume. However, in this section some of the key issues to test selection decisions are discussed.

The first way to approach this issue is to consult the list of recommended functions to assess that have been generated by experts such as Moye (1999) or the

American Bar Association and American Psychological Association (American Bar Assocation Commission on Law and Aging & American Psychological Association, 2005). The second approach is look to the evidence from studies that have examined the relationship between neuropsychological test performances as predictors of capacity decisions. As seen in other chapters, further research of this type is needed because the evidence base comes primarily from studies of financial decision making (e.g., Hoskin, Jackson, & Crowe, 2005), and in some instances the populations studied have been relatively limited. This literature suggests that the relationship between predictors and criterion may be different for different groups. A third approach might be to consider the four elements of decision making (as defined by Grisso and Appelbaum)—communication, reasoning, expression, and choice—and to select neuropsychological measures that target the skills that underlie these abilities (such as expressive language skills or novel problem-solving tasks), either selectively if problems are suspected in relation to communication only, or comprehensively, across all four domains. Finally, using the data from practice surveys is another way of reasoning through test selection decisions.

However, a theme of this chapter is that capacity assessments should be viewed in a manner similar to other neuropsychological assessments, and that the general principles that neuropsychologists use to guide other test selection decisions, including those that are applicable in forensic neuropsychology settings, should also be applied to capacity test selection decisions. Heilbrun's advice on this issue provides some key criteria to consider when choosing a test (Heilbrun, 1992). In addition to these principles, an understanding of the relevant legal precedents is important, since capacity assessments may be resolved in court. These criteria should be brought to bear in the selection of neuropsychological tests as well as the performance-based measures that may be used in capacity assessments.

Advice on Choosing "Performance-Based" Measures of Decision-Making Capacity

In an early attempt to identify performance-based measures of capacity (Sullivan, 2004), 12 measures of capacity to consent to treatment were identified, most of which were structured patient interviews. Since that time, there has been a proliferation of new measures, some diversification of approach, growth in the evidence base for the more established measures, and translation of some tests to languages other than English. Currently, there are performance-based tests for some types of decision making such as financial decision making and driving, but not for others (e.g., testamentary capacity). More detail on these measures is provided in other chapters.

The literature in this area has grown and test reviews are now appearing. There have been several relatively recent reviews of capacity instruments related to medical treatment (Dunn, Nowrangi, Palmer, Jeste, & Saks, 2006; Moye, 2003; Moye, Gurrera, Karel, Edelstein, & O'Connell, 2006; Okai et al., 2007; Sturman, 2005), financial decision making (Pinsker et al., 2010), testamentary capacity

(Roked & Patel, 2008; Shulman, Peisah, Jacoby, Heinik, & Finkel, 2009), and so-called "office-based" or "frontline" tests of driving capacity (Molnar, Patel, Marshall, Man-Son-Hing, & Wilson, 2006). Data on new tests that are in the very early development phase, such as the Test of Everyday Financial Ability (Smith, 2010), are currently being presented at conferences, and these tests may ultimately make their way into the research literature and clinical practice.

The emergence of these reviews is important because they facilitate comparisons across measures. Several of these reviews have noted the dimensions on which these tests, even within a specific area of decision making, differ. For example, a careful mapping exercise of medical and treatment decision-making tests was undertaken by Dunn and colleagues to determine the extent to which 15 measures assessed the four "domains" of understanding, appreciation, reasoning, and expression of a choice. Only nine of the reviewed measures assessed all four domains. The measures varied in terms of their format: eight of these tests use vignettes and almost all of them incorporated an interview of some sort. Training requirements were highly variable, ranging from minimal to well-supported with manuals and a training video. The reporting of the reliability for these instruments was patchy. Although estimates of interrater reliability were available for 12 of the 15 instruments, internal consistency data were less often available and test–retest reliability was reported for only four scales. Validity investigations were mainly comprised of evaluations that used the external criterion of decisional capacity made by physicians (predominant method), family members (in one study), and, in a handful of studies, correlations with cognitive tests.

A key feature of performance-based measures for capacity assessment is that their complexity, format, and sophistication appear to be related to the type of capacity being assessed. For example, performance-based tests of capacity for informed consent may be performed largely by interview. They do not have normative standards as such, and there is no functional task that can be performed to assist with capacity determinations. Tests of financial decision making on the other hand may involve a clinical interview and a performance element, such as the ability to count money or carry out basic arithmetic operations. These performance elements are typically subject to normative comparisons. Tests of the capacity to drive an automobile may involve a more direct observation of the behavior (e.g., an on-road driving test) or under simulated driving conditions than an assessment of testamentary capacity.

The role of performance-based measures in capacity assessments is difficult to characterize succinctly; nevertheless, it is important to consider these roles. A test of handling or counting money might be used as, or as part of, a performance-based measure of financial capacity. The assumption is that it provides a means of demonstrating that financial tasks can be performed. However, the capacity to perform an action must not be confused with decision-making capacity. The ability to count money, add up a bill, count change, and so on may be a component of decision-making capacity, but when decision-making capacity is called into question, it is likely to involve much more complex and unstructured scenarios than can be mimicked in performance-based tasks. The capacity to perform the tasks that are required to action the subtasks of a decision is not the same as making the decision in the first place; the latter challenge is an abstract cognitive/psychological one. Although at the conceptual level a distinction can be made between these aspects of decision making, the true test lies in the evidence. Thus, despite the apparent mismatch at the construct level between decision-making capacity and its operationalization in a performance-based test, evidence on this matter needs to be considered. One should not be swayed by the apparent appeal of so-called direct tests nor should one reject these tests as irrelevant.

Just as there are recommendations that capacity decisions should not be made on the basis of cognitive tests alone, a similar recommendation against the sole reliance on performance-based measures as the basis for recommendations about decision-making capacity may be needed. In the context of capacity assessments, if the neuropsychologist had information on a client only from a performance-based test of capacity, unless that test surpassed the highest standards of almost every other existing measure, this would prove insufficient as a basis for a conclusion about decision-making capacity. Thus, invoking the principle that converging lines of evidence provide the strongest basis for capacity assessment is one way to guide practice, just as this principle would be used to guide assessments in other contexts.

Evaluating a Model of Assessment

It is becoming clear that we now need studies that test the accuracy of our approaches to capacity assessments. This work is beginning to be done and is clearly important. At a number of points in this chapter, this issue has come up, and further research is needed to test the various models that have been suggested. A relevant study is the review article by Okai and colleagues (2007) that highlights some of the key outcome measures that could be included in such work. Based on their review of existing studies, Okai et al. (2007) concluded that using a standardized method of assessing capacity to make treatment decisions resulted in very high interrater reliability, higher, in fact, than agreement among other health professionals (cardiologists) who were asked to interpret data relevant to their clinical decisions. This study also identified a difference between trained raters' assessment of capacity and the treating clinician's assessment. Compared to the relatively independent assessment of the trained rater, clinicians were less like to judge a patient as lacking capacity. This finding is interesting in light of the earlier discussion of who should conduct capacity assessments because it suggests that dual relationships directly impact the outcome of such assessments. It may be possible to work toward testing a model of practice that incorporates a range of variables that are important to capacity assessment.

As Mullaly and colleagues (2007) wrote, "neuropsychologists, lacking any clear processes for translating formal neuropsychological assessment results directly into categorical decisions about the absence or presence of decision-making capacity, often combine a formal assessment approach with an interview that attempts to explore the functional effects of neuropsychological deficits on the reasoning and decision-making process." One may dispute whether it is necessary to arrive at a categorical decision about the absence or presence of decision-making capacity, since such distinctions do not seem to adequately capture probabilistic clinical decision making or the nature of capacity itself (i.e., it is changeable and occurs on a continuum). Nevertheless, this comment highlights a key theme of this chapter, that the ideal way of combining information from multiple sources, of whichever type (interview, neuropsychological test, or performance-based measure) is still unclear. Notwithstanding the arguments about the ends to which an assessment might be put, applying the principle that capacity assessments should be subject to the ordinary rules of assessment, it should be possible to learn from the broader clinical decision-making literature and to subject the various models to an empirical test. Thus, a comparison of decisions made only on the basis of interview, or interview and neuropsychological tests, or any other combination of assessment elements, appears to be a necessary next step.

In this chapter a suggestion has been made that comprehensive assessments provide the ideal evidence base against which recommendations about capacity might be made, but this notion challenges some conceptualizations of capacity and may be seen as poorly targeted and unnecessary. A comprehensive approach to capacity assessment makes sense if decision-making capacity is viewed as related to other factors that also need assessing. It makes less sense when capacity is viewed in a strictly legalistic way or when it is viewed as so specific that it might be measured with a single performance-based test or clinical interview. Even a structured clinical interview, such as the one suggested by Jones and Holden (2004), which has advantages over less standardized interview approaches, does not provide room for assessing some of the other relevant factors, such as undue influence or impairment of higher level cognitive functions. Comprehensive assessments also by their very nature are longer and therefore more difficult to fit into the practice schedule, so the benefits of this approach over briefer, focused assessments need to be demonstrated empirically. This research is important to help practitioners argue for the appropriate level of resourcing for capacity assessments.

RECOMMENDATIONS

Several researchers have made suggestions about the directions for future decision-making capacity research (Moye & Marson, 2007). The recommendations provided in this chapter are not intended to replace those recommendations. Rather, in some cases they add weight to the calls that have already made by others for future directions. In other cases, new recommendations are provided and are the product of this attempt to identify, describe, and learn from the trends evident in the capacity assessment literature.

Benchmark Current Neuropsychological Practice Standards

More needs to be known about current practice standards for assessing capacity among neuropsychologists. The survey by Mullaly and colleagues (2007) highlighted important information about the use of neuropsychological tests in capacity assessments, as well as broader professional issues, such as the time required to perform such assessments. Further data of this type is needed to recognize this growing role, so that neuropsychological services can be adequately resourced. Data on neuropsychologists' use of performance-based tests are also needed to provide a clearer picture of current practice in relation to the use of such instruments.

Conduct Comparative Evaluations of Instruments

Further comparative evaluations of instruments are required to inform test selection. Test selection will be hampered until good comparisons of multiple measures are available to generate estimates of concurrent validity. Studies such as those of Baird et al. (2009) provide a model of how such research could be conducted as they evaluated the relationship between two measures purposed to assess the same capacity. Although there may be debate over the conceptual boundaries implied by this interpretation, the basic premise—that concurrent validity needs to be demonstrated—is sound. As Baird and colleagues note: "concurrent validity studies [of capacity instruments] are crucial" (p. 298). A deeper understanding of the comparative properties of civil capacity tests is vital.

Conduct External Validity Evaluations of Instruments

In addition to furthering our understanding of concurrent validity, it is important to build the evidence base of the external and predictive validity of measures and methods used by neuropsychologists in capacity assessments. Currently, there is debate about the most appropriate standard to use, and the method that is most often used (physician's judgment) is clearly problematic. The use of multiple outcome measures appears to be an important future direction for studies of the predictive and external validity of capacity tests.

Conduct Reliability Studies

More independent investigations of the psychometric properties of tests are needed, in particular studies that report the test–retest reliability of civil capacity instruments. Test–retest reliability is a property of civil capacity tests about which a good deal more evidence will be needed to support efforts to explore the effect of training and educational interventions to remedy limited capacity. The need for such information is also evident given recommendations for the periodic reassessment of capacity in individuals with neurodegenerative conditions such as dementia (Moye et al., 2006).

Further Validate Existing Tools in a Range of Clinical Groups

In their review of performance-based measures of financial decision-making capacity, Pinsker and colleagues articulated the need to examine the psychometric properties of existing tests, many of which were developed for a specific clinical population (e.g., Alzheimer's disease) in other populations (Pinsker et al., 2010). This recommendation is an important one. The utility of tests is highly dependent on the quality of the evidence base developed around a specific measure. Given that the frequency of mental incapacity varies based on setting and population (Hotopf, 2005), it is imperative that the psychometric properties of measures are demonstrated in contexts with different base rates (Moye & Marson, 2007).

Study the Process, Not Just the Test

Moving beyond the properties of individual tests to the direct study of assessment processes and practices also seems important if we are to identify good assessment practices and skills and if, as some have suggested, further training in capacity assessment is needed (Hill et al., 2006). This recommendation reflects the fact that information from multiple sources is used, even if the algorithm for combining them is somewhat unclear. An appropriate methodology may be to conduct scenario-based studies to determine consistency of assessments about decision-making capacity, especially if those scenarios are based on genuine cases in which multiple outcomes are known, including the legal judgment if applicable. Although scenario-based research methodologies that mimic clinical decision making in other areas have been criticized for failing to adequately convey clinical nuances, drawing on well-established methods of studying clinical decision making would seem to be a key way of determining potential pitfalls. Just like all clinical decision making, recommendations about decision-making capacity should be put to the same tests as other clinical judgments (Wedding & Faust, 1989). This approach enables psychologists to bring to these discussion elements of judgment theory and to identify if there is a role for decision-making aids. Training and experience can also be modeled, as they are suggested in the literature as potential modifiers of the accuracy of capacity assessments.

Defining and/or Refine Conceptual Models of Decision-Making Capacity

The suggestion that the development of the conceptual basis of capacity to inform assessment practice is not new (Moye, Butz, Marson, & Wood, 2007; Sullivan, 2004), but it is worth reiterating. The more a theoretical understanding of the factors that are related to capacity can be advanced, the more an assessment of this construct can also be advanced. This effort is critical to further ensuring that research and clinical practice in the area of neuropsychological capacity assessment reflect and are informed by relevant theoretical principles.

CONCLUSIONS

The selection, application, and interpretation of capacity instruments need to be done carefully, and in light of the available evidence. The available elements of an assessment (e.g., the availability of standardized performance-based tests and interviews) and the relationship between these elements and traditional neuropsychological tests are highly variable, depending on the type of capacity in question. For these assessments, as for all other assessments, the rationale for these clinical choices needs to be sound, and if need be, clearly articulated in a legal context. Continued efforts to build the evidence base around the question of how best to assess capacity are important. Until this evidence grows, it is important that practice decisions are informed by the available literature, and, where necessary, that the limits of understanding of capacity instruments are noted.

ACKNOWLEDGMENTS

I would like to acknowledge Mr. Anthony Schnyder, Test Librarian, School of Psychology and Counselling, Queensland University of Technology.

References

American Bar Association Commission on Law and Aging & American Psychological Association. (2005). *Assessment of older adults with diminished capacity: A handbook for lawyers.* Washington, D.C.: American Bar Association and American Psychological Association.

Baird, A. D., Solcz, S. L., Gale-Ross, R., & Blake, T. M. (2009). Older adults and capacity-related assessment: Promise and caution. *Experimental Aging Research: An International Journal Devoted to the Scientific Study of the Aging Process, 35,* 297–316.

Bradshaw, J., Pangnadasa-Fox, L., & McGregor, J. (2010). *Decision making capacity: Improving the quality and appropriateness of referrals to clinical neuropsychology.* Paper presented at the 10th Annual Conference of the Australian Psychological Society College of Clinical Neuropsychologists, Freemantle Perth, Western Australia.

Dunn, L. B., Nowrangi, M. A., Palmer, B. W., Jeste, D. V., & Saks, E. R. (2006). Assessing decisional capacity for clinical research or treatment: A review of instruments. *American Journal of Psychiatry, 163,* 1323–1334.

Edelstein, B., Nygren, M., Northrop, L., Staats, N., & Pool, D. (1993). *Assessment of capacity to make financial and medical decisions.* Paper presented at the American Psychological Association, Toronto, Canada.

Etchells, E., Katz, M. R., Shuchman, M., Wong, G., Workman, S., Choudhry, N. K., et al. (1997). Accuracy of clinical impressions and mini-mental state exam scores for assessing capacity to consent to major medical treatment: Comparison with criterion-standard psychiatric assessments. *Psychosomatics, 38,* 239–245.

Gibson, R. M., & Ferrini, R. (2010). You let them do what??!! Decision-making capacity and the exercise of patient autonomy in LTC. *Annals of Long-Term Care, 18,* 25–30.

Glass, K. C. (1997). Refining definitions and devising instruments: Two decades of assessing mental competence. *International Journal of Law and Psychiatry, 20,* 5–33.

Griffith, H. R., Belue, K., Sicola, A., Krzywanski, S., Zamrini, E., Harrell, L., et al. (2003). Impaired financial abilities in mild cognitive impairment: A direct assessment approach. *Neurology, 60,* 449–457.

Heilbrun, K. (1992). The role of psychological testing in forensic assessment. *Law and Human Behavior, 16,* 257–272.

Hill, S. A., Mather, G. I., & James, A. J. B. (2006). Assessing decision-making capacity: A survey of psychiatrists' knowledge. *Medicine, Science and the Law, 46*, 66–68.

Hoskin, K. M., Jackson, M., & Crowe, S. F. (2005). Can neuropsychological assessment predict capacity to manage personal finances? A comparison between brain impaired individuals with and without administrators. *Psychiatry, Psychology, and Law, 12*, 56–67.

Hotopf, M. (2005). The assessment of mental capacity. *Clinical Medicine, Journal of the Royal College of Physicians of London, 5*, 580–584.

Jacoby, R., & Steer, P. (2007). How to assess capacity to make a will. *British Medical Journal, 335*, 155–157.

Johansson, K., & Lundberg, C. (2008). Assessment of fitness to drive, possession of professional drivers' license, possession of firearms, and pilot's certificate in clients with dementing conditions. In G. Stoppe (Ed.), *Competence assessment in dementia* (pp. 94–101). Vienna: Springer-Verlag.

Johnson-Greene, D. (2010). Informed consent issues in traumatic brain injury research: Current status of capacity assessment and recommendations for safeguards. *Journal of Head Trauma Rehabilitation, 25*, 145–150.

Jones, R. C., & Holden, T. (2004). A guide to assessing decision-making capacity. *Cleveland Clinic Journal of Medicine, 71*, 971–975.

Kapp, M. B., & Mossman, D. (1996). Measuring decisional capacity: Cautions on the construction of a "Capacimeter." *Psychology, Public Policy, and Law, 2*, 73–95.

Leifker, F. R., Patterson, T. L., Bowie, C. R., Mausbach, B. T., & Harvey, P. D. (2010). Psychometric properties of performance-based measurements of functional capacity: Test-retest reliability, practice effects, and potential sensitivity to change. *Schizophrenia Research, 119*, 246–252.

Loeb, P. A. (1996). *Independent Living Scales manual.* San Antonio, TX: The Psychological Corporation.

Lowenstein, D. A., Amigo, E., Duara, R., Guterman, A., Hurwitz, D., Berkowitz, N., et al. (1989). A new scale for the assessment of functional status in Alzheimer's disease and related disorders. *Journal of Gerontology: Psychological Science, 44*, 114–121.

Maeck, L., & Stoppe, G. (2008). Why is competence assessment important? Development of the EDCON Consensus Statement. In G. Stoppe (Ed.), *Competence assessment in dementia* (pp. 1–10). Vienna: Springer-Verlag.

Meyers Sorger, B., Rosenfeld, B., Pessin, H., Kosinski Timm, A., & Cimino, J. (2007). Decision-making capacity in elderly, terminally ill patients with cancer. *Behavioral Sciences and the Law, 25*, 393–404.

Michels, T. C., Tiu, A. Y., & Graver, C. J. (2010). Neuropsychological evaluation in primary care. *American Family Physician, 82*, 495–502.

Miller, S. S., & Marin, D. B. (2000). Assessing capacity. *Emergency Medical Clinics in North America, 18*, 233–241.

Molnar, F. J., Patel, A., Marshall, S. C., Man-Son-Hing, M., & Wilson, K. G. (2006). Clinical utility of office-based cognitive predictors of fitness to drive in persons with dementia: A systematic review. *Journal of the American Gerontological Society, 54*, 1809–1824.

Moye, J. (1999). Assessment of competency and decision making capacity. In P. A. Litchtenberg (Ed.), *Handbook of assessment in clinical gerontology.* (pp. 488–528). New York: John Wiley.

Moye, J. (2003). Guardianship and conservatorship. In T. Grisso (Ed.), *Evaluating competencies* (pp. 309–390). New York: Plenum Press.

Moye, J., Butz, S. W., Marson, D. C., & Wood, E. (2007). A conceptual model and assessment template for capacity evaluation in adult guardianship. *Gerontologist, 47*, 591–603.

Moye, J., Gurrera, R. J., Karel, M. J., Edelstein, B., & O'Connell, C. (2006). Empirical advances in the assessment of the capacity to consent to medical treatment: Clinical implications and research needs. *Clinical Psychology Review, 26*, 1054–1077.

Moye, J., & Marson, D. C. (2007). Assessment of decision-making capacity in older adults: An emerging area of practice and research. *The Journals of Gerontology Series B: Psychological Sciences and Social Sciences, 62*, 3–11.

Moye, J. & Marson, D. C. (2009). Assessment of decision-making capacity in older adults: An emerging area of practice and research. *Journal of Gerontology: Psychological Sciences*, 62B, P3- P11.

Mullaly, E., Kinsella, G., Berberovic, N., Cohen, Y., Dedda, K., Froud, B., et al. (2007). Assessment of decision-making capacity: Exploration of common practices among neuropsychologists. *Australian Psychologist, 42*, 178–186.

Newberry, A. M., & Pachet, A. K. (2008). An innovative framework for psychosocial assessment in complex mental capacity evaluations. *Psychology, Health & Medicine, 13*, 438–449.

O'Connor, D., Hall, M. I., & Donnelly, M. (2009). Assessing capacity within a context of abuse or neglect. *Journal of Elder Abuse & Neglect, 21*, 156–169.

Okai, D., Owen, G., McGuire, H., Singh, S., Churchill, R., & Hotopf, M. (2007). Mental capacity in psychiatric patients. *British Journal of Psychiatry, 191*, 291–297.

Okonkwo, O. C., Wadley, V. G., Griffith, H. R., Ball, K., & Marson, D. C. (2006). Cognitive correlates of financial abilities in mild cognitive impairment. *Journal of the American Geriatrics Society, 54*, 1745–1750.

Okonkwo, O. C., Wadley, V. G., Griffith, H. R., Belue, K., Lanza, S., Zamrini, E. Y., et al. (2008). Awareness of deficits in financial abilities in patients with mild cognitive impairment: Going beyond self-informant discrepancy. *American Journal of Geriatric Psychiatry, 16*, 650–659.

Pinsker, D. M., Pachana, N. A., Wilson, J., Tilse, C., & Byrne, G. J. (2010). Financial capacity in older adults: A review of clinical assessment and considerations. *Clinical Gerontologist, 33*, 332–346.

Querques, J., Kontos, N., & Freudenreich, O. (2010). Determination of capacity: A first step. *Critical Care Medicine, 38*, 1614–1615.

Roked, F., & Patel, A. (2008). Which aspects of cognitive function are best associated with testamentary capacity in patients with Alzheimer's disease? *International Journal of Geriatric Psychiatry, 23*, 552–553.

Shulman, K. I., Peisah, C., Jacoby, R., Heinik, J., & Finkel, S. (2009). Contemporaneous assessment of testamentary capacity. *International Psychogeriatrics, 21*, 433–439.

Smith, L. A. (2010). *Assessment of financial ability in younger onset dementia*. Paper presented at the 10th Annual Conference of the Australian Psychological Society of Clinical Neuropsychologists, Freemantle, Western Australia.

Sturman, E. D. (2005). The capacity to consent to treatment and research: A review of standardized assessment tools. *Clinical Psychology Review, 25*, 954–974.

Sullivan, K. A. (2004). Neuropsychological assessment of mental capacity. *Neuropsychology Review, 14*, 131–142.
Wedding, D., & Faust, D. (1989). Clinical judgment and decision making in neuropsychology. *Archives of Clinical Neuropsychology, 4*, 233–265.
Willner, P., Bailey, R., Parry, R., & Dymond, S. (2010). Evaluation of the ability of people with intellectual disabilities to "weigh up" information in two tests of financial reasoning. *Journal of Intellectual Disability Research, 54*, 380–391.
Wood, S. (2007). The role of neuropsychological assessment in capacity evaluations. In S. H. Qualls & M. A. Smyers (Eds.), *Changes in decision-making capacity in older adults: Assessment and interventions* (pp. 191–204). Hoboken, NJ: John Wiley & Sons.
Zombor, R., Mullaly, E., & Morriss, E. (2010). *Decision making capacity: The multiple roles of neuropsychologists*. Paper presented at the 10th Annual Conference of the Australian Psychological Society of the College of Clinical Neuropsychologists, Freemantle, Western Australia.

11

Other Aspects of Data Collection in Capacity Evaluations

ROBERT RUCHINSKAS

An 83-year-old woman presents for an evaluation of her capacity to manage her finances. Her medical history is relatively unremarkable except for a breast lump removal and past alcohol use, which the patient describes as "one or two drinks a day." Her daughter, who lives in the next state and doesn't see her mother often, believes that her consumption is closer to one to two bottles of wine per day. She was seen by a neurologist who ordered a computed tomography (CT) scan of the head and the traditional laboratory work for reversible causes of dementia and eventually concluded that she has Alzheimer's disease. A Mini-Mental State Examination (MMSE; Folstein, Folstein, & McCugh, 1975) was done the previous month by a nurse at her assisted living facility where she had been living for a year and was 23/30. Closer examination of the MMSE revealed that the three words were apparently randomly chosen and were objects likely in sight in the interview room and that spelling a word backward was used instead of serial 7's. Today she was evaluated in a different town and in an office building previously unknown to her. She was notably anxious and scored a 13/30 on the MMSE-2. Based on the fact that both of her MMSE scores were at or below 23, the neurologist concluded that the patient should not be making medical or financial decisions and recommended that the daughter obtain guardianship.

Conversely, in another evaluation, a 70-year-old woman presents with a 1 year history of a decline in MMSE scores from 24 to 19 with an accompanied decrease in independent daily living skills (although her daughter questioned if this was due to a decreased desire to perform these duties versus reduced ability). She also had neuroimaging and laboratory work and was subsequently diagnosed with Alzheimer's disease by her neurologist who started her on an anticholinesterase inhibitor. The neurologist noted during the next visit that the patient appeared depressed due to the diagnosis of dementia and prescribed an antidepressant.

He also completed paperwork to appoint her family as guardian for financial affairs. On today's visit she scored a 28 on the MMSE. The neurologist again diagnosed Alzheimer's disease and made no comment regarding reevaluating her capacity for financial management despite this marked "improvement" in her cognitive abilities.

Both of these cases dramatize some of the issues facing clinicians conducting capacity evaluations in that the accuracy of multiple pieces of history, interview, and measurement must be considered. The clinician must evaluate both the veracity of outside data that was obtained prior to the evaluation and also the reliability of interviews and observations done at the time of the evaluation. Still, while evaluating the past and present is a daunting task, the clinician must also examine the future in terms of defining the exact amount of risk(s) inherent in allowing a person to continue to decide independently. As each decision is unique and carries its own level of risk(s), different degrees of decision-making ability are possible. It is only after determining potential risk(s) that the "sliding scale" (i.e., the degree of understanding, reasoning, and communication needed versus the level of inherent risk in the decision) can be established. Once the sliding scale is realized, the clinician can then properly integrate the history, current neuropsychological results, behavioral observations, and other data to reach an opinion regarding capacity. Although underresearched, the challenges of evaluating the past, present, and the future will be reviewed in this chapter.

HISTORY GATHERING AND COGNITIVE SCREENING

There are many purposes for completing a record review including obtaining a rudimentary timeline regarding the onset of difficulties, discerning contributing factors (medical, psychological, and social) related to the referral question, examining prior patterns of behavior, etc. The concept that "the best predictor of future behavior is past behavior" drives some of the review process. Capacity evaluations often challenge this maxim because many individuals have acted in a functional manner for some time and yet their current behavior (and the decisions that drive such behavior) is now in question. Hence, knowledge of behavior prior to a neurological event such as a cerebrovascular accident, traumatic brain injury, or dementia is valuable in determining a person's values and how they likely would have acted in the past. The challenge to the clinician is that they must determine how the person is acting, thinking, choosing, and behaving at present and integrate this new set of patterns with the past in order to predict the future.

The first step in the process involves a review of records, which can be an intimidating task that involves pouring over volumes of material from different clinicians without knowledge of their clinical acumen or decision-making strategies. As noted in the case examples, the accuracy of medical records should not be assumed. In fact, many factors regarding the accuracy of prior records must be considered and could comprise a chapter all of its own. For the sake of brevity, however, this review will highlight two prominent areas that can affect capacity evaluations: diagnostic reliability and error in measurement or interpretation.

There are numerous instances in psychology, neuropsychology, psychiatry, and neurology in which a definitive diagnosis is not possible, but rather opinions regarding the degree of diagnostic certainty are offered. In clinical experience, however, once even a provisional diagnosis is offered it can take on a life of its own and reappear in subsequent medical records with little regard as to where this information was obtained, the criteria used to make the diagnosis, or the degree of diagnostic certainty. Even when well documented, the veracity of the original diagnosis must still be questioned as many conditions have multiple and sometimes competing diagnostic formulas. For example, the diagnosis of Alzheimer's or vascular dementia can vary significantly based on whether standard psychiatric, neurological, or other criteria are utilized (Chui et al., 2000; Kukull, Larson, Reifler, Lampe, Yerby, & Hughes, 1990). Even when one criterion was utilized by a research group, those criteria itself may be biased. For instance, researchers have long known that some diagnostic criteria tend to overdiagnose dementia if ethnicity or lower education levels are not considered (Pittman et al., 1992). That being said, these authors found that low education may also work the opposite way, as lower rates of dementia diagnoses were found if a physician-based semi-structured neurological examination was utilized without psychometric testing.

Similarly, even while agreeing on standardized criteria, the diagnosis itself may still have poor interrater reliability. The last major revision of the *Diagnostic and Statistical Manual* engendered criticism as some diagnostic classifications had poor kappa statistics (e.g., schizoaffective disorder, various anxiety disorders) yet were still included (Brown & Leyfer, 2009; Maj, Pirozzi, Formicola, Bartoli, & Bucci, 2000). Difficulties with diagnostic classification are not only restricted to psychiatric diagnosis but can affect many areas of collateral data that are considered during capacity evaluations. For example, Mäntylä et al. (1997) examined interpretation of the degree of periventricular and deep white matter hyperintensities on magnetic resonance imaging (MRI) scans on 13 rating scales. Not surprisingly, they found that degree of white matter compromise, a factor that can potentially affect the diagnosis of a dementia, varied considerably based on which visual rating scale was utilized.

That being said, an equally robust body of research has found that clinicians utilizing the same criteria can reliably arrive at similar diagnostic conclusions, even with methods such as chart review without interview, assuming that a uniform standard set of criteria is utilized. Kasner et al. (1999) found that reliable results could be obtained for a common stroke scale (National Institute of Health Stroke Scale) simply through chart review (interrater reliability of 0.82). Similarly, Keilp et al. (1995) reported similar agreement rates for retrospective chart review of schizophrenia or dementia diagnoses using the *Diagnostic and Statistical Manual of Mental Disorders, III, Revised* (*DSM-III-R*) criteria. Overall, however, diagnostic opinions must often be recognized as that—just opinions—unless evidence regarding the criteria and diagnostic process is available. In fact, additional records may provide evidence that challenges prior diagnoses, such as finding that the label of dementia that has followed the patient was given in the midst of a documented episode of delirium while the patient was hospitalized for an infection.

Hence, chart review includes the opinions and diagnoses of many professionals who may have used various diagnostic criteria to reach their conclusions. The methods of arriving at diagnoses must also be considered, as these opinions are sometimes rendered in the absence of standardized measurement forms. For example, research with nonpsychiatric professionals found that they are not proficient at detecting cognitive dysfunction or diagnosable psychiatric illness and may either overdiagnose or underdiagnose these conditions if they have not used standardized screening instruments (e.g., Guilmette, Snow, Grace, & Giuliano, 1992; Cushman & Dikjers, 1990). Basically, the commonly heard clinical maxim that "if I was in that situation I'd be depressed also" allows for both the exaggeration of the base rate depression and the "normalization" of the minority of individuals (even those with life-threatening medical conditions) who do have major depression. The research appears to apply not only to individuals who have had a one-time evaluation but also to those who were observed over time. For example, rehabilitation professionals who worked with a patient for an average of 6 to 10 days correctly identified only about 37% of those with cognitive impairment and between 0% and 14% of those with significant depressive symptoms (Ruchinskas, 2002). These results suggest that opinions from those who are not utilizing some form of validated screening instrument can often miss underlying cognitive and emotional dysfunction. In addition, this suggests that those referred for capacity evaluations will likely be individuals who have the most significant compromise, whereas many others with questionable capacity will not be identified until they make an odd decision that is "out of character" or display unexpected behavior.

A second common source of possibly misleading information comes from the administration of diagnostic instruments that lack standardization or those that are standardized and mistakenly interpreted. A common example of such an error in measurement can be seen with the Mini-Mental State Examination (MMSE; Folstein et al., 1975). Although it has been in the public domain for over 35 years and remains the most widely used cognitive screening instrument in the United States, no other measure may be as widely misinterpreted or have so many unstandardized variations (Tombaugh & McIntyre, 1992). The instrument has been recently copywritten and revised. Yet clinical practice still finds many individuals using a version that was in the public domain for years, was part of a drug study, or was published in a geriatric nursing guidebook. The 2000 standardized version of the MMSE (Folstein, Folstein, & Fanjiang, 2000) cites interrater reliability studies that range from 0.83 to 0.95 and 24-hour test–retest correlations of 0.85 to 0.92, which decline as the time between administrations increases. Although these reliability statistics are adequate, the clinician must determine which form of the MMSE was utilized as various versions in the public domain prescribe different words (or leave them up to the examiner), have different subtraction tasks, determine that orientation needs to be to the exact day/date or can be within 1 or 2 days, have different scoring for the design drawing, or have less than adequate normative data (Tombaugh & McIntyre, 1992). Perhaps the largest source of measurement differences, no matter which version is utilized, comes from the use of the serial subtraction task versus the easier spelling "world" backward (Ganguli et al., 1990; Watkins, Gouvier, Callon, & Barkemeyer, 1989). Although the standardized MMSE states that serial 7's must be administered unless the patient refuses, in our clinical experience, these directions are often purposefully ignored or not followed out of ignorance. Often only the easier "world" task is given or both tasks are administered and the best score is recorded. Interchanging these two tasks can cause a large difference in scoring as they comprise 17% (5/30) of the total MMSE score.

In addition variations in administration, differences in interpretation are common with various "cutting scores," particularly 23/30, having been proposed for all individuals. The use of a blanket cut-off score can lead to an overdiagnosis of incapacity. For example, one study reported that 36% of individuals in a long-term care facility who had significant cognitive compromise (MMSE score of less than 15) displayed the capacity to designate consistently a healthcare proxy or state a decision to not name one (Sansone, Schmitt, & Nichols, 1998). In addition, the difficulties with using this instrument with older individuals, a cohort that is less likely to have a high school education, has been well recognized and several large-scale normative databases have been published to correct for age and education effects (i.e., Crum, Anthony, Bassett, & Folstein, 1993). Despite this fact, clinical experience shows that "below 23 means dementia" and "dementia means incapacity" still hold fast in the mind of many clinicians.

There is also little recognition that variability and practice effects are present on the MMSE. For example, little research has been performed to provide reliable change indicators for the MMSE. Hensel, Angermeyer, and Riedel-Heller (2007) argued that small differences in MMSE scores must be interpreted with caution and at least three point differences between scores are necessary over short intervals between testing to document that a true change has occurred. Still, as noted in the case examples above, a decline of three points or more on the standardized MMSE can easily occur if the examinee is at a new office in a new town (thereby possibly losing orientation points), is anxious, or is not exerting full effort.

Artificial inflation of scores can occur. Given the fact that the MMSE is so widely used and often routinely readministered, it is not surprising that practice effects are present (Galasko, Abramson, Corey-Bloom, & Thal, 1993). Lastly, it must be noted that some change in scores or inflation of an original MMSE score may come through the form of "coaching." Gofton and Weaver (2006) found that approximately 18% of their small sample in a memory disorder clinic may have been coached on the MMSE prior to the evaluation (often within an hour prior to the appointment). This was determined because when asked to spell the word "worm" backward they instead spelled "world," revealing that they knew this test item either because they had previously taken the test or had been coached. Forty-two percent of caregivers in this study also admitted reviewing part or all of the MMSE prior to arrival. The authors conclude that significant caution must be exercised when evaluating MMSE scores due to the test's availability in the public domain.

Hence, an MMSE score may be neither accurate nor stable, which certainly argues for investigating exactly which version of the MMSE was administered and how exactly the score was determined. In addition, the possible instability of MMSE scores also argues for an often ignored concept that capacity may need to be determined over a series of observations in order to ensure that the samples of behavior obtained are consistent across time. Overall, the research presented so far suggests caution, as difficulties with diagnostic agreement and errors in test measurement and interpretation exist.

THE CLINICAL INTERVIEW

In addition to record review and a brief cognitive screening examination, much of the information regarding past history and current status is attained in interviews of the person, his or family, significant others, caregivers, and staff. The fact that individuals may overreport symptoms is well documented in the literature (i.e., Schrag, Brown, & Trimble, 2004) and the base rate of "unexplained" or exaggerated symptoms can range from small to the majority of patients based on the nature of the practice. For example, Nimnuan, Hotopf, and Wessely (2001) surveyed new patients at seven specialty clinics and found the number of patients with at least one unexplained medical symptom ranged from 26% (dentistry) to over 60% (neurology). Interestingly, gynecology (54%) was the next highest specialty for medically unexplained symptoms, although this result may have been influenced by different response rates across clinics. Although this tendency to exaggerate cannot be ignored, it is generally not seen in those attempting to prove their capacity as they will likely underreport any experienced difficulties.

Before the possibility of downplaying or denying difficulties is considered, however, it must first be established if willing examinees are able to accurately report their history. In general, the evidence suggests that individuals are able to accurately report most of their history. For example, many studies have found strong agreement between self-report of medical conditions or medication compliance when compared with objective evidence (Solomon et al., 2007; Choo et al., 2007; Bush, Miller, Golden, & Hale, 1989). That being said, complete accuracy should not be expected as other studies have reported moderate or poor accuracy of self-report versus objective measures (Lim et al., 2010; Volk & Cass, 2002; Gordon, Hiatt, & Lampert, 1993). For example, Gordon, Hiatt, and Lampert (1993) found strong agreement for reports of medical procedures that generated a report such as a mammogram and Pap smear, but lower agreement for those generating a physician note such as clinical breast and digital rectal examinations. In addition, mitigating factors such as increased age can reduce the veracity of self-reported histories. For instance, although Goebeler, Jylha, and Hervonen (2007) found that, unlike previous research on younger old participants, those over the age of 90 years less accurately reported their medical histories and tended to report higher rates of depression and dementia than were documented in their medical charts.

In addition to variable rates of recall accuracy, there are many other behaviors that are traditionally assumed to be downplayed, such as alcohol usage. As Del Boca and Noll (2000) state, the clinical maxim of "never trust an alcoholic (as) he or she will always underestimate consumption" (p. S353) is frequently invoked in clinical settings and rules of thumb such as automatically doubling the amount of alcohol intake reported have been around for years. Research, however, suggests that those actively using alcohol to the point of alcoholism can and will provide accurate accounts of their consumption (Killeen, Brady, Gold, Tyson, & Simpson, 2004; Barbor, Brown, & Del Boca, 1990). Yet the authors note that similar to the literature regarding reporting medical conditions, individuals may not be completely accurate. Factors such as the severity of dependence and the stage of recovery appear to affect reporting accuracy (Barbor, Steinberg, Anton, & Del Boca, 2000; Brown, Kranzler, & Del Boca, 1992) as those with greater levels of addiction and individuals early in the recovery process tend to be less reliable reporters. In addition, reports of consumption amounts for those who are actively drinking and have cognitive impairments at baseline or as a result of their alcohol abuse did not correspond with blood and urine toxicology findings in one study (Brown et al., 1992).

Thus, the common belief that alcoholics consistently misrepresent their alcohol consumption does not appear to be supported in the literature, although they, like most individuals, will likely offer some information that is not fully accurate. In addition, it is unrealistic to expect that examinees will be completely forthcoming in every circumstance. The exact degree of exaggeration and defensiveness during the clinical interview has to be determined by corollary information such as agreement between self-report and objective findings or through examination of other sources of data. For example, there is a growing body of research in personality assessment that instructs clinicians to expect a degree of wariness, if not outright defensiveness, in regards to admitting psychological difficulties in certain evaluative settings. Ruchinskas, Combs, Riley, and Broshek (2006) found that nearly two-thirds of presurgical candidates adopted either a mildly defensive stance or an outright defensive response style on the Minnesota Multiphasic Personality Inventory-2 (MMPI-2). The authors note that similar findings are present across a variety of evaluations including preemployment screening, child custody evaluations, and other presurgical consultations and argue that a degree of defensiveness is to be expected when performing such psychological evaluations. Perhaps the strongest of this evidence is from Long, Rouse, Nelsen, and Butcher (2004) who cluster analyzed MMPI-2 profiles of claimants of sexual harassment. Although openly admitting psychological distress would likely strengthen the evidence of their legal cases, the modal validity profile of these claimants was defensive.

Given that self-report is often not fully accurate, gathering collateral data is frequently utilized to obtain multiple perspectives. The research on how well a family reports its family's medical history or the medical history of a living family member is, not surprisingly, mixed. Some studies have suggested that conditions such as dementia and depression can be reliably assessed via structured family interviews and questionnaires, although this method is not reliable for all psychiatric conditions such as phobias and other anxiety disorders (Heun, Muller, Freyberger, & Maier, 1998). Accuracy of recalling personal and family medical history has also been found to be good, but less than perfect, for most cognitively intact individuals (Parent, Ghardirian, Lacroix, & Perret, 1997) as patients were 91% accurate about reporting the presence of breast cancer in a first-degree relative and 97% accurate for the absence of a family history of cancer. They were less correct for reporting the histories of multiple family members. As noted previously in regard to personal medical history, decreased accuracy of recall of family medical history as a function of increasing age was noted even in cognitively intact individuals (Murabito, Nam, D'Agostino, Lloyd-Jones, O'Donnell, & Wilson, 2004; Parent, Ghardirian, Lacroix, & Perret, 1997). As with other aspects of self-report, however, decreased self-report can occur as a function of age but should not be expected as the norm as the literature (e.g., Bush, Miller, Golden, & Hale, 1989) also indicates that accurate histories can be given at most any age. Overall, however, history gathering and clinical interview must be as empirically scrutinized as neuropsychological data during the capacity evaluation process.

RISK ASSESSMENT

While gathering reliable information about the past is challenging, an integral yet overlooked aspect of capacity evaluations is the prediction of future risk. Capacity questions are essentially framed in terms of "if/then," whereby "if" the individual is incapable yet is allowed to choose "then" an undesired outcome(s) may occur. These statements tend to be emotionally charged such as "if they are allowed to drive it's only a matter of time before they hit a child who is running after a ball." In reality, capacity evaluations usually do not contain concrete evidence outcome ratios such as "if you undergo this treatment then there's a 95% chance you will be illness free for the next five years." Rather, as seen in the above statement about driving risk, there are numerous "if" statements that are typically not voiced and need to occur in order for the unwanted outcome to result. It is the clinician's responsibility to determine how many "if" statements are present and to also determine the likelihood of "then" occurring.

The reason risk assessment is integral to capacity evaluation is that most theoretical models of capacity utilize the concept of a sliding scale, whereby the necessary levels of understanding, reasoning, and communication are adjusted based on the amount of risk inherent in the decision. Two popular views guide the standard when utilizing a sliding scale. The first viewpoint suggests that as risk increases so does the need for higher levels of decisional capacity (e.g., greater abstract reasoning skills are needed when making life or death decisions than when making decisions that are less risky). This standard has been criticized as it may automatically declare incapable a proportion of the population that lacks such high-level thinking, abstraction, or vocabulary skills at baseline. Another viewpoint suggests the level of evidence for determining decisional capacity rises with increased risk. Thus, as risk rises, the level of evidence that the person has basic abilities for understanding, appreciation, reasoning, and communication (Beauchamp & Childress, 2001) also increases. This standard shifts the burden from the need for higher cognitive skills as risk increases to greater confidence in the evaluator that these basic skills are in fact present. The use of this standard decreases the chance for inappropriate restraint of autonomous behavior, but also increases the chance for informed yet idiosyncratic decisions. These standards are certainly not exclusive nor is there a "gold standard." Clinical practice often finds that aspects of both can be utilized in the conceptualization of capacity.

Regardless of the standard utilized, risk must be evaluated and quantified in order to evaluate the core components of autonomous decision making. As is seen elsewhere in this volume, the process of evaluating a patient's core components of capacity has been the main focus of research. Conversely, determining risk ratios and gauging the accuracy of an evaluator's judgment of the inherent level of risk for a particular decision have been essentially ignored in the literature. Macciocchi and Stringer (2001) state that "We are ethically obliged to provide scientifically sound data when constraining autonomy or, absent such data, to state the basis for our predictions" (p. S19). Because there is not a large body of research, however, risk assessment often relies solely on clinical judgment, which, as clinicians from Meehl (1973) on have shown, is far from perfect.

Risk is difficult to quantify, in part, because clinicians are often trying to predict relatively rare events (i.e., getting into a car accident, squandering a substantial savings, etc.). Base rates greatly affect our ability to quantify risk. One study (Ruchinskas, 2003) looked at predictions by physical and occupational therapists, considered to be experts in gait dysfunction, of patient falling during the first month after discharge from acute rehabilitation. Therapists were accurate 34% of the time when identifying those who eventually fell and 82% of the time predicting those who did not fall. This accuracy rate was no greater than if those with a prior history of falling or the presence of a neurological disorder were classified as likely fallers, meaning that clinical judgment added no incremental validity. As seen above, the clinician was incorrect more often than correct when trying to predict an infrequent event (only 12% of the sample actually fell), which is partly due to the fact that variables that have poor predictive power tend to be utilized alongside or in place of data with stronger empirical foundations (Ruchinskas, Macciocchi, Howe, & Newton, 2001; Macciocchi & Eaton, 1995). Despite generally poor predictive accuracy in clinical settings, opinions regarding future events were made with great confidence and were often offered as "fact" with little realization that the clinician's judgment could be faulty.

Base rates can also reduce the efficacy of instruments designed to improve decisional accuracy. For example, Macciocchi and Stringer (2001) used the example of a test that has 95% sensitivity and specificity to driving problems after a traumatic brain injury. If the base rate of a crash in the first year following a traumatic brain injury is low, such as 5/1000, a Bayesian analysis reveals that a person with a positive sign on the test has only a 9% likelihood of getting into a car accident. Although this instrument adds value over the base rate, clinicians who utilizes this instrument may not realize that they still will likely be incorrect more than correct due to the infrequent nature of this event. Thus, despite societies' continued push toward requiring that professionals protect the public from negative events, research reveals that clinicians have difficulties in predicting dangerous behaviors such as suicide (Hughes, 1995) and dangerousness to others (Serin & Amos, 1995; Litwack, Kirschner, & Wack, 1993).

The literature reinforces the fact that behavior is driven by numerous complex factors and the ability to predict most behaviors by utilizing only one or two predictors (which is our natural tendency) or by using suboptimal predictive variables is unacceptably low. The only exception may be with patients who are severely incapacitated. For example, a person who is completely bed ridden is unlikely to fall, and a person diagnosed with severe intellectual disability is unlikely to have a high-income profession (Fisher, 1959). The challenge is that many capacity and risk evaluations are conducted on patients who are in the "gray area," where either capacity or incapacity is not grossly obvious.

Our knowledge of the limitations in quantifying risk and of trying to predict infrequent behaviors suggests that a cautious stance should be the norm when questions of restricting autonomy arise. In fact, given that the entire capacity assessment process is currently more often driven by clinical judgment than science should give the clinician pause. Rather than being disheartened, however, our lack of ability to scientifically quantify risk can be liberating when faced with the prospect of an ethically and scientifically challenging capacity evaluation. Because risk helps determine the "sliding scale" that guides the evaluation of cognitive and emotional capabilities, modifying risk may in fact eliminate the need for a capacity determination. There are at least two obvious alternatives: either improve a person's abilities in order to meet the demands of his or her environment (improve capacity) or decrease the demands of the environment (reduce risk) in order to meet a person's current capabilities. Practical examples of the first solution can be viewed in attempts to provide more information concerning the views of others regarding the perceived risk of the situation. In clinical practice, there are times when concerns are voiced among the treatment staff or within families, but these never get shared with the individual until a capacity evaluation is requested. If individuals are unaware of the legal system and are unable to participate in their proceedings, then a solution could be to educate them regarding the roles of lawyers, judges, and juries as a means of improving their capacity. Similarly, enrolling a person in cognitive rehabilitation to improve either the general or specific cognitive abilities that are thought to underlie capacity can be attempted before initiating a formal capacity evaluation.

More often than not, however, it may be easier to modify the demands being placed on an individual. "Safety-proofing" a home to reduce the likelihood of a fall, providing home nursing to increase medication compliance, naming a trusted family member as Power of Attorney for finances, and convincing the individual to allow the family to supervise money management are all practical solutions that can allow the individual's capabilities to meet the environmental demands and eliminate the need for a capacity evaluation. Given that every capacity evaluation is unique to the person, the situation, and the question to be decided, the possibilities for remediation and accommodation are limited only by the clinician's imagination and skill in dealing with individuals in conflict.

In summary, this chapter highlights the difficulty in obtaining reliable data for use in capacity evaluations and the challenges of determining the level of risk involved in allowing for continued autonomous decision making. Other chapters in this volume echo similar themes regarding the nascent state of our science in regard to evaluating specific cognitive capacities and the lack of a "gold standard" for capacity. Thus, searching for workable alternatives that improve capacity or reduce risk to allow the individual's capabilities to match the environmental demands should be considered well before entering into the ethically and scientifically challenging world of capacity evaluations.

References

Barbor, T., Brown, J., & Del Boca, F. (1990). Validity of self-reports in applied research on addictive behaviors: Fact or fiction? *Behavioral Assessment, 12,* 5–31.

Babor, T., Steinberg, K., Anton, R., & Del Boca, F. (2000). Talk is cheap: Measuring drinking outcomes in clinical trials. *Journal of Studies in Alcohol, 61,* 55–63.

Beauchamp, T., & Childress, J. (2001). *Principles of biomedical ethics* (5th ed.). New York: Oxford University Press.

Brown, J., Kranzler, H., & Del Boca, F. (1992). Self-reports by alcohol and drug abuse inpatients: Factors affecting reliability and validity. *British Journal of Addiction, 87,* 1013–1024.

Brown, T., & Leyfer, O. (2009). Classification of anxiety disorders. In D. Stein, E. Hollander, & B. Rothbaum (Eds.), *Textbook of anxiety disorders* (pp. 17–34). Arlington, VA: American Psychiatric Publishing, Inc.

Bush, T., Miller, S., Golden, A., & Hale, W. (1989). Self-report and medical record report agreement of selected medical conditions in the elderly. *American Journal of Public Health, 79,* 1554–1556.

Choo, P., Rand, C., Inui, T., Lee, M., Cain, E., Cordeiro-Breault, M., et al. (2007). Validation of patient reports, automated pharmacy records, and pill counts with electronic monitoring of adherence to antihypertensive therapy. *Arthritis and Rheumatism, 57,* 234–239.

Chui, H., Mack, W., Jackson, E., Mungas, D., Reed, B., Tinklenberg, J., et al. (2000). Clinical criteria for the diagnosis of vascular dementia. *Archives of Neurology, 57,* 191–196.

Crum, R., Anthony, J., Bassett, S., & Folstein, M. (1993). Population-based norms for the Mini-Mental State Examination by age and education level. *Journal of the American Medical Association, 269,* 2386–2391.

Cushman, L., & Dijkers, M. (1990). Depressed mood in spinal cord injured individuals: Staff perceptions and individual realities. *Archives of Physical Medicine and Rehabilitation, 71,* 191–196.

Del Boca, F., & Noll, J. (2000). Truth or consequences: The validity of self-report data in health services research on addictions. *Addiction, 95(Suppl. 3),* S347–360.

Fisher, J. (1959). The twisted pear and the prediction of behavior. *Journal of Consulting Psychology, 23,* 400–405.

Folstein, M., Folstein, S., & Fanjiang, G. (2000). *Mini-Mental State Examination: Clinical guide.* Lutz, FL: Psychological Assessment Resources, Inc.

Folstein, M., Folstein, S., & McHugh, P. (1975). Mini-mental state: A practical method for grading the cognitive state of patients for the clinician. *Journal of Psychiatric Research, 12,* 189–198.

Galasko, D., Abramson, I., Corey-Bloom, J., & Thal, L. (1993). Repeated exposure to the Mini-Mental State Examination and the Information-Memory-Concentration Test results in practice effects in Alzheimer's disease. *Neurology, 43,* 1559–1563.

Ganguli, M., Ratcliff, G., Huff, F., Belle, S., Kancel, M., Fischer, L., et al. (1990). Serial sevens versus world backwards: A comparison of the two measures of attention from the MMSE. *Journal of Geriatric Psychiatry & Neurology, 3,* 203–207.

Goebeler, S., Jylha, M., & Hervonen, A. (2007). Self-reported medical history and self-rated health at age 90. Agreement with medical records. *Aging Clinical and Experimental Research, 19,* 213–219.

Gofton, T., & Weaver, D. (2006). Challenges in the clinical diagnosis of Alzheimer's disease: Influence of "family coaching" on the Mini-Mental State Examination. *American Journal of Alzheimer's Disease and Other Dementias, 21,* 109–112.

Gordon, N., Hiatt, R., & Lampert, D. (1993). Concordance of self-reported data and medical record audit for six cancer screening procedures. *Journal of the National Cancer Institute, 85,* 566–570.

Guilmette, J., Snow, M., Grace, J., & Giuliano A. (1992). Emotional dysfunction in a geriatric population: Staff observations and patients' reports. *Archives of Physical Medicine and Rehabilitation, 73,* 587–593.

Hensel, A., Angermeyer, M., & Riedel-Heller, S. (2007). Measuring cognitive change in older adults: Reliable change indices for the Mini-Mental State Examination. *Journal of Neurology, Neurosurgery, and Psychiatry, 78,* 1298–1303.

Heun, R., Muller, H., Freyberger, H., & Maier, W. (1998). Reliability of interview information in a family study in the elderly. *Social Psychiatry & Psychiatric Epidemiology, 33,* 140–144.

Hughes, D. (1995). Can the clinician predict suicide? *Psychiatric Services, 46,* 449–451.

Kasner, S., Chalela, J., Luciano, J., Cucchiara, B., Raps, E., McGarvey, M., et al. (1999). Reliability and validity of estimating the NIH stroke scale score from medical records. *Stroke, 30,* 1534–1537.

Keilp, J., Waniek, C., Goldman, R., Zemishlany, Z., Alexander, G., Gibbon, M., et al. (1995). Reliability of post-mortem chart diagnoses of schizophrenia and dementia. *Schizophrenia Research, 17,* 221–228.

Killeen, T., Brady, K, Gold, P., Tyson, C., & Simpson, K. (2004). Comparison of self-report versus agency records of service utilization in a community sample of individuals with alcohol use disorders. *Drug and Alcohol Dependence, 73,* 141–147.

Kukull, W., Larson, E., Reifler, B., Lampe, T., Yerby, M., & Hughes, J. (1990). Interrater reliability of Alzheimer's disease diagnosis. *Neurology, 40,* 257–260.

Lim, K., Rank, M., Li, J., Patel, A., Volcheck, G., Branda, M., et al. (2010). How well does patient self-report predict asthma medication possession? Implications for medication reconciliation and adherence assessment. *Journal of Asthma, 47,* 878–882.

Litwack, T., Kirschner, S., & Wack, R. (1993). The assessment of dangerousness and predictions of violence: Recent research and future prospects. *Psychiatric Quarterly, 64,* 245–273.

Long, B., Rouse, S., Nelsen, R., & Butcher, J. (2004). The MMPI-2 in sexual harassment and discrimination litigants. *Journal of Clinical Psychology, 60,* 643–657.

Macciocchi, S., & Eaton, B. (1995). Decision and attribution bias in neurorehabilitation. *Archives of Physical Medicine and Rehabilitation, 76,* 521–524.

Macciocchi, S., & Stringer, A. (2001). Assessing risk and harm: The convergence of ethical and empirical considerations. *Archives of Physical Medicine and Rehabilitation, 82*(Suppl. 2), S15–S19.

Maj, M., Pirozzi, R., Formicola, A., Bartoli, L., & Bucci, P. (2000). Reliability and validity of the DSM-IV diagnostic category of schizoaffective disorder: Preliminary data. *Journal of Affective Disorders, 57,* 95–98.

Mäntylä, R., Erkinjuntti, T., Salonen, O., Aronen, H., Peltonen, T., Pohjasvaara, T., et al. (1997). Variable agreement between visual rating scales for white matter hyperintensities on MRI. Comparison of 13 rating scales in a poststroke cohort. *Stroke, 28,* 1614–1623.

Meehl, P. (1973). *Psychodiagnosis: Selected papers.* Minneapolis: University of Minnesota Press.

Murabito, B., Nam, H., D'Agostino, R., Lloyd-Jones, D., O'Donnell, C., & Wilson, P. (2004). Accuracy of offspring reports of parental cardiovascular disease history: The Framingham offspring study. *Annals of Internal Medicine, 140,* 434–440.

Nimnuan, C., Hotopf, M., & Wessely, S. (2001). Medically unexplained symptoms: An epidemiological study in seven specialties. *Journal of Psychosomatic Research, 51,* 361–367.

Parent, M., Ghadirian, P., Lacroix, A., & Perret, C. (1997). The reliability of recollections of family history: Implications for the medical provider. *Journal of Cancer Education, 12,* 114–120.

Pittman, J., Andrews, H., Tatemichi, T., Link, B., Struening, E., Stern, Y., et al. (1992). A comparison of paradigm-based diagnosis and physician's diagnosis. *Archives of Neurology, 49,* 461–467.

Ruchinskas, R. (2002). Rehabilitation therapists' recognition of cognitive and mood disorders in geriatric patients. *Archives of Physical Medicine and Rehabilitation, 83,* 609–612.

Ruchinskas, R. (2003). Clinical prediction of falls in the elderly. *American Journal of Physical Medicine and Rehabilitation, 82,* 273–278.

Ruchinskas, R., Combs, C., Riley, K., & Broshek, D. (2006). Defensive responding on the MMPI-2 in pre-surgical candidates. *Journal of Clinical Psychology in Medical Settings, 13,* 441–445.

Ruchinskas, R., Macciocchi, S., Howe, G., & Newton, R. (2001). Clinical decision-making in the prediction of falls. *Rehabilitation Psychology, 46,* 262–270.

Sansone, P., Schmitt, L., & Nichols, J. (1998). Determining the capacity of demented nursing home residents to name a health care proxy. *Clinical Gerontologist, 19,* 35–50.

Schrag, A., Brown, R., & Trimble, M. (2004). Reliability of self-reported diagnoses in patients with neurologically unexplained symptoms. *Journal of Neurology, Neurosurgery, & Psychiatry, 75,* 608–611.

Serin, R., & Amos, N. (1995). The role of psychopathy in the assessment of dangerousness. *International Journal of Law and Psychiatry, 18,* 231–238.

Solomon, D., Stedman, M., Licari, A., Weinblatt, M., Maher, N, & Shadick, N. (2007). Agreement between patient report and medical record review for medications used for rheumatoid arthritis: The accuracy of self-reported medication information in patient registries. *Arthritis and Rheumatism, 57,* 234–239.

Tombaugh, T., & McIntyre, N. (1992). The Mini-Mental State Examination: A comprehensive review. *Journal of the American Geriatrics Society, 40,* 922–935.
Volk, R., & Cass, A. (2002). The accuracy of primary care patient's self-reports of prostate-specific antigen testing. *American Journal of Preventive Medicine, 22,* 56–58.
Watkins, P., Gouvier, W., Callon, E., & Barkemeyer, C. (1989). Equivalence of items on the Mini-Mental State. *Archives of Clinical Neuropsychology, 4,* 381–384.

12

Forensic Report Writing and Testimony in Capacity Evaluations

PATRICIA A. ZAPF AND GIANNI PIRELLI

The forensic evaluation report is the primary means by which information, opinions, and conclusions about a forensic examinee are conveyed to other parties. Given the necessity for clear and accurate documentation of a forensic evaluation and the legal context in which the evaluation report is considered, it is important to write the report as if multiple parties will closely scrutinize each and every sentence. All conclusions and opinions should be supported by multiple pieces of relevant data and the reader should be taken through the process of how the data provide the basis for the evaluator's final conclusions and opinions. This chapter will provide an overview of forensic report writing and testimony in capacity evaluation. We begin by highlighting the legal standards for capacity evaluation and the issues involved in addressing the ultimate legal issue. Next, we summarize the nature and purpose of the written forensic evaluation report and discuss the contents of the written report. Finally, we address issues related to expert testimony. The reader is also referred to other sources for more information on this topic [e.g., American Bar Association Commission on Law, Aging & American Psychological Association (ABA/APA), 2005, 2006, 2008; Ackerman, 2006; Allnut & Chaplow, 2000; Conroy, 2006; Melton, Petrila, Poythress, & Slobogin, 2007; Weiner, 2006].

Upon completion of a forensic evaluation, the evaluator will often present his or her opinions in the form of a written forensic report. Before doing so, however, the evaluator must determine whether a written report is, in fact, required. In certain situations, a written report may be neither desired nor required. For example, in instances in which the evaluator is retained as an *ex parte* evaluator in a civil or criminal legal matter, the decision regarding whether a written report is required or desired belongs to the retaining attorney. Thus, the evaluator should consult with the retaining attorney before preparing a written report, especially in light of the rules of discovery. In these instances, it is customary for the evaluator to provide an oral report of his or her conclusions and opinions regarding the legal issue to the retaining attorney. Upon consideration of the oral report, the retaining attorney will then be in a position to determine whether the evaluator should prepare a written report.

LEGAL STANDARDS FOR FORENSIC REPORT WRITING

Faust and colleagues (2010) presented a focused review of issues related to the admissibility of behavioral science evidence in court and the interested reader is referred to their article for more detailed information. The following is a brief summary of relevant legal standards for forensic report writing.

In 1993 the U.S. Supreme Court tightened the standards for admissibility of expert evidence in *Daubert v. Merrill Dow Pharmaceuticals.* Prior to *Daubert*, the *Frye* test was used to determine the admissibility of scientific evidence (*Frye v. United States*, 1923). The *Frye* test required that expert opinion be based on a scientific technique that is generally accepted as reliable in the relevant scientific community in order to be admissible as evidence. *Daubert* served to raise the bar from *general acceptance* in the hopes of eliminating junk science. As such, *Daubert* requires that the court consider a number of criteria in determining the admissibility of evidence on a particular theory or technique, including (1) whether the theory or technique can be or has been tested; (2) whether the theory or technique has been subjected to peer review and publication, as such review "increases the likelihood that substantive flaws in the methodology will be detected"; (3) in the case of the particular technique, the known or potential rate of error; and (4) whether the theory or technique enjoys general acceptance within the relevant scientific community (pp. 593–594). The inquiry is a flexible one, and its focus must be solely on principles and methodology, not on the conclusions that they generate.

The Court has since decided two cases that, along with *Daubert*, are referred to as the *Daubert* trilogy. In *General Electric Co. v. Joiner* (1997) the Court made it clear that the trial judge is the gatekeeper with respect to the evidence to be admitted at trial and that courts could scrutinize the reliability of an expert's reasoning process as well as the expert's general methodology, making it clear that "nothing in either *Daubert* or the Federal Rules of Evidence requires a district court to admit opinion evidence that is connected to existing data only by the *ipse dixit* of the expert" (p. 146). Instead, *Joiner* specified that courts were free to conclude that "there is simply too great an analytical gap between the data and the opinion proffered" (p. 146). In *Kumho Tire Co. v. Carmichael* (1999), the Court considered whether *Daubert* applied solely to scientific evidence, as opposed to technical or other specialized knowledge or testimony. The Court in *Kumho* acknowledged that that distinction between scientific and technical knowledge is not always clear and extended *Daubert's* gatekeeping function beyond scientific evidence to encompass all expert testimony, including nonscientific testimony.

Although *Daubert* applies only in Federal court and about half the states, the most conservative approach is to adhere to the Daubert standard regardless of jurisdiction and refrain from including anything in a written report that cannot be supported by research or professional literature. As Ackerman noted, "The basic message that should be taken from the Daubert standard is that it is no longer acceptable to say something is true based merely on anecdote or simply because it is the opinion of the expert" (Ackerman, 2006, pp. 60–61).

THE "ULTIMATE ISSUE" ISSUE

The ultimate issue is the specific question at hand in a legal proceeding, such as whether a defendant is competent/incompetent to stand trial (in criminal cases) or whether an elderly individual is competent to manage his or her financial affairs or in need of a guardian (in a civil context). The determination of the ultimate legal issue is the purview of the trier of fact; however, medical and mental health professionals are often called upon to *assist* the court in making such determinations by providing clinical conclusions and opinions. The debate about whether medical and mental health professionals should speak to the ultimate legal issue (i.e., the "ultimate issue" issue) refers to whether the professional should explicitly address (answer) the legal question when providing his or her expert opinion regarding related psycholegal issues. Slobogin (1989) noted a differentiation between speaking to the ultimate legal issue and providing testimony using penultimate language, which addresses the components of a specific legal question rather than the question directly. It is important to note that ultimate issue testimony and testimony using penultimate language are both forms of clinical opinion and that the legal determination ultimately rests with the court. As Ganzini and colleagues (2003) noted, confusing legal competence, as decided by a formal judicial proceeding, and clinical determinations of decision-making capacity is one of the most common pitfalls in assessments of decision-making capacity (and suggest that this is an important distinction to make in the education and training of evaluators). Those readers for whom the distinction between legal competence and clinical determinations of capacity is unclear are encouraged to read further and/or obtain further training before proceeding with clinical work in this area. A brief summary of issues relevant to ultimate issue opinions follows.

Expert witnesses have been permitted to present their opinions and inferences to the court since the 1800s, provided the opinions and inferences were based on a particular area of knowledge and expertise (exceeding that of a layperson) and that such testimony would likely aid the trier of fact (Rogers & Ewing, 1989). Rules 702, 703, 704, and 705 of the Federal Rules of Evidence directly address the parameters of expert testimony. Rule 704 specifically pertains to ultimate issue opinions and reads:

> (a) Except as provided in subdivision (b), testimony in the form of an opinion or inference otherwise admissible is not objectionable because it embraces an ultimate issue to be decided by the trier of fact.
> (b) No expert witness testifying with respect to the mental state or condition of a defendant in a criminal case may state an opinion or

> inference as to whether the defendant did or did not have the mental state or condition constituting an element of the crime charged or of a defense thereto. Such ultimate issues are matters for the trier of fact alone.[1]

Although ultimate issue opinions are typically permissible in court, debate about whether to offer ultimate issue opinions has been a part of the professional literature for over 30 years. Much of the focus in the literature has been on providing such opinions within the context of criminal responsibility (i.e., insanity) evaluations; however, the issue is relevant to all areas of forensic mental health assessment. Cogent arguments have been made on both sides of the debate. Some psycholegal scholars (e.g., Grisso, 1986; Melton et al., 2007; Tillbrook, Mumley, & Grisso, 2003; Slobogin, 1989) have generally opposed addressing the ultimate issue on the basis that these opinions are outside of the role and expertise of the mental health professional. Others, however, have argued that testimony lacking such opinions would likely be incomplete and, therefore, unhelpful to the trier of fact (e.g., Rogers & Ewing, 1989, 2003; Slovenko, 2006). A brief review of the specific arguments is delineated below.

Melton and colleagues (2007) have generally been cautious about the role of mental health professionals in this regard and have written that "Despite the fact that such opinions are commonly sought and, unfortunately, are commonly given, *mental health professionals ordinarily should refrain from giving opinions as to ultimate legal issues*" (p. 17, italics in original), citing "near-unanimity among scholarly commentators" against setting forth ultimate issue opinions (p. 17). These authors characterized ultimate issues as legal and moral judgments outside the expertise of mental health professionals. Furthermore, although they acknowledged that such testimony is generally permissible per Rule 704(a), they argue that Rule 702, which bars opinions not based on specialized knowledge, prohibits such testimony. Melton and colleagues further argued that ultimate opinion testimony could usurp the role of the trier of fact and may mislead the trier of fact by suggesting that the (ultimate legal issue) opinions are based on specialized knowledge specific to the profession. They also contended that inferences based on the elements of the legal issue should "generally be avoided" because they would be predicated on legally defined language (p. 17) outside the domain of mental health professionals (for example, the magnitude required to satisfy a legal requirement—how much "knowledge" or "awareness"—is purely a legal issue).

As Grisso (2003) articulated, "Forensic assessment might provide a comparative description of a defendant's abilities and probable trial demands. Yet one makes a moral judgment when one concludes that the degree of incongruency between these two sets of observations is too great to warrant a finding of competence" (p. 89). Tillbrook and colleagues (2003) have also argued that the threshold

1. The second component, Rule 704(b), represents an amendment enacted by Congress in 1984 in response to the verdict held in the case against John W. Hinckley, Jr., the man who attempted to assassinate President Ronald Reagan. Some states have chosen not to adopt this part of the Rule (e.g., Texas and Pennsylvania).

associated with certain penultimate issues (e.g., sufficient present ability, reasonable degree) is not measurable and, therefore, mental health professionals should not offer opinions about such. In addition, Melton and colleagues (2007) expressed concern that opinions on the ultimate issue may not be subject to the adversarial process—because only a small percentage of cases go to trial and experts testify in only a small percentage of those that do—and, as a result, such opinions should be avoided as a matter of professional ethics regardless of a court's decision regarding admissibility.

In contrast to the position that mental health professionals should not speak to the ultimate legal issue, Rogers and Ewing (1989) have characterized the reinstatement of the ultimate issue rule [Rule 704(b)] as "a quick and cosmetic fix—that is, a hasty, ill-conceived, and probably needless effort, the value of which is more apparent than real" (pp. 360–361). They argued that although the rule is ostensibly attractive and satisfying to some, it is unwarranted, unnecessary, and impractical. Rogers and Ewing contended that ultimate opinions are an inevitable outcome of the forensic assessment process and that no meaningful distinction can be made between ultimate opinions and other expert opinions. They delineated four concerns that might be associated with ultimate opinion testimony: professional taint, which refers to the limitation of the role of experts in insanity trials in an effort to avoid "public and collegial disapproval" (p. 361); insufficient clinical data, such that opinions in this regard would be based on insufficient clinical observations, test findings, or empirically based decision making; undue influence, such that ultimate opinion testimony might usurp the role of the trier of fact; and the concern that mental health professionals lack legal and moral expertise.

Rogers and Ewing (1989) challenged the assumptions regarding what comprises a moral question in the legal arena and further questioned the role of morality in other areas of psychology in which ultimate opinions are proffered (e.g., the American Psychological Association's *amicus* brief on adolescent abortion in *Bowen v. Kendrick*, 1988). In addition, they presented three main arguments as to why a prohibition on ultimate opinion testimony is flawed. First, they argued that clinical judgments and clinical observations are inseparable and that denying experts the ability to explicate their judgments will conceal, rather than alter, their influence. Second, ultimate opinions are an inevitable outcome of the forensic assessment process and to disallow ultimate opinion testimony is akin to tasking a mental health expert with working toward a very specific goal that is never explicitly addressed, thereby leading the trier of fact to "read between the lines" (p. 365). Third, no meaningful difference can be made between ultimate opinions and ordinary expert opinions because essentially the same conclusions are made.

In addition to these three arguments, Rogers and Ewing also set forth five potential, albeit unintended, implications of the prohibition of ultimate opinion testimony: (1) oblique opinions might be substituted for explicit opinions, (2) the scope of mental health expert testimony might be paradoxically expanded, (3) mental health experts might exercise less care in their evaluations, (4) the likelihood of experts being influenced by attorneys might increase, and (5) experts might be prevented from offering "no opinion" testimony when its warranted (such as when they are unable to draw conclusory opinions or firm conclusions).

Although strong arguments have been set forth on both sides of the ultimate issue debate, most of these are theoretically or philosophically based rather than empirically driven. In fact, few empirical studies have investigated the effects of ultimate issue testimony. Those that exist were conducted two decades ago and found that such testimony does not significantly affect verdict patterns (Fulero & Finkel, 1991; Rogers, Bagby, Crouch, & Cutler, 1990). More recent studies have investigated the attitudes and perspectives of mental health professionals, attorneys, and judges with respect to ultimate opinion testimony rather than the effects of such testimony per se.

Borum and Grisso (1996) surveyed 102 forensic psychologists and psychiatrists regarding their perspectives on the content of competency and criminal responsibility reports. Of the professionals surveyed, a majority indicated that ultimate opinion testimony was essential, although a few considered it to be contraindicated. Ryba, Cooper, and Zapf (2003) surveyed 82 psychologists across the country who listed their area of expertise as juvenile forensic assessments and found that the majority characterized proffering ultimate issue opinions as essential, whereas only 10% found this practice to be contraindicated. In contrast, Pirelli and Zapf (2008) surveyed 231 licensed forensic psychologists across 41 states and the District of Columbia with respect to their practices and attitudes toward participation in capital (i.e., death penalty) evaluations and found that, although the majority indicated that experts should avoid answering the ultimate legal issue in the course of their courtroom testimony, nearly half of those surveyed found this practice either acceptable or were neutral on the topic. It is worth noting, however, that the relatively high level of opposition to offering an opinion on the ultimate issue found in this study may have been due to the fact that psychologists were asked this question in the context of capital evaluations rather than in forensic assessments more generally. Redding, Floyd, and Hawk (2001) surveyed trial court judges, prosecutors, and defense attorneys throughout Virginia with respect to their opinions on the testimony of mental health professionals and found that judges and prosecutors ranked ultimate opinion testimony as high in importance, whereas defense attorneys ranked it lower in importance. Viljoen, Wingrove, and Ryba (2008) surveyed juvenile and criminal court judges from seven states and found that the majority of judges classified ultimate opinion testimony as essential (in both juvenile and criminal court), whereas almost none deemed such opinions as optional or contraindicated.

In sum, it appears that mental health professionals, attorneys, and judges are generally in favor of experts offering an opinion on the ultimate issue. Although psycholegal scholars continue to debate this specific issue, standards of practice have been delineated for those conducting forensic mental health assessments, which provide the forensic practitioner with a framework from which to proceed. Some jurisdictions require or expect ultimate opinions, whereas others prohibit or discourage them; therefore, the forensic evaluator must familiarize himself or herself with the relevant jurisdictional requirements. If no such requirements exist, it is incumbent on the forensic evaluator to decide whether and how to address the "ultimate issue" issue. Some evaluators might choose to refrain from providing ultimate opinions, but may feel comfortable incorporating penultimate language in their report and/or testimony. Regardless of one's choice in this regard, what is essential is that the evaluation be conducted in accordance with the standards of practice in the particular area of forensic mental health assessment and that the conclusions be clearly and logically drawn from the data available. The thoroughness and transparency of a well-written report and effective testimony based on a competently performed evaluation should not be overshadowed by the evaluator's decision to offer an opinion (or not) on the ultimate issue.

PURPOSE AND NATURE OF THE WRITTEN REPORT

The purpose of the written report is to document relevant information regarding the evaluation and procedures and to communicate the conclusions and opinions formed regarding the referral question. A well-written report may negate the need for testimony at a court hearing if all parties stipulate to the findings in the report; thus, reports should be carefully written and informative. In addition, in those instances in which the expert is called to testify at a capacity hearing, the written report will usually form the basis for direct examination and thus everything in the report will be subject to question on cross-examination. As such, written reports should be thorough yet concise in their scope and focus. In discussing the necessary characteristics of forensic reports, Weiner (2006) indicated that reports should be clear, relevant, informative, and defensible. A brief discussion of the scope and focus as well as the characteristic of the written report follows.

Scope and focus. Relevant ethics codes and guidelines provide guidance regarding the appropriate scope and focus of the written capacity evaluation report. Ethical Standard 4.04(a) of the Code of Conduct of the American Psychological Association (2002) states that "psychologists include in written and oral reports and consultations, only information germane to the purpose for which the communication is made" (p. 1066). In addition, the recently adopted new Speciality Guidelines for Forensic Psychology (in press), states that forensic practitioners "limit discussion of background information that does not bear directly on the legal purpose of the examination or consultation. Forensic practitioners avoid offering information that is irrelevant and that does not provide a substantial basis of support for their opinions, except when required by law". Thus, capacity evaluation reports should focus specifically on the issue in question and any information that is not directly relevant to this issue should be limited.

Clarity. In writing capacity evaluation reports it is necessary to consider the audience for the report and to write accordingly. Legal professionals, the audience for most competency/capacity evaluation reports, are not trained as mental health professionals; therefore,it is inappropriate to assume that technical jargon used to communicate with other mental health professionals will be understood.

Similarly, family members might be another potential audience for a capacity report. Thus, reports should be written in a clear, concise manner using plain English and as little technical jargon as possible. In those (relatively few) instances when technical jargon must be used (such as when the use of a term is necessary to justify its legal or clinical relevance), it is appropriate to include a definition or description of what is meant by the term immediately following its use. Non-mental health professionals often misunderstand even relatively common terms, such as hallucinations or delusions.

Weiner (2006) offered the following advice for written forensic reports: "the written report itself should be as clear and conversational as the psychologist can make it. This means using unstilted and uncomplicated language that will be comfortable for [evaluators] to repeat on the witness stand, that will be comprehensible to judge and jury, and that will limit a cross-examining attorney's opportunities to badger them with questions about what their statements mean" (p. 645). In addition, Weiner cautioned that the evaluator should concentrate on writing about the *person* that was evaluated rather than about psychological processes since "impersonal descriptions of psychological processes often go hand in hand with jargon" (p. 645). For example, a statement such as "concentration was intact" does not communicate as clearly as "Mr. Z was able to demonstrate appropriate concentration by staying focused during a lengthy discussion of his treatment options and contributing detailed information without becoming distracted."

Relevance. Section 10.01 of the recently adopted new Speciality Guidelines for Forensic Psychology (in press), states that "Forensic examiners seek to assist the trier of fact to understand evidence or determine a fact in issue, and they provide information that is most relevant to the psycholegal issue. In reports and testimony forensic practitioners typically provide information about examinee's functional abilities, capacities, knowledge, and beliefs, and address their opinions and recommendations to the identified psycholegal issues". Thus, the written forensic report should address all factors relevant to the issue of capacity. Evaluators should be knowledgeable about relevant legal standards, statutes, and jurisdictional case law regarding competence/capacity and their written reports should address these relevant standards and jurisdictional capacity requirements and provide a distillate of those features of the examinee that bear directly on the issue of capacity at hand.

During the course of a capacity evaluation it is common to accumulate much more information than is needed to address the issue of competence/capacity. As a general rule, only information that bears directly on the issue of competence/capacity should be included in the written report. Grisso (1988) advocated for a "problem-focused" approach to deciding what information to include in a written report: "The examiner can determine the extent to which information from hospital records, [other] records, and a social history must be described in a given case by applying a simple 'problem-focused' question: '*Does the piece of information I am preparing to report act as an important basis for the reasoning I will use in arriving at one of the competency evaluation's objectives?*' If the answer is no, the piece of information usually should not be included" (p. 74, italics in original).

Informative. The written report should be informative and educational. Data and inferences should be presented and explained in a way that is easy to understand by those who are not forensic mental health professionals. The report can be used as a forum to educate the reader about relevant psychological concepts and their relation to the capacity issue. Brief descriptions of psychological tests or forensic assessment instruments and the abilities that they measure can be provided to assist the reader in understanding the relevance of test results for the capacity issue.

To guard against information overkill (and an unnecessarily lengthy report), it is important to carefully consider which pieces of information to include. Those pieces of information that are directly relevant to the issue of competence/capacity or that are relevant to inferences that are made should be included and inferences should be explained. In addition, it is important to indicate the source from which the information was obtained. Informative and educational reports are those that lead the reader through the relevant pieces of information that were considered and weighed by the evaluator and that delineate the expert's thought processes in coming to an opinion or conclusion regarding the examinee's capacity.

Defensible. Written reports are discoverable and may be entered into evidence; thus, evaluators may be held accountable for every statement made in their reports. For this reason, it is imperative that evaluators choose their words carefully and thoughtfully and be able to defend the opinions and conclusions set out in their reports. Weiner (2006) cautioned that "forensic psychologists should limit their written reports to statements they will feel comfortable hearing read aloud in the courtroom and to conclusions they feel able to defend against reasonable challenge" (p. 639).

CONTENTS OF THE WRITTEN REPORT

Although there are a number of different ways in which to organize an evaluation report and the specific contents of a written evaluation report will be dependent upon the type of capacity evaluated, the following provides some general guidelines regarding the types of information to be included. The evaluator should provide relevant information that will assist the requesting party or trier of fact in understanding the current functioning of the examinee and how his or her functioning relates to the specific areas of concern for the particular type of capacity evaluated.

Case and Referral Information

The first part of the written evaluation report typically includes relevant information about the examinee including demographic information such as age, race, gender, and any relevant information about the evaluation, such as case number (if applicable), date(s) of the evaluation, and the date the report was written.

In addition, this section will usually include information regarding the legal background and referral, such as the legal issue at hand, the referral source, the specific referral question, and the specific elements of capacity at issue. The evaluator may choose to reference the relevant legal statutes in either this section of the report or later on when discussing the forensic inquiry or his or her conclusions and opinions.

Notification or Informed Consent

As a general rule, court-ordered evaluations do not require that the evaluator obtain the informed consent of the examinee; however, the evaluator is still required to provide notification of all the information that would typically be divulged to obtain informed consent to the examinee. In those cases in which the evaluation is not ordered by the court but, rather, is requested by a particular party, informed consent procedures should be followed.

This section of the report will provide information regarding how the evaluator provided the notification for the evaluation and obtained assent or informed consent from the examinee, including how the evaluator described the purpose of the evaluation, the examinee's understanding of the evaluation and its risk and benefits, and a statement of the examinee's assent or consent to participate in the evaluation. In situations in which the capacity of the examinee to provide informed consent is questionable, the evaluator should explain all the relevant information about the evaluation, including the purpose of the evaluation, the risks and benefits, the limits on confidentiality, those individuals who will have access to any report that might be written, and the possible consequences that the evaluation results might have for the examinee, and should obtain the assent of the examinee before proceeding. In these instances and if necessary, it is best to obtain informed consent from a guardian or other legally responsible party.

Data Sources and Tests Administered

This section delineates the various data sources that were considered by the evaluator in conducting the evaluation. All sources of data, including interviews with the examinee, collateral interviews with family members or other individuals, records reviewed, interactions observed between the examinee and relevant others (e.g., the examinee's attorney in testamentary capacity inquiries), and test data considered should be reported along with the relevant dates and duration of the interviews as well as whether the interviews occurred in person or by telephone. The full names of any tests administered should be listed in this section, including any tests that the examinee discontinued or was unable to complete, along with the date(s) of administration and the duration of testing for each instrument. Each data source should be listed individually and in chronological order to make it easier for the reader to understand. If an attorney or another individual was present during any of the interviews, this should also be noted.

Background: History of Present Illness/Functioning and Psychosocial History

This section includes a description of the examinee's present illness, including current symptoms and severity, and a psychosocial history. Typically the areas of inquiry for a psychosocial history include the following: developmental history; family history; interpersonal functioning; academic, occupational, military, medical, criminal, and psychiatric history; history of drug and alcohol use; current living situation; and any other information relevant to the issue at hand. As discussed earlier, it is important to carefully consider the amount of information (as well as the amount of detail) provided in this section of the report. Using Grisso's problem-focused approach, wherein only information that provides an important basis for the reasoning used to arrive at an opinion regarding the examinee's competence-related or capacity-related abilities is included, appears to be a useful strategy. Thus, the referral question(s) should guide the nature and extent of the information provided in the psychosocial history section of the report. Finally, it is important to accurately attribute information included in this section of the report to its appropriate source (examinee's self-report, medical records, collateral interview, etc.).

Clinical Assessment: Mental Status and Behavioral Observations

This section of the report includes information on the examinee's current mental status as well as behavioral observations noted during the evaluation. A description of the examinee's appearance and presentation, mood and range of emotional expression, speech and communication abilities, insight and judgment, and motivation is appropriate and relevant in this section. Any indications of neurological impairment or mental illness should be noted including perseveration, flat affect, morbid ideation, paranoid or delusional thinking, hallucinations, confusion or inability to follow task directions, short-term memory loss, or any other symptom that might have an impact upon capacity-related abilities.

The evaluator's observations of the examinee over the course of the evaluation are an important piece of the evaluation process to report as these provide objective information regarding the types of behaviors that are tied to specific clinical impressions of an examinee. In describing his or her observations of the examinee, the evaluator should be cautious about implying stable characteristics (traits) from his or her observations of a sample of the examinee's behaviors and functioning (state). In addition, the evaluator should use concrete descriptors of what he or she observed of the examinee. All information provided in this section of the report should be relevant to the referral question.

Test Results

This section should include a summary of the results for any psychological or neuropsychological tests that were administered. A statement regarding the motivation and test-taking style (i.e., response style) of the examinee, including an opinion regarding the extent to which the test results are valid, should always accompany any description of test results. The evaluator should be clear about the link between the ability or characteristic measured by the test and the examinee's psychological functioning in this section of the report because, in the next section, any psychological testing results will need to be directly tied to inferences regarding the examinee's capacity-related abilities or deficits (that is, his or her ability to engage in the tasks or abilities required to meet the specific capacity at issue).

The distinction between test data and test results is an important point to note. Section 9.04 of the 2002 APA Code of Conduct defines test data as "raw and scale scores, client/patient responses to test questions or stimuli, and psychologists' notes and recordings concerning client/patient statements and behavior during an examination" (p. 1071) and requires psychologists to release test data to the client/patient pursuant to a client/patient release. The Code further notes that test data should be explained to the client/patient upon its release and should be released to other mental health professionals only to guard against misinterpretation or misrepresentation. Given that a wider audience than just other mental health professionals receives forensic reports, Ackerman (2006) noted that "there is no room in any forensic report for the inclusion of test data. . .as defined by the Code. The only time that test data should be included in a report is if it is going to be read exclusively by mental health professionals. Otherwise, it may be a violation of section 9.04, especially because non-mental health professionals and the general public are likely to misuse or misrepresent the data" (pp. 64–65). Others, however, note the expectation that test scores will be included in the test results section of the report (see the ABA/APA Assessment of Capacity in Older Adults Project Working Group's Handbooks). We take the stance that raw test scores should not be included in the forensic evaluation report but, rather, full descriptions of the abilities measured and the examinee's normative performance (that is, in relation to the relevant comparisons groups) should be provided as well as appropriate cautions regarding standard error of measurement, confidence intervals, and test limitations.

Diagnostic Impression and Forensic Issue(s)

This section of the evaluation report includes the evaluator's clinical impressions as well as information regarding the specific capacity at issue. The evaluator may choose to include the relevant legal statutes in this section if these were not included earlier in the report. The evaluator's conclusions regarding diagnosis and current symptoms should be provided as well as a clinical interpretation of test results and psycholegal capacities. It is essential for the evaluator to link the functional assessment of relevant abilities to the examinee's mental illness or cognitive deficits to provide the basis for the conclusions and opinions regarding the examinee's capacity status. Although the legal decision maker will be required to make a dichotomous judgment regarding the examinee's competency (e.g., is the individual competent or not), the forensic evaluator will typically indicate his or her opinion regarding whether, or the degree to which, the examinee possesses particular capacities. Providing the link between the psychiatric, emotional, or cognitive factors and any functional deficits noted in the required capacity-related abilities is the key to providing the courts or other decision makers with the requisite information for making a legal determination of competency. As important as this linkage is to show, it is the one area in which forensic evaluators fall woefully short in their written reports (Robbins, Waters, & Herbert, 1997; Skeem, Golding, Cohn, & Berge, 1998). Using clear language that explicitly denotes the relevant linkage is important for clear communication with a legal decision maker. For example, Mr. Z's thought disorder is characterized by a system of delusions in which he believes that various members of his family have colluded in an attempt to poison him by forcing oral chemotherapy. As such, Mr. Z is strongly opposed to this course of treatment; however, given his delusional belief system, Mr. Z in unable to rationally understand the various treatment options available to him and, therefore, is unable to engage in rational decision making regarding his medical treatment. Nonetheless, Mr. Z is able to demonstrate rational decision making when asked to engage decision-making exercises unrelated to his medical treatment.

This section of the report should provide a complete description of the examinee's capacity-related abilities and deficits. In addition, the issue of the examinee's motivation and response style should be addressed, even if only to indicate that there appeared to be no evidence of malingering. Of course, if malingering or another identifiable response style was indicated (e.g., minimization), more details about response style and any formal evaluation of malingering should be described. If a capacity assessment instrument was used to structure the evaluation or to supplement capacity-related inquiries, a brief description of the instrument(s) used as well as a description of the examinee's performance in terms of his or her capacity-related abilities and deficits should be provided.

To structure the presentation of information regarding the examinee's capacity-related abilities and deficits, it is often helpful to include the jurisdictional definition, standard, or criteria for the capacity at issue. This way, the evaluator can provide a description of the examinee's relevant abilities and deficits for each part of the standard. Once a description of the examinee's capacity-related abilities and deficits has been provided, the evaluator then needs to delineate the cause of any noted deficits (e.g., mental illness, malingering, and/or situational factors) and provide the bases for his or her conclusions or opinions on this matter. Examples of the examinee's inadequate or impaired capacity-related abilities (e.g., in understanding, appreciation, reasoning, and/or decision making) may assist the evaluator in describing these deficits. When the evaluator believes that psychiatric and/or cognitive impairment (mental illness, broadly defined) is the cause of the noted functional deficits, the report should clearly indicate how the psychiatric and/or cognitive impairment accounts for the deficits. It is not sufficient to merely establish that psycholegal deficits and mental illness coexist; a causal connection between the two must be established and should be clearly described in the report. The evaluator should then describe how the noted symptoms would affect the examinee's performance or participation in the activities or decisions in which he or she is expected to engage. In situations in which fluctuations in mental state or cognitive functioning are especially apparent, conditional statements regarding how the examinee's capacity-related abilities might be affected are appropriate.

The nature and logic behind the evaluator's reasoning are critical components of the capacity determination process and must be spelled out accordingly. Careful delineation of the links between (a) mental illness and capacity-related deficits and (b) capacity-related deficits and functional abilities within the context of what is required of the examinee (i.e., financial, medical, or healthcare decision making, testamentary capacity, personal care and independence, driving, etc.) will elevate the quality and the utility of the evaluator's report. As Heilbrun, Marczyk, and DeMatteo (2002) suggested, the evaluator can use contingency statements in the form of "if x, then y; if not x, then z" to assist the audience in understanding the links between clinical observations, the evaluator's reasoning, and the conclusions that he or she reaches (p. 53). As an example, the following would be appropriate: "If Mr. Z receives treatment for his thought disorder and delusional belief system, then he will likely be able to make rationally informed decisions about his medical treatment options. If he does not receive such treatment, it is unlikely that he will be able to engage in rational decision making about medical treatment."

If prescriptive remediation for any noted deficits can be offered, a description of this should be included in this section of the report. For example, if the evaluator determines that an examinee with a low IQ is unable to understand lengthy, complicated descriptions of information but is able to understand short sentences, then including a recommendation that using short sentences with an uncomplicated structure and defining uncommon or large words for the examinee would be appropriate.

This section of the report should also contain the evaluator's conclusions or opinions regarding each of the jurisdictional criteria for the capacity at issue. In addition, if comfortable for the evaluator or required by the jurisdiction, the ultimate issue of capacity can be addressed using appropriate language to convey that the conclusion on the matter is a clinical opinion, not a legal determination. Finally, any information regarding the examinee's prognosis for restoration or remediation of any noted capacity-related deficits can be included here. The evaluator is responsible for knowing whether any legal statutes or jurisdictional requirements demand that certain types of information be included in an evaluation report and for ensuring that all required information is included.

Summary and Recommendations

This final section of the report should offer a brief summary of the evaluator's conclusions and opinions. Brevity is expected in this section, as detailed descriptions of the information provided here should have been included in earlier sections of the report. A brief description of the examinee's competence/capacity-related abilities and deficits should be provided along with the cause of the deficits and their relationship to the defendant's functional abilities (e.g., how these deficits will impact the examinee's participation in whatever activity or decision is implicated). A formal diagnosis would be included here if one is required or expected. In addition, the evaluator may offer an ultimate opinion regarding the examinee's capacity, if acceptable or expected, in this section of the report. Finally, a brief summary of prescriptive remediation or remediation potential should be offered for those examinees with significant competence/capacity-related deficits.

EXPERT TESTIMONY

Although arguably more common for some types of forensic evaluations than others, a forensic evaluator may be called to testify at a hearing on the issue after he or she has conducted a capacity evaluation and produced a written report. Before the forensic evaluator testifies as an expert it is essential that he or she understand the basis of expert testimony as it pertains to attorney work product, the Federal Rules of Evidence, and legal admissibility standards. In addition, it is imperative that the evaluator be versed in the specific requirements of the jurisdiction in which the case is being considered; thus, locating and understanding the jurisdictional statutes and requirements with respect to the specific issue at hand should be one of the first tasks of any forensic evaluator prior to commencing a forensic evaluation.

An evaluator may typically be either subpoenaed by the court or called by the retaining attorney to testify at a hearing on the issue under consideration. Although a defense expert may not be compelled to produce a report or testify if the jurisdictional statutes classify his or her evaluation as part of the attorney work product (*U.S. v. Alvarez*, 1975), the state has the right to access the defense's expert once the issue of mental state is raised (*U.S. ex rel Edney v. Smith*, 1976) because the burden of proof vis-à-vis the defendant's mental state is then assumed by the defense. In civil cases, the burden of proof regarding mental state rests with the petitioner.

In the following sections we will briefly describe information with respect to three areas related to providing expert testimony: preparing to take the stand, being on the witness stand, and facing cross-examination. Given the space limitations, however, the reader is also referred to other sources for more detailed information on this topic (Bank & Packer, 2007; Barsky & Gould, 2002; Blau, 1998; Brodsky, 1991, 1999, 2004; Dvoskin & Guy, 2008; Ewing, 2003, 2008; Gutheil, 1998; Hess, 2006; Tsushima & Anderson, 1996; Ziskin & Faust, 1995).

Preparing to take the stand. Being called to testify can be anxiety provoking for some forensic evaluators. If this is the case, it might be useful to explore the source of the anxiety. Perhaps public speaking, in general, is a worrisome endeavor for the evaluator; perhaps it is the expert's first case; or perhaps the expert has a fear of being "exposed" (i.e., not knowing as much as one's degree and experience would suggest). It is important to recognize that providing effective expert testimony is an acquired skill that requires training, consultation, and practice;

however, it does not have to be a daunting task or one to be feared. In fact, as Dvoksin and Guy (2008) articulated, it can be considered a rather straightforward process:

> expert testimony, at its best, is a simple process. By simply answering questions honestly, telling the court what we know, how we know it, and what we do not know, we will not only abide by our legal oath to be truthful, but also will maintain the credibility that is ultimately the only asset for which we get paid. (p. 202)

Nevertheless, providing effective expert testimony can be challenging at times. The following recommendations, although not exhaustive, are intended to provide experts with a framework for preparing to testify ethically and effectively.

The initial preparatory step is to review the written report, which will serve as the basis for the direct testimony, in its entirety as well as re-familiarize oneself with the individual sources of information included in the report (such as notes from the clinical interview, collateral interview notes, test protocols, file review notes, or any other sources of data from which clinical interpretations and/or opinions have been drawn). The second step is to ensure that one is familiar with the extant empirical literature for the area of inquiry and for any tests or measures used in the evaluation. Although it would be impossible to read every journal article and book published on capacity, the expert should have a reasonable knowledge of the seminal works in the capacity arena as well as the most recent empirical findings and contemporary standards of practice (e.g., ABA/APA, 2005, 2006, 2008; Kim, 2010; Zapf & Roesch, 2009). The expert should also review test manuals for the instruments used in the evaluation, with special attention paid to the administration, scoring, interpretation, and psychometric properties. It would also be prudent to conduct a literature review on the measures used to ensure familiarity with the latest information available.

The third step is to review or be prepared to address general clinical principles that may apply in a given case. For example, forensic evaluators should be prepared to address questions pertaining to clinical diagnoses and symptoms; therefore, familiarity with the *Diagnostic and Statistical Manual of Mental Disorders* (*DSM-IV-TR*; American Psychiatric Association, 2000) and other relevant diagnostic advancements in the field is expected. Attorneys might also inquire about principles from other general clinical areas (such as psychological assessment or clinical interviewing); thus, the expert should be prepared to address such questions if they are relevant to the current case. The fourth step is to review the opposing expert's report if applicable and possible. Close consideration of the opinions of the opposing expert and the sources of information from which such opinions were derived is warranted. For example, if the opposing expert utilized a different assessment measure, it would behoove the psychologist to read the test manual as well as recent publications on the measure.

If the expert was privately retained (*ex parte*), as opposed to court-ordered, the next step would entail engaging in a pretrial or prehearing conference with the retaining attorney. This conference will typically consist of the attorney providing an overview of the presentation of the case, including the way in which the expert's information will be presented and a discussion of how the opposing side may present its case. The attorney may further prepare the expert by discussing the courtroom process, addressing the expert's qualifications (and *curriculum vitae*), and by asking practice questions (from both the direct and cross-examination perspectives); however, in reality, many attorneys expect that their experts have experience in these matters and do not spend a lot of time, if any, in step-by-step preparation of the expert. The well-prepared expert will provide the attorney with relevant information regarding his or her education and experience (two of the three areas that will be considered by the court in qualifying the expert; the third area to be considered is the evaluation procedures used by the expert) as well as a description of his or her opinions and the key pieces of information (data) that form the basis for those opinions. Including a list of questions that will assist the attorney in eliciting this information as part of your testimony is also helpful. In addition, the expert should notify the attorney of any potential weaknesses in the case as they relate to the expert's evaluation and/or opinions as well as those of the opposing expert that may be apparent. Finally, the expert should read the available literature on delivering effective testimony (listed earlier in this section) and should seek professional consultation when necessary.

Being on the witness stand. In general, the evaluator should not be present in the courtroom for anything other than his or her testimony. In some instances the evaluator will be asked to stay in the courtroom and to listen to the testimony of other witnesses, but he or she should not do so unless specifically requested.

There are a number of recommendations for experts to consider when testifying on the witness stand. It is appropriate to dress conservatively in the courtroom and to focus attention on the judge (or the jurors, if applicable). The evaluator should use clear, conversational language and should explain unfamiliar concepts in a clear manner using lay language rather than professional jargon. Deference to the judge and courtesy toward the attorneys and the judge should be displayed. When being questioned, the evaluator should speak loud enough for the judge (or jury) to hear and in a confident manner. If a question is unclear, the evaluator should ask politely that it be repeated or reworded. The evaluator should answer only what has been asked without volunteering additional information. When an objection has been made, the expert should stop speaking and wait for the judge to make a ruling. If the evaluator does not have a particular piece of knowledge, he or she should answer honestly, "I do not know."

The credibility of the evaluator is essential to effective testimony and, as such, it is of the highest priority. As Ewing (2008) noted, forensic mental health professionals testify to their professional opinions, albeit specially weighted opinions, but not facts. A number of internal and external factors can potentially influence the expert to stray from his or her role. The length and stability of his or her career as an expert witness will likely be dependent on his or her reputation. Although a "hired gun" can make money and even do so over a lengthy career, such is accomplished by either rejecting or ignoring the principles of forensic mental health assessment as well as the ethical principles for psychologists more generally. An evaluator's credibility and, ultimately, his or her performance on the stand can be bolstered by being transparent with respect to the bases of opinions, educating the trier of fact with clear language and simple explanations, being truthful, staying as objective as possible, and considering opposing perspectives fairly, seriously, and with an open mind (Dvoskin & Guy, 2008). In his seminal texts on the topic, Brodsky (1991, 1999, 2004) provided numerous guidelines for expert witnesses to follow while testifying. In his most recent book, he presented 10 points relevant to expert testimony, which includes two particularly salient points related to the expert's humility while on the stand: (1) you do not have to have an answer to every question, and (2) it is not about winning. In sum, the purpose of the evaluator's testimony is to educate the fact finder about the relevant issues and to provide data, inferences, and opinions. Just as in the written report, the data should be set out and the inferences explained so that the evaluator's logic in arriving at conclusions and opinions is evident.

Facing cross-examination. Some experts may be comfortable with testifying, whereas others may fear the potential embarrassment accompanied by performing poorly on cross-examination (Dvoskin & Guy, 2008). As Brodsky (2004) articulated in his book, *Coping with Cross-Examination and Other Pathways to Effective Testimony*, "For most witnesses, the cross is the time in a trial that symbolizes whether they are powerful, competent, and masterful—or whether they are weak, incompetent, and ineffectual" (p. 3). Undoubtedly, the cross-examination aspect of a trial is what is most typically dramatized on television and in the movies; indeed, it is when the "Ah-ha!" or "Gotcha" moments occur. The reality of an actual trial (and cross-examination) typically differs greatly from the media portrayals. That is not to suggest that such moments cannot occur, but rather that they are often avoidable when the proper preparation and attitude are employed.

Similar to the approach for direct testimony, the evaluator should maintain a calm and composed demeanor throughout the cross-examination. The ideals of honesty, objectivity, and humility should continue to be embraced during this aspect of the trial or hearing; however, the evaluator can and should continue to be an advocate of his or her opinion and the data. As Brodsky (2004) noted, although there is reason to believe that likeability and credibility are related constructs, "*you do not have to be friendly*" (p. 11). The expert should focus on such and avoid becoming emotional and/or flustered during cross-examination. The role of the expert witness is to educate the trier of fact and to clearly, accurately, and, truthfully present his or her clinical opinions as well as the data from which they were drawn, regardless of which attorney is asking questions at the time. Put differently, although cross-examination testimony differs from that of direct testimony in tone and format (i.e., typically, it is more adversarial and yes/no questions are asked), the role and ultimate goals of the expert witness remain the same.

Cross-examination provides the evaluator with the opportunity to reiterate points made during his or her direct examination testimony. If questions are long or confusing, the evaluator should ask that they be repeated. When asked a hypothetical question, the evaluator should be clear about what data are provided in the question and should state whether more data are needed to answer the question. If the cross-examining attorney misstates a fact, the evaluator should clarify the fact before answering the question (e.g., being careful not to let the attorney put words in the expert's mouth). If the evaluator misspeaks on the stand, the expert should indicate that he or she spoke in error and correct the error. If the cross-examining attorney asks a question for which a yes/no answer is demanded and the evaluator believes that this type of answer is not appropriate, the expert should indicate to the court that a yes/no answer would be misleading.

As a general statement, testimony, whether it be on direct or cross, is most effective when the evaluator presents the data and inferences in a clear, concise manner in language that is easy to understand while focusing attention on the trier of fact. Maintaining a calm composure on the witness stand and speaking in a confident manner about the evaluation and the data offers the evaluator the opportunity to share his or her knowledge and to educate others about relevant issues. The goal for any forensic mental health expert is to present conclusions or opinions as well as the data and inferences on which those conclusions and opinions were based.

SUMMARY AND CONCLUSIONS

Well-written and informative reports are the key to the accurate communication of forensic evaluation results to other relevant and interested parties. Legal determination of an individual's capacities is informed by the clinical evaluation of these capacities and the relevant specific capacity-related abilities. Providing detailed information regarding the bases for one's opinions and conclusions is imperative so that the legal decision maker is able to follow the logic and reasoning used in arriving at a particular opinion or conclusion. The information presented in this chapter provides a general overview of report writing and testimony in capacity evaluations; however, evaluators are strongly encouraged to become familiar with the research literature and best professional practices in their particular area of practice. The various chapters in this book provide a starting point for many of the specific capacities that one might be asked to evaluate.

References

Ackerman, M. J. (2006). Forensic report writing. *Journal of Clinical Psychology, 62*, 59–72.

Allnut, S. H., & Chaplow, D. (2000). General principles of forensic report writing. *Australian and New Zealand Journal of Psychiatry, 34*, 980–987.

American Bar Association Commission on Law, Aging & American Psychological Association. (2005). *Assessment of older adults with diminished capacity: A handbook for lawyers*. Washington, D.C.: American Bar Association and American Psychological Association.

American Bar Association Commission on Law, Aging & American Psychological Association. (2006). *Judicial determination of capacity of older adults in guardianship*

proceedings: A handbook for judges. Washington, D.C.: American Bar Association and American Psychological Association.
American Bar Association Commission on Law, Aging & American Psychological Association. (2008). *Assessment of older adults with diminished capacity: A handbook for psychologists.* Washington, D.C.: American Bar Association and American Psychological Association.
American Psychiatric Association. (2000). *Diagnostic and statistical manual of mental disorders* (Revised 4th ed.). Washington, D.C.: Author.
American Psychological Association. (2002). Ethical principles of psychologists and code of conduct. *American Psychologist, 57*, 1060–1073.
American Psychological Association. (in press). Speciality guidelines for forensic psychology. *American Psychologist.*
Bank, S. C., & Packer, I. K. (2007). Expert witness testimony: Law, ethics, and practice. In A. M. Goldstein (Ed.), *Forensic psychology: Emerging topics and expanding roles* (pp. 421–445). Hoboken, NJ: John Wiley & Sons.
Barsky, A. E., & Gould, J. W. (2002). *Clinicians in court: A guide to subpoenas, depositions, testifying, and everything else you need to know.* New York: Guilford Press.
Blau, T. H. (1998). *The psychologist as expert witness* (2nd ed.). Hoboken, NJ: John Wiley & Sons.
Borum, R., & Grisso, T. (1996). Establishing standards for criminal forensic reports: An empirical analysis. *Bulletin of the American Academy of Psychiatry and the Law, 24*, 297–317.
Bowen v. Kendrick, 487 U.S. 589 (1988).
Brodsky, S. L. (1991). *Testifying in court: Guidelines and maxims for the expert witness.* Washington, D.C.: American Psychological Association.
Brodsky, S. L. (1999). *The expert expert witness: More maxims and guidelines for testifying in court.* Washington, D.C.: American Psychological Association.
Brodsky, S. L. (2004). *Coping with cross-examination and other pathways to effective testimony.* Washington, D.C.: American Psychological Association.
Conroy, M. A, (2006). Report writing and testimony. *Applied Psychology in Criminal Justice, 2*, 237–260.
Daubert v. Merrell Dow Pharmaceuticals, Inc. (1993), 113 S. Ct. 2786.
Dvoskin, J. A., & Guy, L. S. (2008). On being an expert witness: It's not about you. *Psychiatry, Psychology and Law, 15*, 202–212.
Ewing, C. P. (2003). Expert testimony: Law and practice. In A. M. Goldstein (Ed.), *Handbook of psychology: Forensic psychology* (Vol. 11, pp. 55–66). Hoboken, NJ: John Wiley & Sons.
Ewing, C. P. (2008). Ethical expert testimony, an uneasy "moral adventure": A grateful response. *Journal of Psychiatry & Law, 36*, 653–658.
Faust, D., Grimm, P. W., Ahern, D. C., & Sokolik, M. (2010). The admissibility of behavioral science evidence in the courtroom: The translation of legal to scientific concepts and back. *Annual Review of Clinical Psychology, 6*, 49–77.
Frye v. United States (D.C. Cir. 1923), 293 F.1013.
Fulero, S. M., & Finkel, N. J. (1991). Barring ultimate issue testimony: An "insane" rule? *Law and Human Behavior, 15*, 495–507.
Ganzini, L., Volicer, L., Nelson, W., & Derse, A. (2003). Pitfalls in assessment of decision-making capacity. *Psychosomatics, 44*, 237–243.

General Electric Co. v. Joiner (1997), 522 U.S.136.

Grisso, T. (1986). *Evaluating competencies: Forensic assessments and instruments.* New York: Kluwer Academic/Plenum Publishers.

Grisso, T. (1988). *Competency to stand trial evaluations: A manual for practice.* Sarasota, FL: Professional Resource Press.

Grisso, T. (2003). *Evaluating competencies: Forensic assessments and instruments* (2nd ed.). New York: Kluwer Academic/Plenum Publishers.

Gutheil, T. G. (1998). *The psychiatrist as expert witness.* Washington, D.C.: American Psychiatric Press.

Heilbrun, K., Marczyk, G. R., & DeMatteo, D. (2002). *Forensic mental health assessment: A casebook.* New York: Oxford University Press.

Hess, A. K. (2006). Serving as an expert witness. In I. B. Weiner & A. K. Hess (Eds.), *The handbook of forensic psychology* (3rd ed., pp. 652–697). Hoboken, NJ: John Wiley & Sons.

Kim, S. Y. H. (2010). *Evaluation of capacity to consent to treatment and research.* New York: Oxford University Press.

Kumho Tire Co. v. Carmichael (1999), 526 U.S.137.

Melton, G. B., Petrila, J., Poythress, N. G., Slobogin, C., with Lyons, P. M., Jr., & Otto, R. K. (2007). *Psychological evaluations for the courts: A handbook for mental health professionals and lawyers* (3rd ed.). New York: Guilford Press.

Pirelli, G., & Zapf, P. A. (2008). An investigation of psychologists' practices and attitudes toward participation in capital evaluations. *Journal of Forensic Psychology Practice, 8,* 39–66.

Redding, R. E., Floyd, M. Y., & Hawk, G. L. (2001). What judges and lawyers think about the testimony of mental health experts: A survey of the courts and bar. *Behavioral Sciences & the Law, 19,* 583–594.

Robbins, E., Waters, J., & Herbert, P. (1997). Competency to stand trial evaluations: A study of actual practice in two states. *Journal of the American Academy of Psychiatry and Law, 25,* 469–483.

Rogers, R., Bagby, R. M., Crouch, M., & Cutler, B. (1990). Effects of ultimate opinions on juror perceptions of insanity. *International Journal of Law and Psychiatry, 13,* 225–232.

Rogers, R., & Ewing, C. P. (1989). Ultimate opinion proscriptions: A cosmetic fix and a plea for empiricism. *Law and Human Behavior, 13,* 357–374.

Rogers, R., & Ewing, C. P. (2003). The prohibition of ultimate opinions: A misguided enterprise. *Journal of Forensic Psychology Practice, 3,* 65–75.

Ryba, N. L., Cooper, V. G., & Zapf, P. A. (2003). Juvenile competence to stand trial evaluations: A survey of current practices and test usage among psychologists. *Professional Psychology: Research and Practice, 34,* 499–507.

Skeem, J., Golding, S. L., Cohn, N., & Berge, G. (1998). Logic and reliability of evaluations of competence to stand trial. *Law and Human Behavior, 22,* 519–547.

Slobogin, C. (1989). The "ultimate issue" issue. *Behavioral Sciences & the Law, 7,* 259–266.

Slovenko, R. (2006). Commentary: Deceptions to the rule on ultimate issue testimony. *Journal of the American Academy of Psychiatry and the Law, 34,* 22–25.

Tillbrook, C., Mumley, D., & Grisso, T. (2003). Avoiding expert opinions on the ultimate legal question: The case for integrity. *Journal of Forensic Psychology Practice, 3,* 77–87.

Tsushima, W. T., & Anderson, R. M., Jr. (1996). *Mastering expert testimony: A courtroom handbook for mental health professionals.* Mahwah, NJ: Erlbaum.

U.S. ex rel Edney v. Smith (1976), 425 F. Supp. 1038 (E.D. N.Y.).

U.S. v. Alvarez (1975), 519 F.2d 1036 (3rd Cir.).

Viljoen, J. L., Wingrove, T., & Ryba, N. L. (2008). Adjudicative competence evaluations of juvenile and adult defendants: Judges' views regarding essential components of competence reports. *The International Journal of Forensic Mental Health, 7*, 107–119.

Weiner, I. B. (2006). Writing forensic reports. In I. B. Weiner & A. K. Hess (Eds.), *The handbook of forensic psychology* (3rd ed., pp. 631–651). Hoboken, NJ: John Wiley & Sons.

Zapf, P. A., & Roesch. R. (2009). *Guide to best practices for forensic mental health assessments: Competency to stand trial.* New York: Oxford University Press.

Ziskin, J., & Faust, D. (1995). *Coping with psychiatric and psychological testimony.* Beverly Hills, CA: Law and Psychology Press.

13

Ethical Issues in Capacity and Competency Evaluations

PAUL J. MOBERG AND SANJAY SHAH

STANDARDS FOR NEUROPSYCHOLOGISTS IN THE ASSESSMENT OF COMPETENCY STATUS

Currently, there is no consensus in the field for the evaluation of capacity or competency (Moberg & Gibney, 2005; Lai et al., 2008). Indeed, there has been debate in the medical and psychological communities as to whether such a standard needs to exist with some arguing against formal testing (American Medical Directors Association, 2003) and others arguing in favor of establishing clinical practice parameters (Kapp & Mossman, 1996). Despite the absence of any clear consensus on this important topic, neuropsychologists are bound by the ethical obligations of practicing within their area of expertise, using empirically derived assessment instruments, and protecting the autonomy as well as the safety of their patients.

It should be noted that the terms "competency" and "capacity" are sometimes used interchangeably to describe the same phenomena despite the fact that these terms have somewhat different meanings. Indeed, Marson (2001) defined capacity as a *clinical status* as judged by a healthcare professional (e.g., a neuropsychologist), whereas competency reflected a *legal status* as judged by a legal professional (e.g., a judge). Regardless of the terms used, neuropsychologists are often asked to make competency judgments. In this chapter, the term competence will be used to refer to a judgment, either by a healthcare professional or legal professional, as to whether a person is able to provide informed consent or is capable of carrying out the activity in question. The ultimate competency decision is made by the trier of fact, such as a judge, magistrate, or clerk. In contrast, capacity will refer to the cognitive and emotional resources that a patient utilizes to provide informed consent or to perform functional tasks and is thought to lie on a continuum. In this light, abilities are treated as task-specific dimensions that inform the legal standards of competency. Consistent with this general definition, according to Denny and Wynkoop (2000), competency refers to an individual's capacity to decide or to perform activities of daily living. Included in this overarching definition are the capacities to work, drive, parent, make medical decisions, provide informed consent in treatment and research settings, care for oneself or one's property, and enter into legal contracts (e.g., designate a will). Although neuropsychologists may be specifically asked to perform such assessments by the court for civil or criminal matters, most often these questions arise in the course of daily clinical practice. Indeed, a recent on-line survey of practicing neuropsychologists found that only 30% of respondents reported that they regularly perform civil or criminal capacity evaluations specifically referred from the court or attorneys. However, capacity issues were raised in up to 75% of standard clinical examinations; the three most common types of cases in which these issues were raised were dementia, traumatic brain injury, and stoke or cerebrovascular disease. In contrast, capacity issues were significantly lower in pediatric referrals (i.e., 0–25%).

Ethics Provisions

The Ethical Principles of Psychologists and Code of Conduct ["Ethics Code," American Psychological Association (APA), 2002] details a number of issues central in the civil competency assessment. Foremost among these is the precarious balancing of respect for individuals' rights and autonomy with the ethical obligation to do no harm (Principles A and E).

Additionally, adherence to the APA Ethical Standards governing assessment (9.01, Bases for Assessment) and professional competence (2.01, Boundaries of Competence) is made particularly difficult by the lack of empirical evidence as to the ecological validity and predictive ability of neuropsychological tests and by the absence of an agreed-on standard of assessment or training in capacity evaluations. Despite this, there are ways to ensure that a competency assessment follows best clinical practice with regard to the ethical standards.

Standard and Structured Competency Assessment Procedures

As noted in Standard 9.02 of the APA Ethics Code, Use of Assessments: (a) "Psychologists administer, adapt, score, interpret, or use assessment techniques, interviews, tests, or instruments in a manner and for purposes that are appropriate in light of the research on or evidence of the usefulness and proper application of the techniques." We have previously suggested four elements thought to be essential for a comprehensive and ethically sound competency evaluation (Moberg & Gibney, 2005; Moberg & Kniele, 2006). First, a comprehensive and structured clinical/diagnostic *interview* with the patient and collateral informants should be undertaken. Collateral informants can include the patient's spouse, relatives, treating physician, hospital staff, co-workers, etc. Such interviews give the neuropsychologist detailed information regarding the patient's mood, cognition, and functional abilities as well as provide information about medical, social, and environmental limitations. Notably, the use of structured interviews designed to specifically assess competency [e.g., Assessment of Capacity for Everyday Decision Making (ACED; Lai & Karlawish, 2007), MacArthur Competence Assessment Tool (MacCAT-T; Grisso et al., 1997); Capacity to Consent to Treatment Instrument (CCTI; Marson, Ingram, Cody, & Harrell, 1995)] is a crucial addition to the standard clinical interviews performed by most clinicians. Specifically, Standard 9.02(b) indicates that "Psychologists use assessment instruments whose validity and reliability have been established for use with members of the population tested. When such validity or reliability has not been established, psychologists describe the strengths and limitations of test results and interpretation." With this Standard in mind, the onus is on the neuropsychologist to ensure that a reliable and valid competency scale is used. Although an exhaustive review of the available competency measures is beyond the scope of this chapter, Table 13.1 lists a number of published and validated competency scales/interviews that can be employed in a given competency examination to ensure that the stated Ethical Standards are being addressed.

Second, we suggest the use of *neuropsychological measures* that have been empirically shown to be sensitive to the cognitive constructs underlying specific capacities. Marson and colleagues have performed some groundbreaking research examining how neuropsychological measures interface in the competency assessment process (Marson, Cody, Ingram, & Harrell, 1995; Marson, Chatterjee, Ingram, & Harrell, 1996). For example, Dymek and colleagues (2001) assessed individuals with Parkinson's disease (PD) with overall mild cognitive impairment and healthy controls using the CCTI and a brief battery of neuropsychological instruments. Five legal standards for capacity to consent to medical treatment were investigated: (1) knowing that a decision is to be made, (2) making a reasonable decision, (3) understanding the personal and future impact of the choice selected, (4) demonstrating logical reasoning in the decision making, and (5) comprehension of the treatment context and choices. Results revealed that healthy controls were competent for all legal standards using a statistical determination, whereas the PD group demonstrated increasing impairment as the complexity of the standard rose (e.g., 30% were statistically determined to be marginally incapable or incapable for the first standard, and 80% for the fifth). The authors noted that individuals with declines in simple executive function, and to a lesser extent memory abilities, appeared to be particularly vulnerable. Third, we propose the use of *functional ability* measures that target the capacity-specific ability in question and that provide an ecologically valid picture of the patient's competency. An important consideration in determining competency is how well the patient meets the specific demands of his or her environment. Indeed, some state laws have questioned the ecological validity of neuropsychological testing and subsequently have required an additional evaluation of everyday living skills in judging competency (Moberg & Rick, 2008). Such an assessment can be

Table 13.1 Published Scales for the Assessment of Various Competencies and Capacities

Instrument	**Source Citation**
Assessment of Capacity for Everyday Decision Making (ACED)	Lai, J. M., & Karlawish, J. H. (2007). Assessing the capacity to make everyday decisions: A guide for clinicians and an agenda for future research. *American Journal of Geriatric Psychiatry, 15*, 101–111.
Aid to Capacity Evaluation (ACE)	Etchells, E., Darzins, P., Silberfeld, M., Singer, P. A., McKenny, J., Naglie, G., et al. (1999). Assessment of patient capacity to consent to treatment. *Journal of General Internal Medicine, 14*, 27–34.
California Scale of Appreciation (CSA)	Saks, E. R., Dunn, L. B., Marshall, B. J., Nayak, G. V., Golshan, S., & Jeste, D. V. (2002). The California Scale of Appreciation: A new instrument to measure the appreciation component of capacity to consent to research. *American Journal of Geriatric Psychiatry, 10*, 166–174.
Capacity Assessment Tool (CAT)	Carney, M. T., Neugroschl, J., Morrison, R. S., Marin, D., & Siu, A. L. (2001). The development and piloting of a Capacity Assessment Tool. *The Journal of Clinical Ethics, 12*, 17–23.
Capacity to Consent to Treatment Instrument (CCTI)	Marson, D. C., Ingram, K. K., Cody, H. A., & Harrell, L. E. (1995). Assessing the competency of patients with Alzheimer's disease under different legal standards. A prototype instrument. *Archives of Neurology, 52*, 949–954.
Competency Interview Schedule (CIS)	Bean, G., Nishisato, S., Rector, N. A., & Glancy, G. (1994). The psychometric properties of the Competency Interview Schedule. *Canadian Journal of Psychiatry, 39*, 368–376.
Evaluation to Sign Consent (ESC)	Deronzo, E. G., Conley, R. R., & Love, R. (1998). Assessment of capacity to give consent to research participation: State of the art and beyond. *Journal of Health Care Law and Policy, 1*, 66–87.
Financial Capacity Instrument (FCI)	Marson, D. C., Sawrie, S. M., Snyder, S., McInturff, B., Stalvey, T., Boothe, A., Aldridge, T., Chatterjee, A., & Harrell, L. E. (2000). Assessing financial capacity in patients with Alzheimer disease: A conceptual model and prototype instrument. *Archives of Neurology, 57*, 877–884.
Hopemont Capacity Assessment Interview (HCAI)	Edelstein, M., Nygren, L., Northrop, N., Staats, N., & Pool, D. (1993). Assessment of capacity to make financial and medical decisions. Paper presented in August at the meeting of the American Psychological Association, Toronto, Canada.
Hopkins Competence Assessment Tool (HCAT)	Janofsky, J. S., McCarthy, R. J., & Folstein, M. F. (1992). The Hopkins Competency Assessment Test: A brief method for evaluating patients' capacity to give informed consent. *Hospital and Community Psychiatry, 43*, 132–136.

(Continued)

Table 13.1 Published Scales for the Assessment of Various Competencies and Capacities (Cont'd)

Instrument	**Source Citation**
MacArthur Competence Assessment Tool—Clinical Research (MacCAT-CR)	Appelbaum, P. S., & Grisso, T. (1996). *The MacArthur Competence Assessment Tool—Clinical Research*. Sarasota, FL: Professional Resource Press.
MacArthur Competence Assessment Tool—Treatment (MacCAT-T)	Grisso, T., Appelbaum, P. S., & Hill-Fotouhi, C. (1997). The MacCAT-T: A clinical tool to assess patient's capacities to make treatment decisions. *Psychiatric Services*, *48*, 1415–1419.
Measure for Assessing Awareness of Financial Skills (MAFS)	Cramer, K., Tuokko, H. A., Mateer, C. A., & Hultsch, D. F. (2004). Measuring awareness of financial skills: Reliability and validity of a new measure. *Aging & Mental Health*, *8*, 161–171.
Structured Interview for Competency/Incompetency Assessment Testing and Ranking Inventory (SICIATRI)	Tomoda, A., Yasumiya, R., Sumiyama, T., Tankada, K., Hayakawa, T., Kimimori, M., et al. (1997). Reliability and validity of structured interview for competency/incompetency assessment testing and ranking inventory. *Journal of Clinical Psychology*, *53*, 443–450.

achieved via direct observation or the use of structured functional assessments [e.g., Vineland Adaptive Behavior Interview (Sparrow, Cicchetti, & Balla, 2005); Scales of Independent Behavior-Revised (Bruininks, Woodcock, Weatherman, & Hill, 2005); Observed Tasks of Daily Living (Diehl et al., 2005)]. Lastly, evaluators should perform a careful review of the *legal standards* of the state in which they are practicing to ensure that the civil and/or criminal competency evaluation presents evidence that is relevant to the legal standards of determination where the patient resides. The evaluator is also responsible for identifying and recommending adaptations and environmental supports that may enable compromised persons to perform the task/decision at issue in the evaluation. For example, a severe memory deficit may impair decision-making ability, though written cues and other environmental manipulations may enable a person to successfully make certain decisions. Because interventions may require a trial period to establish efficacy, final decisions regarding capacity may need to be deferred until interventions are tested.

OBTAINING INFORMED CONSENT OF POSSIBLY INCOMPETENT INDIVIDUALS

As noted in the 2002 APA Standard 9.03 entitled Informed Consent in Assessments: "(a) Psychologists obtain informed consent for assessments, evaluations, or diagnostic services, as described in Standard 3.10, Informed Consent, except when (1) testing is mandated by law or governmental regulations; (2) informed consent is implied because testing is conducted as a routine educational, institutional, or organizational activity (e.g., when participants voluntarily agree to assessment when applying for a job); or (3) one purpose of the testing is to evaluate decisional capacity." Although the ability to consent to treatment is routinely addressed in the psychotherapeutic context, there has been less attention to the issue of consent in the arena of competency assessment. An ethical approach to the assessment of competence demands that the patient be informed of the scope and nature of the assessment, the terms of confidentiality, and how feedback and dissemination of information will be handled. If the clinician is faced with a patient who has questionable capacity, additional safeguards, beginning with special consideration of the patient's ability to consent to assessment [Standards 9.03, Informed Consent in Assessments, subsection (b) and 3.10, Informed Consent, subsection (b); APA, 2002] are required. Most neuropsychologists disseminate this information in an informal way prior to testing, but the 2002 Ethical Standards now give an explicit mandate to formally engage and inform patients about the assessment process and provide them with information and reassurances if needed. For example, if a clinician is asked to perform a competency assessment of a patient via a court order, the neuropsychologist would be exempt under the APA Ethical Standards from obtaining formal consent [Standard 9.03, subsections (a)(1) and (a)(3)] because the evaluation was (1) ordered by the court [9.03 (a)(1)] and (2) designed to assess competence to undergo treatment [9.03 (a)(3); APA, 2002]. Despite this, the clinician still strives to attain some form of consent or assent in this situation as it establishes respect for the patient's rights and dignity and concern for his or her well-being (General Principles A and E).

As noted in Standard 9.03, subsection (b) (APA, 2002), informed consent for an assessment of competency involves an "explanation of the nature and purpose of the assessment, fees, involvement of third parties, and limits of confidentiality and sufficient opportunity for the client/patient to ask questions and receive answers."

With the basic tenets of this standard in mind, in a civil competency examination the neuropsychologist must, at a minimum, ensure that the examinee can (1) understand the nature of the evaluation and of his or her participation in the examination, (2) appreciate the consequences of their participation, including personal consequences, (3) show the ability to consider alternatives, including the option not to participate, and (4) show the ability to make a reasonably reasoned choice. At the outset of the evaluation, the neuropsychologist should discuss with the patient the purpose and parameters of the examination, its significance, and the patient's options. Because of cognitive impairment, poor health literacy, and individuals coming from culturally and linguistically disadvantaged backgrounds, the vocabulary used in this discussion should be simple and avoid any medical jargon. In essence, "keep it simple, yet accurate."

The Impaired Patient

The largest problem arises when it is determined that the patient lacks the capacity to consent to the specific clinical examination. As noted in part (b) of Standard

3.10 (Informed Consent) (APA, 2002): "For persons who are legally incapable of giving informed consent, psychologists nevertheless (1) provide an appropriate explanation, (2) seek the individual's assent, (3) consider such persons' preferences and best interests, and (4) obtain appropriate permission from a legally authorized person, if such substitute consent is permitted or required by law. When consent by a legally authorized person is not permitted or required by law, psychologists take reasonable steps to protect the individual's rights and welfare." In the scenario of the impaired patient, it may be necessary to obtain permission from a proxy with both actual capacity and legal authority to give it, as well as assent to participate from the patient. Permission means obtaining the proxy's informed consent to the proposed evaluation.

Identifying a Proxy. In the patient with significant cognitive compromise, the neuropsychologist must rely on proxy decision makers, usually a spouse, child, caregiver, or other trusted individual, for decisions of everyday life or medical care. This permission should be sought from someone who, under state law, has the right to be the participant's legally authorized representative. The following hierarchy of priority may be followed when choosing a proxy decision maker: (1) legal guardian, (2) proxy (healthcare agent) named in an advance directive or durable power of attorney for healthcare, or (3) family member or other surrogate identified by the state law on healthcare decisions (e.g., spouse, adult children, parents, adult siblings, other relative, or friend). The types of proxy decision makers will vary from state to state, and clinicians should be aware of the requirements of the law in their specific jurisdiction.

Assent from the Patient. If the client is judged to be incapable of providing informed consent and a proxy is used, the patient should be informed in the presence of the proxy that he or she is about to undergo a competency assessment. The procedures, risks, benefits, and alternatives involved should be explained in a simple fashion. Once this information is presented, patients should be asked whether they agree to the assessment and their response should be explicitly documented. When the patient is so impaired so as to be incapable of providing affirmative agreement to participate, then assent (or dissent) should be judged behaviorally based on cooperativeness with the study procedures (e.g., do they refuse to engage in testing?).

Readers interested in more detail concerning the issues surrounding surrogate decision making are directed to Buchanan and Brock's (1990) excellent text: *Deciding for Others: The Ethics of Surrogate Decision Making.*

PRACTICING WITHIN THE SCOPE OF EXPERTISE

As noted above, most capacity evaluations arise within the context of standard clinical assessments. Neuropsychologists in clinical practice may find themselves called upon (often unexpectedly) to determine whether individuals can manage their affairs independently or whether they can manage their finances or other task(s). In addition, a clinician may be asked by the courts to present information related to competency or decision-making status when a family is unable to manage their loved one's behavior, as in cases of patients with severe dementia, who sometimes refuse to give up control of their finances, the privilege of driving, etc. As these scenarios may result in the neuropsychologist's assessment being used in court determinations of competency, it is important for the clinician to appreciate the legal standards of competency [Standard 2.01, Boundaries of Competence, subsection (f); APA, 2002]. Grisso (1986) noted that mental health experts have been criticized on several levels for ignorance and irrelevance in the courtroom, insufficiency and incredibility of information provided to courts, and intrusion into legal matters. Neuropsychologists can avoid a similar criticism if they ensure that they have knowledge of the legal standards for different domains of competency and that they adhere to ethical standards governing practicing within one's domain of expertise. As discussed previously, this is difficult in competency assessment as there are no agreed-on clinical guidelines. Standard 2.01(e) (APA, 2002) recognizes that there are not always established methods of practice, but nonetheless charges practitioners with the duty to "take reasonable steps to ensure the competence of their work." This charge to clinicians can be at least partly addressed by the use of specific capacity/functional assessment scales and neuropsychological tests that have shown at least some ecological validity with regard to the question at hand. This is particularly difficult, though, when as reviewed below, there is a paucity of empirical evidence as to the ecological validity of standardized neuropsychological assessments and when there is considerable variability even among experts as to what constitutes a "competent" assessment of competency. There are a number of approaches, however, that can be used by the neuropsychologist to ensure that their evaluations are meeting scientific and ethical requirements. First, if an issue lies outside of an individual's realm of expertise (e.g., psychological autopsy or child custody), it may be necessary for the clinician to refer the patient to another provider, work under the supervision of a peer who has expertise in this type of evaluation, or gain the needed expertise and experience through structured and supervised education/training. Second, neuropsychologists should stay abreast of the scientific literature with regard to issues to ecological validity of given tests, research on methods used to assess a given competency area (e.g., driving or financial capacity), and other clinically relevant topics. Third, close examination and understanding of the legal standards in clinicians' specific jurisdiction will also ensure that their assessments are meeting the essential standards of the law. In many cases, it may be helpful to discuss the legal requirements of competency with a local attorney who is experienced or specializes in competency-related work. Many states have agencies specifically chartered to protect the rights of incompetent individuals such as the elderly, mentally retarded, or psychiatrically ill. Lastly, the best way of attaining expertise in competency evaluation is to perform evaluations, preferably under supervision. Although there is no real standard of preparatory training in this area of practice, practitioners are advised to seek information on the topic and obtain supervision by a colleague experienced in performing such evaluations.

ECOLOGICAL VALIDITY OF NEUROPSYCHOLOGICAL TESTS IN PREDICTING COMPETENCY

With the advent of structural and functional neuroimaging technologies, neuropsychology has moved away from lesion localization and toward an emphasis on a patient's functional or everyday cognitive abilities or disability (Chaytor & Schmitter-Edgecombe, 2003). This emphasis translates nicely into many of the same questions asked during a typical competency examination such as whether a patient is able to live independently, manage his or her personal finances, drive, or make health or life-care decisions (Heinrichs, 1990; Long & Kibby, 1995; Sbordone & Long, 1996; Wilson, 1993). Despite this increased awareness, the question remains whether the standard neuropsychological measures used by most clinical neuropsychologists have "ecological validity" or "real-life" application and consequences (Standards 9.01, Bases for Assessments, and 9.02, Use of Assessments; APA, 2002). Ginsberg, Kibby, and Long (1995) defined such ecological validity as the "functional and predictive relationship between the client's performance on a set of neuropsychological tests and the client's behavior in a variety of real-world settings (e.g., at home, work, school, community, etc.)." A number of researchers have sought to improve the real-world translation of neuropsychological tests by obtaining self or informant reports or behavioral observations (e.g., Everyday Memory Questionnaire, Sunderland, Harris, & Baddeley, 1983) and combining them with neuropsychological data. In addition, a number of neurocognitive measures have been specifically developed to more closely resemble everyday behaviors or experiences. Examples of this approach include standardized tests such as the Rivermead Behavioral Memory Test (Wilson, Cockburn, & Baddeley, 1985) or the Test of Everyday Attention (Robertson, Ward, Ridgeway, & Nimmo-Smith, 1994). A recent study by Higginson, Arnett, and Voss (2000) found that the aforementioned Rivermead Behavioral Memory Test and the Test of Everyday Attention were better predictors of functional impairment in multiple sclerosis patients than either standard neuropsychological tests or attention and memory questionnaires completed by the patient or a significant other. In contrast, a meta-analytic study by Reger et al. (2004) concerning prediction of driving ability in dementia found that within a sample of patients with dementia, neuropsychological test results correlated relatively poorly with real-world on-road driving performance. Notably, aggregate measures of attention were only weakly associated with on-road tests ($r = 0.25$), and measures of executive function were not significantly related to driving performance. These findings raise concerns about the translation of findings on standardized measures of neurocognitive function into real-life situations.

As noted above, the inclusion of more ecologically valid neuropsychological tasks in conjunction with well-validated functional competency measures tapping the area of concern (i.e., use of the Financial Capacity Instrument in a case in which with financial management concerns) can help tie the results of the neuropsychologist's standard assessment more closely to the actual day-to-day behavior and functioning of the patient. Such efforts are crucial to the ethical competency assessment. For more in-depth coverage concerning the neuropsychological prediction of everyday functioning and ability, the reader is directed to an excellent text by Marcotte and Grant (2006) entitled the *Neuropsychology of Everyday Functioning.*

ISSUES OF TEST SECURITY

Civil competency evaluations may use a variety of general ability tests and more specialized tools designed to specifically address competency. This section describes the ethical concern of maintaining test security and the considerations a neuropsychologist must make when asked to release test data and/or test materials. The most immediate practical and ethical issue from the perspective of the neuropsychologist is the potential misuse of test data or materials. The concern does not end with the evaluation. The dissemination of testing information may lead to the decreased validity of tests, which subsequently affects test authors and publishers, as well as neuropsychologists who may have to face the prospect of examinees who have previously been exposed to tests or even coached on them. A simple solution is to provide the attorney with a report containing standardized results, interpretations, and conclusions based on the forensic question of competency. Unfortunately, it may not be this simple. At some point during the legal process, it is not uncommon for requests to obtain test data or test materials to be made to the evaluating neuropsychologist by attorneys or judges. The dilemma arises from conflicting goals and ethical standards of two professions—psychologists and lawyers. This section further elaborates on relevant ethical standards, the problems neuropsychologists may face, and potential solutions to dealing with these issues.

Ethics Provisions

It is important to note that the current Ethics Code (APA, 2002) makes a distinction between test data and test materials not made by the previous version of the Ethics Code. "Test data," in Standard 9.04 (APA, 2002) refers to "raw and scaled scores, client/patient responses to test questions or stimuli, and psychologists' notes and recordings concerning client/patient statements and behavior during an examination" (p. 1071)." This is in contrast to "test materials," for which Standard 9.11 (APA, 2002, p. 1072) includes "manuals, instruments, protocols, and test questions or stimuli and does not include *test data* as defined in 9.04."

Subsection (b) of Standard 9.04 (APA, 2002) takes into consideration the role of the law by stating, "In the absence of a client/patient release, psychologists provide test data only as required by law or court order." Standard 9.11 (APA, 2002, p. 1072) appears to go further as it asserts that "Psychologists make *reasonable efforts* [emphasis added] to maintain the integrity and security of test materials and the other assessment techniques consistent with law and contractual obligations, and in a manner that permits adherence to this Ethics Code" (APA, 2002, p. 1072). Looking at these Standards, it appears that 9.11 would require the neuropsychologist to be more proactive and take affirmative steps in securing testing materials. However, in a further interpretation of these two standards, the National Academy of Neuropsychology (NAN) explains that test data may overlap with test materials when test responses (i.e., test data) are embedded in test materials such as within test forms, or the two may overlap when test materials can be inferred from test data (NAN, 2003a). In addition, NAN (2003a) states that the release of test responses without materials can be misleading. Therefore, it appears that NAN calls for affirmative steps and safeguards to be used in the case of both test data and test materials.

Neuropsychologists involved in forensic evaluations should also be attentive to the Specialty Guidelines for Forensic Psychologists ["Specialty Guidelines," Committee on Ethical Guidelines for Forensic Psychologists (CEGFP), 1991]. The Specialty Guidelines offer an aspirational model for psychologists of any subdiscipline of psychology when representing themselves as experts in the context of legal evaluations. The Specialty Guidelines are similar to that of the Ethics Code (APA, 2002) in that efforts should be made to maintain test security. Guideline VII(A)(a) (CEGFP, 1991, p. 664) states that "When required to disclose results to a nonpsychologist, every attempt is made to ensure that test security is maintained and access to information is restricted to individuals with a legitimate and professional interest in the data." In addition, the Specialty Guidelines emphasize that psychologists working in a forensic context should be knowledgeable of laws that affect their evaluation and subsequent disclosures to legal representatives. Specifically, Guideline V(A)(2) (CEGFP, 1991, p. 660) explains that "Forensic psychologists maintain active control over records and information. They only release information pursuant to statutory requirements, court order, or the consent of the client." In addition, Section V(D) (CEGFP, 1991, p. 660) states that legal representatives who have access to information should also be provided with "a meaningful explanation of that information, consistent with existing Federal and state statutes, the *Ethical Principles of Psychologists*, the *Standards for Education and Psychological Testing*, and institutional rules and regulations."

Problems with Lack of Test Security

A central problem when test security is compromised is the potential for misuse of data by unqualified individuals and the future effect this may have on neuropsychologists and test publishers. The immediate problem is that attorneys who obtain test data or test materials may draw incorrect or misleading conclusions regarding their client's competency. Going further, testing information drawn from a previous evaluation may be used to benefit subsequent clients. Tests used during competency evaluations, like all neuropsychological evaluations, depend on examinees unfamiliarity with test items. Familiarity with tests or specific testing items inevitably leads to decreased validity. Neuropsychologists would then be left with having to make adjustments in testing protocols based on the realistic fear that an examinee may be familiar with a test or specific test questions, or was even given the opportunity to determine their answers in advance. An additional effect of dissemination of tests may be a decreased incentive for test authors and publishers to produce new and innovative measures since the development of tests takes a great deal of financial resources and time. A primary measure of a "good" test is its validity, which becomes compromised once parts of the test or the entirety of it reach those who are unqualified to use and interpret it.

The potential of attorneys coaching their clients does not appear to be an irrational fear for psychologists conducting forensic evaluations. Wetter and Corrigan (1995), in a survey of attorneys and law students, asked the following questions: (1) Should an attorney discuss psychological testing with their client prior to testing? (2) How much detail should an attorney give about the testing process? and (3) Should the attorney be responsible for informing clients of scales on psychological tests designed to detect exaggerated or faked responses? Most of those surveyed thought that the attorney should discuss what psychological testing involves and many responded that they would provide as much specific and detailed information as possible. Regarding the final question, 50% of attorneys and over 33% of law students thought that their clients should always or usually be informed of validity scales.

In another study, Essig, Mittenberg, Petersen, Strauman, and Cooper (2001) found that 29% of surveyed attorneys reviewed the Minnesota Multiphasic Personality Inventory-2 (MMPI-2) with their clients. The authors also reported that 75% of surveyed attorneys spent 15 to 60 minutes preparing clients for forensic neuropsychological examinations (Essig et al., 2001). It is also interesting that this study found the discrepancy that 44% of attorneys received raw data in 75% to 100% of their brain injury cases, while 32% of neuropsychologists indicated providing raw data in 25% or less of their forensic cases. The authors suggest the difference could be attributed to attorneys wanting to appear as an advocate for their clients and neuropsychologists wanting to appear mindful of ethical standards. Studies such as these may provide a reflection of attorneys' motives and training, but beyond this, it may reflect an ethical obligation for attorneys to advocate for their clients and to guide them with great specificity. This adds to the importance of neuropsychologists being forthcoming regarding their own ethical obligations.

Another inquiry is whether examinees coached by their attorneys are more likely to reach their desired outcomes compared to those who have not been coached. In a comparison between normal controls, uncoached malingerers, coached malingerers, and head-injured participants, coached malingerers were better able to avoid detection on measures of malingering compared with those who were uncoached (Rose, Hall, Szalda-Petree, & Bach, 1998). In another study, warned participants were more likely to recognize the forced choice portion of the Auditory Verbal Learning Test (AVLT) as a measure of malingering (Suhr & Gunstad, 2000). The "warning" in this study was vague. It stated that "At least one of the tests you will be given is designed to catch you faking, because it's easier than it looks. Be careful" (Suhr & Gunstad, 2000, p. 424). This simple warning ultimately led to decreased sensitivity of the forced choice portion of the test. The authors indicated that although the warning affected performance on the more obvious forced choice portion, the pattern of performance on memory tests was not altered.

There are cautionary adjustments that neuropsychologists could make in their testing protocols if they believe an examinee has been coached to some extent. One is to obtain multiple measures in a single neuropsychological domain. This provides a pattern of functioning that likely provides more accurate information compared to a solitary test of which an examinee may have prior knowledge. In addition, multiple symptom validity tests could be used since it is less probable that an examinee would have knowledge of several different measures. Finally, in addition to stand-alone symptom validity measures, a neuropsychologist should actively seek to examine imbedded measures that could indicate malingering. Of course, there is a difference between examinees being evaluated for competence and, for instance, those being evaluated as part of a personal injury lawsuit. It is more likely that those in a civil competency evaluation would put forth their best effort and would not have an external incentive to perform poorly. Scales on measures such as the MMPI-2 could still provide some evidence of an attempt to present oneself in a favorable manner. Nevertheless, neuropsychologists should be aware that coaching of clients by attorneys does occur and that this coaching could have an effect on test performance.

Despite the above disadvantages of providing test data and materials to attorneys, some advantages have been previously proposed (Freides, 1993). For instance, displaying all quantitative data may actually reduce the need for even more extensive discovery by attorneys or allow opposing neuropsychologists to reach their own conclusions when presented with data (Freides, 1993). In addition, a longitudinal comparison of results could be made with future evaluations (Freides, 1993). For instance, in competency evaluations, interested parties may want to know whether capacity has diminished and, if so, how much and at what rate. Providing data may easily allow for these sorts of comparisons. Nevertheless, the disadvantages of unqualified individuals having access to and misusing data, and maintaining the integrity and validity of tests, still weigh more heavily than the potential advantages.

What Constitutes Reasonable Efforts?

As noted above, Standard 9.11 (APA, 2002, p. 1072) provides that psychologists should make "reasonable efforts" to maintain test security. Standard 1.02 (APA, 2002, p. 1072) also states that when there is a conflict between ethical responsibilities and law, "psychologists clarify the nature of the conflict, make known their commitment to the Ethics Code, and take reasonable steps to resolve the conflict." The question that follows is what efforts or actions are "reasonable" and will satisfy the Ethics Code? Reasonableness should take into account discovery rules and the manner in which requests are made such as informal requests from attorneys, subpoenas, and court orders.

Neuropsychologists should generally be aware of what may be discoverable in the jurisdiction in which they are operating so as to anticipate what may be asked of them. The obligation of attorneys is to follow the rules of procedure in the relevant jurisdiction. For the federal jurisdiction, the Federal Rules of Civil Procedure ("FRCP"), Rule 26(b)(1) states that unless limited by a court order, "Parties may obtain discovery regarding any nonprivileged matter that is relevant to any party's claim or defense--including the existence, description, nature, custody, condition, and location of any books, documents, or other tangible things." Specifically regarding the disclosure of expert testimony, the FRCP states that an expert report must contain "the data or other information considered by the witness in forming them [opinions]" and "any exhibits that will be used to summarize or support them [opinions]" [Rules 26(a)(2)(B)(ii)–(iii)]. However, a neuropsychologist can also find options in Rule 26(a)(2)(B) in the form of stipulations or orders by the court. In other words, the neuropsychologist may ask the referring attorney to stipulate with opposing counsel that test data or materials not be discoverable or obtain a court order that would limit discoverable materials.

When a request for test data or materials is made, neuropsychologists should attempt to educate attorneys and judges on relevant ethical standards and official statements such as those from NAN. Another option is to offer to send data and/or materials directly to the psychologist on the opposing side who is trained to interpret the assessment data. Caution must still be exercised if this route is taken. It is possible that the Ethics Code does not apply to psychologists retained by the opposing party if they are not a member of APA. Whether or not the psychologist adheres to the Ethics Code, assurances that materials and data will be secure and protected should be obtained. Specifically, written assurance would be preferable (NAN, 2000a).

NAN (2000a), in the appendix ("Handling Requests to Release Test Data, Recording And/Or Reproductions of Test Data"), provides a series of steps that neuropsychologists should take when a request for information is made. These steps will not be outlined here but a few points are highlighted. One is the form in which the request is made (i.e., informal request, subpoena, or court order). A formal subpoena or court order requires a timely response. NAN (2000a) states that a response to a subpoena should provide information regarding conflicts with professional practice guides, the Ethics Code, and NAN's test security position. This may be followed with possible solutions such as release only to a qualified professional, forming a written agreement that includes elements for the protection of test materials, or a court order that contains elements for protection. Regarding the latter solution, those protective orders that may benefit the neuropsychologist include "forbidding the disclosure or discovery" [Rule 26(c)(1)(A)], "specifying terms, including time and place, for the disclosure or discovery" [Rule 26(c)(1)(B)], "designating the persons who may be present while the discovery is conducted" [Rule 26(c)(1)(E)], "requiring that a trade secret or other confidential research, development, or commercial information not be revealed or be revealed only in a specified way" [Rule 26(c)(1)(G)], and "requiring that the parties simultaneously file specified documents or information in sealed envelopes, to be opened as the court directs" [Rule 26(c)(1)(H)]. In contrast, neuropsychologists may be faced with a court order to provide test data or materials, which could lead to serious legal consequences (e.g., contempt of court) if disobeyed. NAN offers two suggestions in this circumstance. One is to release the data but to request that "appropriate safeguards be put in place to maintain test security" (NAN, 2000a, p. 386). Safeguards for test data or materials could include limited circulation, no reproductions/copies, limited courtroom presentation, and/or the destruction of test records upon completion of the legal proceedings. A second suggestion is to obtain legal counsel and, with prior approval from the attorney, state to the court the potential problems that release of test data or materials may create (NAN, 2000a).

A Note on Third Party Observers

The issue of third party presence during a neuropsychological examination is usually discussed in the context of jeopardizing the validity and reliability of test results. For instance, NAN's Official Statement on third party observers explains that this can cause distractions to the examinee and that normative data are not standardized with the presence of a third party (NAN, 2000b). The third party observer is a variable unaccounted for by test publishers during the development of normative data.

The presence of third party observers also raises issues of test security. Threats to test security can occur when in-person observation is made, but also when viewing the evaluation through a one-way mirror, or recording the evaluation using audio and/or visual devices. The American Academy of Clinical Neuropsychology (AACN) defines "involved" third parties as "those who, directly or indirectly, have some stake in the outcome of an examination of a particular plaintiff in civil litigation" (AACN, 2001, p. 433). An attorney is an example of an involved third party. An attorney can have various motivations for observing the examination such as making certain the neuropsychologist appropriately administers the tests or that he or she does not unfairly question the examinee regarding certain issues (NAN, 2000b). The neuropsychologist has limited control during test administration as to whether notes are being taken and whether specific test questions and answers are being written down by the lawyer (AACN, 2001). These notes may be used later to draw conclusions that the lawyer does not have the background or training to do. In addition, attorney's notes or observations can be used to coach subsequent clients. Prior to the evaluation (and preferably prior to agreeing to conduct an evaluation), neuropsychologists should discuss and make known their adherence to the Ethics Code and also help educate attorneys on how their presence during the evaluation could hinder the examinee and test results.

CONFLICTS OF INTEREST AND MAINTAINING OBJECTIVITY

A crucial component of all competency evaluations is the maintenance of objectivity. The official statement provided by (NAN 2003b, p. 2) on independent and court-ordered forensic neuropsychological examinations emphasizes the goal of determining cognitive status "as accurately as possible whether or not the conclusions advance or compromise the examinee's interests." This involves limiting preconceived ideas and biases to the fullest extent possible. This section will highlight relevant ethical provisions and elaborate on how bias may come into play during an evaluation, specifically if the neuropsychologist was in a previous or concurrent treatment role with the examinee.

Ethics Provisions

Standard 3.05(a) (APA, 2002, p. 1065) states that "A psychologist refrains from entering into a multiple relationship if the multiple relationship could reasonably be expected to impair the psychologist's objectivity, competence, or effectiveness in performing his or her functions as a psychologist." Standard 3.06 (APA, 2002, p. 1065), entitled Conflict of Interest, also emphasizes the maintenance of objectivity by asserting that psychologists should not take on roles that may "impair their objectivity, competence, or effectiveness in performing their functions as psychologists." In addition, Guideline IV(D)(1) (CEGFP, 1991, p. 1065) of the Specialty Guidelines specifically states that "forensic psychologists avoid providing professional services to parties in a legal proceeding with whom they have a personal or professional relationships that are inconsistent with the anticipated relationship." Guideline IV(D)(2) (CEGFP, 1991, p. 659) continues: "When it is necessary to provide both evaluation and treatment services to a party in a legal proceeding (as may be the case in small forensic hospital settings or small communities), the forensic psychologist takes reasonable steps to minimize the potential negative effects of these circumstances on the rights of the party, confidentiality, and the process of treatment and evaluation."

Treatment versus Assessment

At first glance, it may seem that a treating neuropsychologist may be well suited to provide an opinion on the competence of a patient. To make clinical determinations, the treating neuropsychologist may have already interviewed the patient and family members, conducted a thorough examination that included measures related to capacity, and formulated conclusions and recommendations. These contacts may have made the neuropsychologist keenly aware of the patient's abilities. However, this familiarity may backfire as it actually could impede objectivity. Moye (1999) asserted that those involved in the care of clients may experience conflicting dual roles and may not be able to maintain objectivity when making judgments of capacity. The desire or even expectation of the neuropsychologist by the examinee may be to offer "help" in legal proceedings and a motivation of the neuropsychologist might be to provide this "help." Efforts should be made to limit bias and make interpretations without "preconceived ideas about the examinee" (NAN, 2003b, p. 2).

Biases, whether conscious or not, could occur if neuropsychologists allow themselves to be both treatment provider as well as forensic evaluator. If a treatment role is converted into an evaluative role for an attorney, it is possible that the neuropsychologist will still view the examinee as a patient, and the examinee may have expectations based on the previous relationship that existed with the neuropsychologist. This is problematic because different conclusions are made when evaluating the decisional ability of an individual with dementia for the purposes of commencing or adjusting ongoing treatment versus conducting this evaluation to address a legal question. At the most basic level, the "treating" neuropsychologist will presumably make decisions with the patient's best interest in mind. In the treatment context, the neuropsychological evaluation will help ascertain options and effectiveness for various targeted interventions that might improve the patient's decision-making ability (Kim, Karlawish, & Caine, 2002). A beneficial alliance is naturally formed in this relationship. In contrast, the forensic neuropsychologist's purpose is to determine the examinee's decision-making status impartially, without regard to whether the conclusions advance the examinee's goals or without suggesting treatment options. Goals may be classified as awards (e.g., financial compensation) or favorable outcomes (Sweet, Grote, & van Gorp, 2002). In civil competency evaluations, examinees will generally be seeking the favorable outcome that they have the cognitive capacity to make decisions regarding various issues. Here, it is the neuropsychologist's duty to provide on objective opinion without regard to the examinee's goals. Ultimately, prior to changing roles from a treating to a forensic neuropsychologist, the neuropsychologist must decide whether he or she can provide these objective services consistent with the Ethics Code.

Dual roles should be clarified with the examinee. Examinees are especially likely to be confused if the neuropsychologist is no longer acting in their interest. Even in a situation in which the treatment role has been completed, it is possible for a former patient to still view his or her former neuropsychologist as a treatment provider. It is therefore likely that a conflict of interest will arise. Standard 3.07 (APA, 2002, p. 1065) states that "When psychologists agree to provide services to a person or entity at the request of a third party, psychologists attempt to clarify at the outset of the service the nature of the relationship with all individuals or organizations involved." Guideline IV(E) (CEGFP, 1991, p. 659) provides that "Forensic psychologists have an obligation to ensure that prospective clients are informed of their legal rights with respect to the anticipated forensic service, of the purposes of any evaluation, of the nature of the procedures to be employed, of the intended uses of any product of their services, and of the party who has employed the forensic psychologist." The neuropsychologist who is providing treatment should also explain to the former or current patient how there may be a perceived conflict of interest between the examinee and the neuropsychologist (NAN, 2003b).

Clarification of roles is also an important component of initial contacts with the attorney (Heilbrun, 2001). Standard 3.07 (APA, 2002), as discussed above, also applies in this scenario. It is possible for the treating neuropsychologist to play the role of a fact witness or an expert witness. Fact witnesses may provide testimony based on their observations and what they have experienced. An expert, however, may offer opinions based on specialized knowledge, training, and experience.

Neuropsychologists who act as witnesses who have had a previous or ongoing role as a treatment provider (i.e., treating expert) as well as neuropsychologists who were retained solely for a forensic evaluation (i.e., forensic expert) can act as experts provided they have the appropriate knowledge, training, and experience. Greenberg and Shuman (1997) explain that a therapist, "if requested to do so by a patient or ordered to do so by a court, properly testify to facts, observations, and clinical opinions for which the therapy process provides a trustworthy basis." In the same manner, the treating neuropsychologist can provide facts, observations, and clinical opinions regarding cognitive functioning using a previous neuropsychological evaluation as the basis. The problem occurs when the treating neuropsychologist takes on the role of a forensic expert to speak to legal issues. For instance, regarding testamentary capacity, many state statutes require that for the testators to be competent they must be "of sound mind." Experts in general should refrain from speaking to ultimate legal questions directly (see Heilbrun, 2001). Although both treating and forensic experts should not directly address whether the testator is "of sound mind," the treating expert should also not offer opinions regarding elements of this ultimate legal determination (e.g., knowing at the time of making a will they are making a will, knowing the nature and extent of property, knowing the manner in which their wills distribute property) [see Spaulding (1985) for a further discussion of testamentary capacity and the role of an expert witness]. It has also been argued that treating mental health experts should not just be prohibited from speaking to psycholegal issues, but should be barred from testifying altogether (Shuman, Greenberg, Heilbrun, & Foote, 1998).

Maintaining Objectivity in an Adversarial Environment

Objectivity can be threatened if a neuropsychologist decides to take on a forensic role or even simply an expert role for the same individual that they are treating. Difficulty in maintaining objectivity may also arise simply due to the adversarial nature in which the neuropsychological evaluation occurs. Incentives may be clearer and more overt for neuropsychologists in a forensic role. These incentives, among others, may be financially related. Fee arrangements should be clarified at the outset and preferably be put in writing especially if the forensic mental health expert is privately retained (Heilbrun, 2001). In other circumstances, fee amounts and schedules may be established by the court. A major threat to objectivity is providing services on a contingency basis. Guideline IV(B) (CEGFP, 1991, p. 659) states that "Forensic psychologists do not provide professional services to parties to a legal proceeding on the basis of 'contingent fees,' when those services involve the offering of expert testimony to a court or administrative body, or when they call upon the psychologist to make affirmations or representations intended to be relied upon by third parties." This sort of fee arrangement provides a tangible reward if a favorable opinion is reached and therefore creates "a significant temptation" to offer a particular opinion as well as the appearance that "the clinician is selling his or her opinion" (Melton, Petrila, Poythress, & Slobogin, 2007, p. 90).

Even without immediate financial incentives, there may be a desire to please the attorney not only in the current evaluation, but also to obtain subsequent referrals. An attorney's obligation is to provide zealous advocacy from the moment the client is retained until the client's case has been completely resolved. Various points have been identified as times when the neuropsychologist may feel pressure to provide favorable opinions to the attorney (van Gorp & McMullen, 1997). These include the initial contact between attorney and neuropsychologist, reviewing of records, the evaluation itself, the postevaluation phase, and during the time of deposition and/or testimony [see van Gorp & McMullen (1997) for a detailed discussion of these time points]. The neuropsychologist may act to minimize potential bias in each of these situations. First, simple awareness that an attorney, perhaps as part of his or her own responsibility, may emphasize strong facts and downplay weaker facts will help the neuropsychologist maintain a healthy skepticism when initial contacts are made. Records, whether deliberate or not, may be incomplete if the attorney decides to purposely omit certain harmful records or omits records considered to be obstructive or unhelpful for the neuropsychologist. The neuropsychologist should make it clear that he or she needs all relevant records, whether they advance the attorney's objectives of not. From here, an appropriate test battery may be chosen depending primarily on the legal question to be addressed and less on the opinions and desires of the attorney. It is then the neuropsychologist's duty to interpret findings without minimizing or maximizing certain strengths or weaknesses of the examinee at the behest of the attorney. Again, when direct communication with the attorney is made during deposition, trial preparation, or direct examination during the trial, the neuropsychologist should be aware that lawyers may inevitably emphasize beneficial aspects of their side, while minimizing areas that are harmful to their case. It is also important to note that the opposing counsel may act in the contrary manner by attempting to disprove and discredit the expert's opinions. In any case, maintenance of objectivity is necessary per the Ethics Code and Specialty Guidelines. In addition, relying on factual information and data from an objective evaluation should enhance the neuropsychologist's credibility. It is then the responsibility of the fact-finder, whether judge or jury, to ultimately make a determination of competency.

EVALUATING INDIVIDUALS WITH DIVERSE BACKGROUNDS

Ethics Provisions

Principle A (APA, 2002) of the Ethics Code, Beneficence and Nonmaleficence, offers general guidance when a neuropsychologist is conducting an evaluation with an individual within a diverse population, particularly as related to race, ethnicity, and language. The potential benefits and harms to the examinee should be weighed prior to agreeing to conduct a competency evaluation. When a neuropsychologist is less familiar with a particular race or ethnicity, or if there are language barriers, the most obvious harm that may result is an invalidation of the testing. For instance, differences in language may lead to overstating an individual's lack of cognitive abilities and concluding that there are impairments in decision making when there are in fact limited or no deficits. Another example is determining whether an examinee has malingered or whether there are cultural differences in response style. Conversing with the examinee regarding a cultural explanation of the illness may be helpful here (Poreh, 2002). In contrast, harm may be done by refusing to evaluate an individual based solely on his or her background without providing alternative solutions. A blanket refusal of services would have implications for Principle D (APA, 2002, p. 1062), Justice, which states that all persons should have "access to and benefit from the contributions of psychology and to equal quality in the processes, procedures, and services being conducted by psychologists." Refusing services can be especially harmful if neuropsychological services are limited in particular geographic locations. The potential examinee would then be deprived of the objective data that a neuropsychological evaluation could provide with respect to competency, which could ultimately lead to a less informed legal decision.

Principle E (APA, 2002, p. 1063), Respect of People's Rights and Dignity, states that "Psychologists are aware that special safeguards may be necessary to protect the rights and welfare of persons or communities whose vulnerabilities impair autonomous decision making." Autonomy may be jeopardized at various points before, during, and after a neuropsychological examination. Obtaining prior consent may be a concern, especially if the examinee is not a native speaker of English or is not fluent in the language. During the examination, the actual process and purpose may not be well understood as the examinee is faced with different tasks that use different skills. A paternalistic feeling may arise if the examinee is simply following the neuropsychologist's instructions without fully understanding the purpose. Finally, the neuropsychological examination may help lead to an erroneous legal decision that the individual is not competent, when in reality, linguistic and cultural issues factored into test performance. Autonomy here would be jeopardized at a much larger scale than before and during the examination. Principle E (APA, 2002, p. 1063) further states that psychologists are aware of individual differences and "try to eliminate the effect on their work of biases based on those factors." The elimination of biases ideally goes beyond eliminating prejudice. An interpretation of this Principle is a need to understand the biases inherent in a neuropsychological examination and proactively taking steps and providing the "special safeguards" aimed at minimizing bias in order to enhance validity.

The neuropsychologist should evaluate the possible available resources when balancing the costs and benefits of accepting an expert role involving individuals of varying background. One consideration is whether there are avenues to educate oneself about a specific ethnicity such as formal education or continuing education. Even simply questioning laypeople or other professionals who have worked frequently with individuals of a particular background may provide helpful information. Consultation with another neuropsychologist familiar with the relevant culture is another possible option if this solution is acceptable to the attorney. However, more formal measures should strongly be considered if the neuropsychologist intends to have continued communications and evaluations with a particular group. These suggestions follow Ethical Standard 2.01(c) (APA, 2002): "Psychologists planning to provide services, teach, or conduct research involving populations, areas, or techniques, or technologies new to them undertake relevant education, training, supervised experience, consultation, or study." If resources are unavailable or if the neuropsychologist decides more harm would arise from administering the evaluation, the neuropsychologist may try to refer the attorney to another neuropsychologist. In particular, NAN provides a database of neuropsychologists who can conduct evaluations in various languages.

If the neuropsychologist decides to conduct the evaluation, one of the first decisions is how informed consent will be obtained if language is an issue. Obtaining an informed consent form in the respective language would be the best option. An interpreter may also be considered. This is an option not only for informed consent, but also in assisting with the clinical interview. However, use of an interpreter for a word-for-word translation of test instruments should not be done (Harris, 2002, p. 232): "A direct translation of a stimulus item may change the difficulty level of the item, change its intent, or make it irrelevant." Instead, efforts should be made to identify some measures that may have versions in different languages. It should also be noted that the presence of an interpreter during testing, which constitutes third party presence, could influence the validity of the testing.

Use of Standardized Measures and Norms

Interpretation of test results is another area in which validity of an evaluation is questionable when serving diverse groups. The possibility of language or culture being a source of error is present when test manuals do not provide norms based on race. The construct validity of a test is threatened when a neuropsychologist uses norms that were originally developed for a different population. However, if norms are not provided by test publishers, relevant norms may be obtained from various research studies. This is especially common for African-American and Hispanic-American populations [see Poreh (2002) for a list of articles and manuals that provide norms for these populations].

Neuropsychological evaluations in general benefit from the ability to be flexible when developing a test battery. In addition, it is possible to give a "predeveloped" battery to address the growing need of providing adequate services when evaluating an individual from a minority population. For instance, the Cross-Cultural Neuropsychological Test Battery (CCNB) has been studied using a sample consisting of five ethnic groups including African-American, white, Chinese, Hispanic, and Vietnamese (Dick, Teng, Kempler, Davis, & Taussig, 2002). The battery included 11 tests (two developed by the authors) in seven domains including mental status, memory, language, visuospatial, attention, reasoning, and psychomotor speed. The authors found that compared to controls, demented patients scored significantly worse on the battery overall, and therefore cognitive impairments in minority groups were detected by the battery. Ultimately, the neuropsychologist must balance the need to choose the appropriate measures to address the referral question with how accurate the results will be considering the adequacy of available norms. If appropriate norms are unavailable, this should be noted in the discussion of test results as well as in the analysis of the referral question.

CONCLUSIONS

Neuropsychologists possess a unique set of skills that make them ideally suited to assess competency in both neuropsychiatric and neurological illness. In general, an ethical approach to any competency assessment demands the use of reliable and valid assessment strategies that cover the broad domains of (1) neuropsychological functioning, (2) decisional capacity, (3) psychiatric and emotional factors, and (4) functional capacity. The issues raised above highlight the need to use standardized, reliable, and ecologically valid measures for the assessment of competency. The use of these tools is crucial in that there is clear evidence that informal assessments often performed by clinicians may be idiosyncratic and unreliable (Marson et al., 1997). Specifically, neuropsychologists are bound by the ethical obligations of practicing within their areas of expertise, using empirically derived assessment instruments, and protecting the autonomy as well as the safety of their patients.

References

American Academy of Clinical Neuropsychology. (2001). Special presentation: Policy statement on the presence of third party observers in neuropsychological assessments. *The Clinical Neuropsychologist, 15*, 433–439.

American Medical Directors Association. (2003). White paper on surrogate decision-making and advance care planning in long-term care. Retrieved March 20, 2011, from http://www.amda.com/governance/whitepapers/surrogate/.

American Psychological Association. (2002). Ethical principles of psychologists and code of conduct. *American Psychologist, 57*, 1060–1073.

Appelbaum, P. S., & Grisso, T. (1996). *The MacArthur Competence Assessment Tool—Clinical Research*. Sarasota, FL: Professional Resource.

Bean, G., Nishisato, S., Rector, N. A., & Glancy, G. (1994). The psychometric properties of the Competency Interview Schedule. *Canadian Journal of Psychiatry, 39*, 368–376.

Bruininks, R. H., Woodcock, R. W., Weatherman, R. E., & Hill, B. K. (2004). Scales of Independent Behavior–Revised (SIB-R). Itasca, IL: Riverside Publishing.

Buchanan, A. E., & Brock, D. W. (1990). *Deciding for others: The ethics of surrogate decision making*. Cambridge, UK: Cambridge University Press.

Carney, M. T., Neugroschl, J., Morrison, R. S., Marin, D., & Siu, A. L. (2001). The development and piloting of a capacity assessment tool. *The Journal of Clinical Ethics, 12*, 17–23.

Chaytor, N., & Schmitter-Edgecombe, M. (2003). The ecological validity of neuropsychological tests: A review of the literature on everyday cognitive skills. *Neuropsychology Review, 13*, 181–197.

Committee on Ethical Guidelines for Forensic Psychologists. (1991). Specialty guidelines for forensic psychologists. *Law and Human Behavior, 15*, 655–665.

Cramer, K., Tuokko, H. A., Mateer, C. A., & Hultsch, D. F. (2004). Measuring awareness of financial skills: Reliability and validity of a new measure. *Aging & Mental Health, 8*, 161–171.

Denney, R. L., & Wynkoop, T. F. (2000). Clinical neuropsychology in the criminal forensic setting. *Journal of Head Trauma Rehabilitation, 15*, 804–828.

Deronzo, E. G., Conley, R. R., & Love, R. (1998). Assessment of capacity to give consent to research participation: State of the art and beyond. *Journal of Health Care Law and Policy, 1*, 66–87.

Dick, M., Teng, E., Kempler, D., Davis, D., & Taussig, I. (2002). The cross-cultural neuropsychological batter (CCNB): Effects of age, education, ethnicity, and cognitive status on performance. In F. R. Ferraro (Ed.), *Minority and cross-cultural aspects of neuropsychological assessment* (pp. 17–41). Lisse, NL: Swets & Zeitlinger.

Diehl, M., Marsiske, M., Horgas, A. L., Rosenberg, A., Saczynski, J. S., & Willis, S. L. (2005). The Revised Observed Tasks of Daily Living: A performance-based assessment of everyday problem solving in older adults. *Journal of Applied Gerontology, 24*, 211–230.

Dymek, M. P., Atchison, P., Harrell, L., & Marson, D. C. (2001). Competency to consent to medical treatment in cognitively impaired patients with Parkinson's disease. *Neurology, 56*, 17–24.

Edelstein, M., Nygren, L., Northrop, N., Staats, N., & Pool, D. (1993). Assessment of capacity to make financial and medical decisions. Paper presented in August at the meeting of the American Psychological Association, Toronto, Canada.

Essig, S., Mittenberg, W., Petersen, R., Strauman, S., & Cooper, J. (2001). Practices in forensic neuropsychology: Perspectives of neuropsychologists and trial attorneys. *Archives of Clinical Neuropsychology, 16*, 271–291.

Etchells, E., Darzins, P., Silberfeld, M., Singer, P. A., McKenny, J., Naglie, G., et al. (1999). Assessment of patient capacity to consent to treatment. *Journal of General Internal Medicine, 14*, 27–34.

Freides, D. (1993). Proposed standard of professional practice: Neuropsychological reports display all quantitative data. *The Clinical Neuropsychologist, 7*, 234–235.

Ginsberg, J. P., Kibby, M. Y., & Long, C. J. (1995). Ecological validity of neuropsychological data as indicated by interrelationships with vocational data. Poster presented at the Annual Meeting of the National Academy of Neuropsychology, San Francisco.

Greenberg, S., & Shuman, D. (1997). Irreconcilable conflict between therapeutic and forensic roles. *Professional Psychology: Research and Practice, 28*, 50–57.

Grisso, T. (1986). *Evaluating competencies: Forensic assessment instruments*. New York: Plenum.

Grisso, T., Appelbaum, P. S., & Hill-Fotouhi, C. (1997). The MacCAT-T: A clinical tool to assess patient's capacities to make treatment decisions. *Psychiatric Services, 48*, 1415–1419.

Harris, J. (2002). Ethical decision making with individuals of diverse ethnic, cultural, and linguistic backgrounds. In S. S. Bush & M. L. Drexler (Eds.), *Ethical issues in clinical neuropsychology* (pp. 223–241). Lisse, NL: Swets & Zeitlinger.

Heilbrun, K. (2001). *Principles of forensic mental health assessment*. New York: Kluwer Academic/Plenum.

Heinrichs, R. W. (1990). Current and emergent applications of neuropsychological assessment: Problems with utility and validity. *Professional Psychology: Research & Practice, 21*, 171–176.

Higginson, C. I., Arnett, P. A., & Voss, W. D. (2000). The ecological validity of clinical tests of memory and attention in multiple sclerosis. *Archives of Clinical Neuropsychology, 15*, 185–204.

Janofsky, J. S., McCarthy, R. J., & Folstein, M. F. (1992). The Hopkins Competency Assessment Test: A brief method for evaluating patients' capacity to give informed consent. *Hospital and Community Psychiatry, 43*, 132–136.

Kapp, M. B., & Mossman, D. (1996). Measuring decisional capacity: Cautions on the construction of a "capacimeter." *Psychology, Public Policy and Law, 2*, 73–95.

Kim, S., Karlawish, J., & Caine, E. (2002). Current state of research on decision-making competence of cognitively impaired elderly persons. *American Journal of Geriatric Psychiatry, 10*, 151–164.

Lai, J. M., Gill, T. M., Cooney, L. M., Bradley, E. H., Hawkins, K. A., & Karlawish, J. H. (2008). Everyday decision-making ability in older persons with cognitive impairment. *American Journal of Geriatric Psychiatry,* 16, 693–696.

Lai, J. M., & Karlawish, J. H. (2007). Assessing the capacity to make everyday decisions: A guide for clinicians and an agenda for future research. *American Journal of Geriatric Psychiatry, 15*, 101–111.

Long, C. J., & Kibby, M. Y. (1995). Ecological validity of neuropsychological tests: A look at neuropsychology's past and the impact that ecological issues may have on its future. *Advances in Medical Psychotherapy, 8*, 59–78.

Marcotte, T. D., & Grant, I. (2006). *Neuropsychology of everyday functioning*. New York: Guilford.

Marson, D. C. (2001). Loss of competency in Alzheimer's disease: Conceptual and psychometric approaches. *International Journal of Law and Psychiatry, 24*, 267–283.

Marson, D. C., Chatterjee, A., Ingram, K. K., & Harrell, L. E. (1996). Toward a neurologic model of competency: Cognitive predictors of capacity to consent in Alzheimer's disease using three different legal standards. *Neurology, 46*, 666–672.

Marson, D. C., Cody, H. A., Ingram, K. K., & Harrell, L. E. (1995). Neuropsychological predictors of competency in Alzheimer's disease using a rational reasons legal standard. *Neurology, 52*, 955–959.

Marson, D. C., Ingram, K. K., Cody, H. A., & Harrell, L. E. (1995). Assessing the competency of patients with Alzheimer's disease under different legal standards. A prototype instrument. *Archives of Neurology, 52*, 949–954.

Marson, D. C., McInturff, B., Hawkins, L., Bartolucci, A., & Harrell, L. E. (1997). Consistency of physician judgments of capacity to consent in mild Alzheimer's disease. *Journal of the American Geriatrics Society, 45*, 453–457.

Marson, D. C., Sawrie, S. M., Snyder, S., McInturff, B., Stalvey, T., Boothe, A., Aldridge, T., Chatterjee, A., & Harrell, L. E. (2000). Assessing financial capacity in patients with Alzheimer disease: A conceptual model and prototype instrument. *Archives of Neurology, 57*, 877–884.

Melton, G., Petrila, J., Poythress, N., & Slobogin, C. (2007). *Psychological evaluations for the courts* (3rd ed.). New York: Guilford.

Moberg, P. J., & Gibney, M. (2005). Decision-making capacity in the impaired older adult. In S. Bush & T. A. Martin (Eds.), *Geriatric neuropsychology: Practice essentials* (pp. 491–506). Lisse, NL: Swets & Zeitlinger.

Moberg, P. J., & Kniele, K. (2006). Evaluation of competency: Ethical considerations for neuropsychologists. *Applied Neuropsychology, 13*, 101–114.

Moberg, P. J., & Rick, J. H. (2008). Assessing competency in the elderly: A clinical and neuropsychological perspective. *NeuroRehabilitation, 23*, 403–413.

Moye, J. (1999). Assessment of competency and decision making capacity. In P. A. Lichtenberg (Ed.), *Handbook of assessment in clinical gerontology* (pp. 488–528). New York: John Wiley & Sons.

National Academy of Neuropsychology. (2000a). Test security: Official position statement of the National Academy of Neuropsychology. *Archives of Clinical Neuropsychology, 15*, 383–386.

National Academy of Neuropsychology. (2000b). Presence of third party observers during neuropsychological testing: Official statement of the National Academy of Neuropsychology. *Archives of Clinical Neuropsychology, 15*, 379–380.

National Academy of Neuropsychology. (2003a). *Test Security: An update*. Official statement of the National Academy of Neuropsychology. Retrieved October 3, 2010 from http://www.nanonline.org/nan/ResearchPublications/PositionPapers.aspx.

National Academy of Neuropsychology. (2003b). *Independent and court-ordered forensic neuropsychological examinations*. Retrieved October 3, 2010 from http://nanonline.org/nan/ResearchPublications/PositionPapers.aspx.

Poreh., A. (2002). Neuropsychological and psychological issues associated with cross-cultural and minority assessment. In F. R. Ferraro (Ed.), *Minority and cross-cultural aspects of neuropsychological assessment* (pp. 329–343). Lisse, NL: Swets & Zeitlinger.

Reger, M. A., Welsh, R. K., Watson, G. S., Cholerton, B., Baker, L. D., & Craft, S. (2004). The relationship between neuropsychological functioning and driving ability in dementia: A meta-analysis. *Neuropsychology, 18*, 85–93.

Robertson, I. H., Ward, T., Ridgeway, V., & Nimmo-Smith, I. (1994). *The Test of Everyday Attention*. Suffolk, UK: Thames Valley Test Company/Gaylord, MI: National Rehabilitation Services.

Rose, F., Hall, S., Szalda-Petree, A., & Bach, P. J. (1998). A comparison of four tests of malingering and the effects of coaching. *Archives of Clinical Neuropsychology, 13*, 349–363.

Rule 26. Federal Rules of Civil Procedure.

Saks, E. R., Dunn, L. B., Marshall, B. J., Nayak, G. V., Golshan, S., & Jeste, D. V. (2002). The California Scale of Appreciation: A new instrument to measure the appreciation component of capacity to consent to research. *American Journal of Geriatric Psychiatry, 10*, 166–174.

Sbordone, R. J., & Long, C. J. (1996). *Ecological validity of neuropsychological testing*. Delray Beach, FL: GR Press/St. Lucie Press.

Shuman, D., Greenberg, S., Heilbrun, K., & Foote, W. (1998). Special perspective an immodest proposal: Should treating mental health professionals be barred from testifying about their patients? *Behavioral Sciences and the Law, 16*, 509–523.

Sparrow, S. S., Cicchetti, D. V., & Balla, D. A. (2005). *Vineland Adaptive Behavior Scales, Second Edition (Vineland-II)*. AGS, Circle Pines, MN.

Spaulding, W. (1985). Testamentary competency: Reconciling doctrine with the role of the expert witness. *Law and Human Behavior, 9*, 113–139.

Suhr. J., & Gunstad, J. (2000). The effects of coaching on the sensitivity and specificity of malingering measures. *Archives of Neuropsychology, 15*, 415–424.

Sunderland, A., Harris, J. E., & Baddeley, A. D. (1983). Do laboratory tests predict everyday memory? A neuropsychological study. *Journal of Verbal Learning and Verbal Behavior, 22*, 341–357.

Sweet, J., Grote, C., & van Gorp, W. (2002). Ethical issues in forensic neuropsychology. In S. S. Bush & M. L. Drexler (Eds.), *Ethical issues in clinical neuropsychology* (pp. 103–133). Lisse, NL: Swets & Zeitlinger.

Tomoda, A., Yasumiya, R., Sumiyama, T., Tankada, K., Hayakawa, T., Kimimori, M., et al. (1997). Reliability and validity of structured interview for competency/incompetency assessment testing and ranking inventory. *Journal of Clinical Psychology, 53*, 443–450.

van Gorp, W., & McMullen, W. (1997). Potential sources of bias in forensic neuropsychological evaluations. *The Clinical Neuropsychologist, 11*, 180–187.

Wetters, M., & Corrigan, S. (1995). Providing information to clients about psychological tests: A survey of attorneys' and law students' attitudes. *Professional Psychology: Research and Practice, 26*, 474–477.

Wilson, B. A. (1993). Ecological validity of neuropsychological assessment: Do neuropsychological indexes predict performance in everyday activities? *Applied and Preventative Psychology, 2*, 209–215.

Wilson, B. A., Cockburn, J., & Baddeley, A. (1985). *The Rivermead Behavioral Memory Test*. Reading, UK: Thames Valley Test Company/Gaylord, MI: National Rehabilitation Services.

PART FOUR

Conclusions

14

A Legal Consumer's Perspective on Competency Evaluations

FREDERICK R. BENSON AND M. JOANNE ROMANO

In North Carolina the Clerk of Superior Court is also the *ex officio* Judge of Probate. As such, the Clerk of Court has exclusive jurisdiction to hear all competency and guardianship cases. By statute, an Assistant Clerk of Court has the same authority as the Clerk of Court. In the most populous counties in North Carolina, such as Mecklenburg County, case volume dictates that Assistant Clerks, referred to as Legal Hearing Officers, conduct incompetency/guardianship hearings. The authors of this chapter practiced as attorneys in the area of incompetency and guardianship before assuming their positions as Assistant Clerks, and have participated in hundreds of these cases.

The significant rise in incompetency cases can be attributed to the aging of the U.S. population as well as to an increased recognition of the rights of persons with disabilities. Historically, people with dementia, other cognitive disabilities, or mental illness often had decisions made for them on an informal basis by family members, medical staff, or other care providers. Over time, statutory recognition of the need for due process of law before assigning the decision-making role to another individual has resulted in an increase in incompetency case filings. With the combination of statutory safeguards and the aging of the "baby boomers" on the horizon, the number of incompetency cases will continue to increase. As the number of cases increases, so will the need for court-ordered evaluations. It is important that these evaluations meet the needs of the court. They should be understandable to the court, relevant to the particular case, and properly supported by testing and appropriate background information.

LEGAL ISSUES AND PROCEDURES

Persons below the age of majority are presumed by law to be incompetent. Except for emancipated minors, parents or persons who stand in *loco parentis* make residential, medical, and financial decisions for the minor. The focus of this chapter is on adult incompetency and guardianship.

The court is the ultimate consumer of psychological or neuropsychological evaluations in competency determinations. The court may be a judge sitting alone, a jury, or some other official designated by applicable statute to make the decisions relating to competency and guardianship. To understand the needs of the court, it may be helpful to understand the manner in which competency and guardianship cases come before the court and how a case progresses.

The procedures, standards of proof, and laws of evidence for incompetency cases are state specific. Even the terminology used in state statutes varies across states. Some states use the term "competency" whereas others use the term "capacity" to express the same concept. The definition of "incompetent adult," "person lacking capacity," or "person with incapacity" also varies from state to state, but is essentially the same [American Bar Association Commission on Law and Aging: Capacity definition and initiation of guardianship proceedings]. The term used to describe the person appointed as guardian also varies. In some states the person appointed to manage a ward's finances is referred to as the "guardian of the estate" and in other states the person is referred to a "conservator." The person appointed to make healthcare, residential, and other personal decisions is referred to as the "guardian of the person" or simply the "guardian." For purposes of clarity and consistency, the terms "competency," "guardian of the person," and "guardian of the estate" are used in this chapter.

It is also important to note that different legal standards are applied, depending on the type of case. The legal standard for an adjudication of incompetence is different from the legal standard applied in a criminal case in which the defendant's capacity to stand trial is in question. The incompetency legal standard is also different from the capacity standard in a domestic case in which an evaluation identifying the individual's parenting skills is needed to assist the court in determining parenting capacity.

An incompetency case is commenced by the filing of an initial pleading with the court. The pleading may be styled as a petition, complaint, motion, or any other document allowed by state law. The pleading alleges that another person, typically termed the "respondent," is an incompetent adult. A pleading may be filed by anyone, including a family member, friend, neighbor, facility, social service agency, or any other person or entity allowed by the laws of the state in which the pleading is filed (American Bar Association Commission on Guardianship and Aging: Capacity definition and initiation of guardianship proceedings). The term "petitioner" is used in this chapter to indicate the individual or entity filing the pleading. When the petitioner is a social service agency, it is not uncommon for the pleading to be accompanied by a consultative evaluation report performed by a psychologist or physician. Those preliminary evaluations range from comprehensive testing reports to one-sentence conclusions hand-written on prescription pads.

The reasons for filing a case are varied and sometimes not apparent on the face of the initial pleading. The petitioner may file solely for the benefit of the respondent, such as the filing by the parents of a respondent with mental retardation who has reached the age of majority. However, in some cases the petitioner, family members, parties, or interested persons have hidden agendas and conflicting motives. Examples include a dispute rooted in sibling rivalry among the children of an aging parent regarding the parent's healthcare and/or finances, or a petitioner's desire for appointment as guardian of the person or estate in order to ensure his own continued exploitation of the respondent. On occasion, multiple petitioners file separate pleadings, each for their own reason. The timing of the case filings also varies; some filings are not anticipated by petitioners, whereas others are. A petitioner sometimes initiates an incompetency proceeding by filing a pleading when a respondent's physical and/or cognitive functioning deteriorates suddenly or slowly over time, when a family member discovers a respondent's self-neglect or exploitation, when an elderly person is discovered squandering his or her own assets, or when a respondent's medical problem triggers the need for medical consents that cannot otherwise be obtained. Some cases are filed at more predictable times. For example, filing often occurs when a disabled minor reaches the age of majority.

Once the case is filed, the court may appoint a person to represent or otherwise assist the respondent. Both the requirement for this appointment and the nomenclature used for this appointee vary widely from state to state. The appointee may be a guardian *ad litem* (who may or may not be an attorney), both an attorney and a guardian *ad litem*, or in some jurisdictions a "visitor." Some states make these appointments automatically, whereas others do so only upon the request of a party or at the court's discretion (American Bar Association Commission on Law and Aging: Representation and investigation in guardianship proceedings). When the court orders an evaluation of the respondent, the evaluator should be familiar with both the appointment procedure in the state in which the case is pending and the state statutes identifying to whom the evaluation report can be released prior to the hearing. The court, as well as the guardian *ad litem*/attorney/visitor and court-appointed evaluator, must abide by statutory and procedural safeguards that ensure the confidentiality of the evaluation results.

Another feature of the judicial process that varies from state to state is the hearing or trial of the matter before the court. Most state statutes allow for jury trials, if requested (American Bar Association Commission on Law and Aging: Conduct and findings of guardianship proceedings). Some state statutes are silent on the issue. In one state, jury trials are mandatory (Kentucky Revised Statutes 387.570.1). It is in dispute as to whether incompetency cases are well suited for jury trials. Taken as a whole, a jury is a small group of lay people without extensive knowledge of the issues confronting a court in an incompetency case. Jurors may be influenced by their own prejudice, bias, and misconceptions about mental illness and mental retardation. The challenge for the evaluator in an incompetency case to be decided by a jury is to sufficiently educate the jury about the respondent's impairment so that the jury's decision is based solely upon facts and not upon misinformation.

The length of an incompetency proceeding depends upon the complexity of the issues, the number of witnesses, and whether the case is presented to a jury or an individual trier of fact. The individual trier of fact may be a judge, magistrate, clerk, or assistant clerk of court. Hearings can be scheduled when needed or when exigent circumstances are alleged. Although most cases come before the court at one setting that is scheduled within the time set forth in the applicable state statute, emergency, preliminary, or interim hearings can be scheduled when exigent circumstances are alleged. An emergency hearing dictates a subsequent final hearing for the determination of the ultimate competency issue. An evaluation may not be feasible for a quickly scheduled emergency, preliminary, or interim hearing because of time constraints, but needs to be completed and available to the court for the final hearing.

Unlike traditional civil or criminal cases, competency cases may be scheduled for subsequent hearing after a respondent has been declared incompetent. Common reasons for subsequent proceedings include a petitioner's allegations that the incompetent person, now referred to as a "ward," has regained some or all of his or her competency and is no longer in need of a guardian, or a petitioner's request that the court appoint a successor guardian due to the guardian's wrongdoing, infirmity, death, or resignation. These subsequent proceedings may also be for good cause, as when a ward with mental illness or brain injury has regained the capacity to handle his or her affairs, or may simply be a continuation of family conflict regarding issues with the ward's treatment, visitation, or finances. The court may enter an order for an evaluation to determine the extent of the ward's recovery or to determine other issues that have not previously come before the court.

COMPETENCY REPORT WRITING FOR THE COURT

Having described the manner in which incompetency cases come before the court and the basic procedure involved in the process, the focus of the remainder of this chapter is on the needs of the court and the factors that the evaluator should consider in performing the evaluation and writing the report. The court considers multiple factors before entering an order for an evaluation, including the number of qualified evaluators available for appointment and the time in which an evaluator can complete the evaluation. Especially in jurisdictions in which large numbers of evaluations are ordered, the court may not have a tracking system to follow the progress of the evaluation process. To further complicate tracking, the court order in some jurisdictions does not specifically name an evaluator, but, instead, directs the area mental health system or some other entity to perform the evaluation. In those cases, the appointed entity then assigns a specific evaluator to perform the evaluation. Where this system of appointment is the practice, it is especially helpful to the court when the assigned evaluator sends written communication to the court that the evaluator has received the appointment, scheduled the evaluation for a certain day and time, and anticipates releasing the evaluation report on a certain date. This communication is important, as the scheduling of court proceedings is often based upon the projected release date of the evaluation report.

The final evaluation report should be the signed and dated original with numbered pages bearing the respondent's name on each page. The report should include the following: evaluator's name, address, and phone and fax numbers; respondent's name, date of birth, and court file number; reason for the evaluation; evaluation methods; tests administered; medical and psychological records reviewed; names and relationships of collateral contacts; method of contact with the respondent and collateral sources; results of the clinical interview with the respondent and collateral sources; behavioral observations regarding all contacts; test results; the evaluator's conclusions regarding competency and guardianship; and the evaluator's recommendations.

The foremost consideration for the evaluator is that the court, whether a judge presiding at a bench trial or a jury in a jury trial, as the consumer of an evaluation report, is not a medical or mental health professional. In addition, judges presiding in incompetency cases have varying degrees of experience in hearing competency cases. Although some judges in incompetency cases are not attorneys, most are. However, their undergraduate or postgraduate studies and experience prior to law school are likely to be in fields other than psychology and medicine. Therefore, their knowledge base in these areas may be limited. Some may have had experience in incompetency cases before becoming judges and others may be experienced in criminal, civil, or domestic law. Therefore, it is important that the evaluation report be written in plain language and in a manner that is understandable by a person who has no scientific or mental health background.

For optimum value to the court, the evaluator should explain, and not simply name, the tests used in the evaluation. The evaluator should not assume that a court will know that MMSE, WISC-IV, and MMPI-2 are acronyms for Mini-Mental State Examination, Wechsler Intelligence Scale for Children–4th Edition, and Minnesota Multiphasic Personality Inventory-2, respectively. It is helpful to the court to have an evaluation report that names the tests, what the tests measure, why these tests are appropriate in that particular case, and the results of the tests.

In the evaluation report, it is also important to include an explanation of the conditions under which the evaluation tests were administered. For example, if the alleged incompetent individual is speech-impaired, sight-impaired, or hearing-impaired, the court will benefit from knowing whether each test was written or oral. A surprising number of tests are administered to alleged incompetent persons who, due to a physical impairment, have difficulty taking or completing the tests. The usefulness of the evaluation and the resulting report are negatively affected when this occurs. When physical impairment exists, it is helpful to the court that the evaluator, to the extent that he or she can express an opinion, states how the respondent's impairment affected the test results and the resulting validity of the test. To guard against the submission of an evaluation report that the court questions on this issue, the evaluator should attempt to ascertain any physical limitations existing at the time of the testing, the extent to which these limitations are accommodated by the evaluator, and, ultimately, the validity of the testing if adequate accommodation is not possible.

Another consideration that the evaluator in a court-ordered evaluation should keep in mind is that the court is, and must remain, objective and neutral. All court-ordered evaluations should be the same. Although the parties in the case may have an agenda, the court and the evaluator must begin their respective processes with no preconceived opinions of the eventual outcome. Sometimes when a party to the case retains an evaluator, as opposed to the court appointing an evaluator, the retained evaluator's report and live testimony have the hallmarks of being prepared and presented by a "hired gun" in favor of the retaining party in the case. The retained evaluator's bias may come to light when the opposing party questions the evaluator in live testimony. In situations in which the evaluator submits only a written report, the evaluator's bias can often be perceived when the evaluator's opinion too closely matches the position and desire of the party that retained the evaluator. The court sometimes finds an almost verbatim match between the position of a party to the case and the opinion of the evaluator retained by that party. Although there is nothing in and of itself wrong with this development if the retained evaluator's opinion and testimony are supported by the facts, the court may have a certain level of wariness in these cases.

Court-ordered evaluators can also avoid court skepticism and vulnerability to criticism by stating the facts upon which the report and conclusions are based. Any conversations with family members, social workers, friends, or other persons should be described, as should all prior medical and psychological records that were reviewed in the preparation of the report. If necessary and appropriate in the state in which the case is pending, the evaluator should seek to ascertain collateral sources for all available information and attempt to obtain information from those sources. The evaluator should include the collateral's name and relationship to the respondent and the method of contact (i.e., interview in person, by telephone, or in writing). For example, if it is an allowable practice for the evaluator to gather the respondent's medical and psychological history from family members or other persons, the evaluator should attempt to contact as many sources as possible. Thoroughness in gathering information from varied sources is important, as some individuals who know the respondent may be aware of only a portion of the respondent's history or may dissemble for their own purposes. It is not uncommon for family members or friends to deny or misstate known facts because of embarrassment, family conflict, or other personal agenda. Some level of denial by family members, especially parents, is common when the respondent has mental retardation or mental illness. The authors have presided at hearings in which the petitioning parent of a soon-to-be-18-year-old respondent with mental retardation told the court that the respondent is actually "pretty smart" or just has a "learning problem." One respondent with a vocabulary of only 20 words was described as "actually pretty bright."

Similarly, petitioning parents of a respondent with mental illness will sometimes attribute the respondent's behavior problems to physical conditions that are nonexistent or of little significance, while insisting that the mental illness component is nothing other than a misdiagnosis or a condition long since cured. More nefarious are the misstatements made by exploiters aiming to continue their exploitation of the respondent by denying that the respondent has dementia symptoms or delusional thought processes. The challenge for the evaluator is to obtain enough information from allowable sources to be able to present a report that the court finds to be thorough, credible, and as free of bias as possible given the sometimes limited information with which the evaluator begins the process.

The thoroughness of the evaluation report is made even more important by the limits of the information that the court has at the beginning of the legal process. Although the amount of information in the initial pleading varies from state to state, it is not unusual for it to be a bare bones statement of the alleged incompetent person's condition. As many of these cases are not filed by experienced attorneys, social workers, or other persons familiar with the incompetency process, the initiating pleadings are sometimes lacking in relevant detail. Petitioners often state in their petitions and come to court to testify simply that the alleged incompetent person has "mental retardation," "mental illness," or "dementia." The degree of impairment is not described. This situation may be a result of the petitioner being unaware of the need for a more complete description, or it may be the result of the petitioner being unaware of the level of impairment. Sometimes the condition is relatively recent in origin, as with a traumatic brain injury, cardiovascular accident, or mental illness, and no testing or evaluation has yet taken place. A petitioner who has recently become a full-time caregiver is often without knowledge of the exact diagnosis or degree of disability. The lack of detailed information in the court file makes the thoroughness of the court-ordered evaluation all the more important, as it is sometimes the only record of substance that the court has before it.

The court may also struggle with the validity of a diagnosis appearing in the respondent's medical records that are presented for the court's consideration. Medical records may contain statements such as a "history of mental illness" or "history of schizophrenia." Upon the court's inquiry about the origin of those statements, it may become apparent that the statements have been repeated from record to record over time, without recent clinicians questioning where and when the original diagnosis was made. The information may come from well-meaning but ill-informed relatives. In one case, the court traced a "history of schizophrenia" statement to a verbal diagnosis made by a hospital emergency department physician almost 20 years prior to the filing of the incompetency case and never subsequently confirmed by a psychiatrist or psychologist. The statement had been repeated multiple times in the patient/respondent's medical records based upon statements made by the respondent's family to various physicians during the course of the patient's adult life. An evaluator assists the court when the evaluator looks closely at all the respondent's records, weighs the validity of the information in the record, and performs a new evaluation without undue reliance upon past records.

Another stumbling block for courts is a case in which the respondent has conflicting diagnoses. An evaluator can greatly assist the court in these cases. On occasion, an alleged incompetent person is presented to the court with past medical or psychological records containing different diagnoses from different sources.

The diagnoses may conflict, be a case of dual diagnoses, or may have changed over time. The court's determination of competency is based upon the respondent's condition at or around the time of the competency hearing. However, the respondent's history may be relevant in the case of chronic or recurring conditions. The authors are familiar with a case in which the respondent had been given five different diagnoses by five different mental health professionals. The mental health professional testifying at the hearing explained that the court should accept his diagnosis as the correct one and disregard the diagnoses of the others because he was the most experienced professional. Fortunately, given the degree of incapacity the respondent displayed during the course of the hearing, the court was not required to decide which of the multiple diagnoses, if any, was correct, as the respondent was incompetent based on any of the diagnoses and other evidence that met the statutory standard. In a case of conflicting diagnoses, it is helpful to the court if the evaluator acknowledges the conflict, states the basis for his or her conclusions, and explains how those conclusions were reached.

The evaluation in competency cases focuses on both the respondent and the proposed guardian. First, the issue for the evaluator is whether the respondent has the ability to make and communicate decisions and function independently. When the evaluator selects tests to administer to the respondent and prepares the evaluation report, it is helpful to the court if the evaluator keeps in mind that the purpose of the report is to assist the court in determining the respondent's capacity to make decisions and function without a guardian, without confusing this type of case with others that exist in the court system. If the evaluator determines that the respondent cannot make and communicate decisions, the issue then becomes assessing a proposed guardian's suitability to assume the responsibilities of appointment as guardian of the respondent.

Given the fact that the ultimate result of a determination of incompetence is the loss of rights of the alleged incompetent person, most states have set high standards of proof. Most states require that the proof of incompetence be "clear and convincing" (American Bar Association Commission on Law and Aging: Conduct and findings of guardianship proceedings). Wyoming uses the lower standard of "preponderance of the evidence" [Wyoming Statutes 3-2-104(a)], whereas New Hampshire stands alone in requiring the even higher standard of "beyond a reasonable doubt" (New Hampshire Revised Statutes 464-A: 8). Thirteen states have no statutory level of required proof.

All other factors being equal, the court places greater weight on a current evaluation than on a past evaluation. The court may consider past evaluations, but generally assigns less value to them as old evaluations have limited usefulness to the court in determining the issues of current competency and guardianship. This is especially true in cases in which the respondent's alleged incompetency is based upon mental illness or a brain injury and his or her condition has either improved or deteriorated over time. Similarly, although dementia is progressive, an older evaluation report may not pinpoint the respondent's condition at or near the time of the hearing; old reports are also not likely to document a respondent's recent improvement due to medication or other treatment. Even in cases in which past testing has determined that a person functions in the severe and profound range of mental retardation, recent testing is useful to the court. These cases may come before the court at the initial hearing to determine competency and select a guardian, or at a hearing to replace a guardian. In either of these instances, the court relies upon a recent evaluation to determine whether the parent/caregiver/applicant has been providing appropriate care and accessing needed services for the respondent and is, therefore, an appropriate guardian. This information assists the court in selecting the appropriate guardian.

Beyond the general purpose of evaluations in competency cases, the court sometimes needs specific information from the evaluation in that particular case. It is most helpful to the court when the evaluation is not based upon a "cookie-cutter" approach. The evaluator should determine, if possible, the basis for the specific allegations of the respondent's alleged incapacity in the case. To the extent allowed by state law and court procedure, the evaluator should review the initial pleadings before selecting the tests to be administered to the respondent. For example, in a case involving a college professor's or other professional's mental illness, an intelligence test may not be helpful to the court. However, if the initial pleadings simply state that the basis of alleged incompetency is "mental retardation," an intelligence test is a necessity, as the degree of impairment will be the issue. In dementia cases, the court may benefit from the results of memory tests. With some disabilities, attendant conditions may affect capacity and should be considered when selecting tests for the respondent's evaluation. The following examples illustrate this: respondents with mild or moderate mental retardation may have problems with anxiety that may interfere with their functioning; some respondents with autism have obsessive-compulsive traits that impact their ability to make decisions and function effectively; and some respondents with mental illness have high levels of suspicion and paranoia that may affect the ultimate issue of competence. In such cases, the court will benefit from an evaluation that has been tailored to the individual respondent.

The court will also benefit from knowing the respondent's limitations to the testing, and how those limitations have affected the validity of the results. Limitations may include the respondent's degree of literacy, fatigue, and anxiety; reaction to the evaluation setting; and the effect of medications on the respondent's functioning at the time of testing. In addition, suspicion and paranoia may make the respondent's participation in the testing problematic. It is frustrating for the court to review the evaluation of a respondent with these types of limitations without being able to determine if the limitations have rendered the results invalid. An evaluation of a respondent with any type of limitation, including limitations previously addressed in this chapter, without the evaluator's acknowledgment of the respondent's limitations and explanation of how the tests were administered, challenges the court to determine whether the evaluation results are valid. For the evaluation to have maximum usefulness for the court, the evaluator should advise the court of any limitations the evaluator discovered, report how the tests were administered to accommodate those limitations, and explain what effect, if any, the limitations had on the test's validity.

It may also be helpful for the court to receive information in the evaluation report regarding the respondent's socioeconomic status as well as history in the areas of criminal involvement, housing, family affiliation, employment, academics, and social relationships. Medical and mental health histories are also helpful. Events in the respondent's history such as multiple divorces, military history, and traumatic past episodes round out the test results. Frequently the initial pleadings do not contain any of that helpful information. Having as complete a picture of the respondent as possible assists the court in weighing important known factors in order to facilitate a holistic view of the respondent.

Equally important to the court in obtaining an understanding of the respondent is to determine if ethnic or cultural factors affect either the respondent's test results or ability to function independently. In some cultures, providing personal information to a stranger, a person of the opposite sex, or a person of a different religion or ethnic group is done with great reluctance, if at all. Respondents holding such beliefs may appear guarded and uncooperative, but not necessarily because of mental illness or other defects. Similarly, in some cultures a senior family member or community leader is responsible for speaking to authority figures on behalf of others in the group. For a respondent, refusing to share information with the evaluator may not be a sign of incapacity or inability to handle his or her own affairs, but of cultural differences. Respondents from countries in which fewer civil liberties are protected may not understand the nature of court proceedings that triggered the evaluation and be reluctant or fearful to participate fully in the evaluation. Although these factors may challenge an evaluator's ability to produce a thorough and accurate evaluation of the respondent's capacity, both the court and evaluator should use patient inquiry and explanation of the process in an effort to minimize or alleviate these problems.

Another challenge for the evaluator is to ensure that the respondent's uniqueness is considered in order to determine the proper weight to assign the respondent's long-held personal beliefs. Some respondents have acquired unique beliefs through family or community influence. These beliefs are not so much delusional as simply inaccurate or culturally different. Some people, for example, do not believe in the legitimacy of paper currency or believe they can communicate with deceased relatives through séances. Although these beliefs may seem odd or idiosyncratic to a majority of the population, they do not rise to the level of psychosis. The authors are aware of a case in which an elderly respondent "put weeds" on another person with whom she had recently argued. In the part of the United States in which she grew up, it was a common belief in her community that one could put a curse on another person by empowering dried vegetation with an incantation. The respondent's actions, although odd to the court and all other parties to the case, were not abnormal for her and many of her generation from her community of origin. In that respondent's case, the act of putting weeds on her neighbor was merely an act rooted in cultural belief and/or religion, and not an act generated by a delusional thought process.

The evaluator may also assist the court by including a report of the respondent's views. For example, the evaluator should include the respondent's own account of the court proceeding and the reason for the evaluation as well as his or her description of family conflict, current assets, medical problems, current mood, sleep or appetite disturbances, suicidal/homicidal ideations, energy level, medical and psychiatric history, past and present medications, alcohol and drug use, education, and past and present employment. In cases in which the respondent has executed a power of attorney, the court benefits from the evaluator's inclusion of the respondent's account of when the document was executed, who was present when the document was executed, and the circumstances surrounding the execution. The authors are aware of a case in which an exploiter, alleging that the respondent had a long history of significant dementia, petitioned the court for appointment as guardian of the respondent's estate. Testimony revealed that the exploiter had arranged for the respondent to execute a power of attorney only a few weeks prior to the initiation of the incompetency proceeding. The respondent had no memory of executing the power of attorney.

The evaluation report should indicate whether the respondent canceled testing appointments prior to the testing session and/or appeared confused about the evaluation appointment day and time. Adding to the list of useful information is inclusion of the evaluator's observations about the respondent's memory, language expression, and comprehension; orientation as to person, place, and time; and displays of odd behavior, hallucinations, or delusions. Where the respondent admits to hallucinations, the evaluation should include the degree to which the respondent is impaired as a result of the hallucinations.

The court benefits from any observations and insights that the evaluator has gleaned from the session or sessions with the respondent. The evaluator's visual observations can be helpful. For example, whether the respondent is disheveled or neat, appropriately or inappropriately dressed for the season, and well groomed or lacking adequate hygiene are all helpful observations. It is important for the evaluator to ascertain, if possible, the real reason for the described observation. For example, ill-fitting clothes may be a sign of recent intentional weight loss and not necessarily a manifestation of self-neglect or another sinister condition. It may be helpful to the court for the evaluator to note clothing with logos or slogans, although some clothing may be simply the result of personal inclinations or a gift giver's poor gift selection. Although the Nike "swoosh" and sports team logos are ubiquitous among young men and are usually without relevance, a black tee-shirt with a depiction of a human skull and the words "Kill Them All And Let God Sort Them Out," as recently seen by one of the authors, is worth noting in the evaluation report. Slogans on clothing that defy legitimate authority, communicate strange opinions, or describe or advocate dangerous or illegal behavior may give some insight into the wearer's thought process or personality.

It is important to note the identity of the person who accompanied the respondent to the evaluation session. In an incompetency case in which exploitation of a disabled respondent is alleged, the exploiter may accompany the respondent to the evaluation. Although the evaluator may have read in the initial pleading that exploitation is alleged, the evaluator may not know the identity of the person accused of the exploitation. Similarly, when the identity of the alleged exploiter is not apparent of the face of the pleadings, it may assist the court to learn in the evaluation report that the alleged exploiter accompanied the respondent to the evaluation session. It may also be helpful to the court to learn from the evaluation report the identity of any person who accompanied or attempted to accompany the respondent into the testing room or answered or attempted to answer questions for the respondent. However, in some cases, answers from a person accompanying the respondent may be necessary. For example, when a respondent does not have the ability to answer questions, it may be necessary for the evaluator to obtain information from the person accompanying the respondent. When that occurs, the evaluation report should reflect that information. Another situation in which a collateral source may appropriately answer questions on behalf of the respondent in the testing process is when a young parent-dependent respondent who lacks self-confidence prefers for the parent to answer on his or her behalf. For example, it is not uncommon for a young adult with mental retardation to exhibit dependence and shyness in an unfamiliar situation and rely on parents to speak on his or her behalf. It is helpful to the court to have that information included in the evaluation report.

Once the background and individuality of the respondent are set out in the evaluation report, the court can address the issue of whether the person's condition rises to the level of the legal definition of incompetence. At this stage, the court needs the information in the evaluation report to determine whether the respondent can remember, understand directions, communicate, reason, solve problems, and weigh the risks and benefits of his or her choices. If the respondent cannot fully function in some way, the court needs assistance from the evaluator to determine how this affects the respondent's ability to make rational decisions and adequately carry them out. For this determination the court relies on testimony, past records of various kinds, and the court-ordered evaluation.

The most important feature of the evaluation for the court at this stage is that it be based on functional capacities. The decision the court must make does not rest on a diagnosis; the decision rests on how the respondent functions with that diagnosis. For example, a respondent, although delusional, may still go to work every day, pay bills, obtain appropriate medical treatment, practice good hygiene, and otherwise successfully tend to activities of daily living. The resulting court decision in a case with these factors may well be that the delusional respondent is adequately handling his or her own affairs and is not incompetent. The court looks to the evaluator to document how the respondent's impairment results in a lack of adequate functioning, either by the respondent's inability to make important decisions or the inability to carry them out.

Although the court does not determine competency based upon a diagnosis alone, the court does rely upon the evaluator for a diagnosis. The diagnosis is the context for understanding the respondent's impairment, but the court relies upon the evaluator to go beyond the diagnosis and inform the court how this condition results in a respondent's lack of capacity. For example, the result of a respondent's mental retardation may affect the respondent's ability to read and/or understand how to count or manage money. Similarly, a respondent's dementia may result in a degree of memory loss that renders the respondent's decision-making ability impaired, financial understanding diminished, and safety awareness compromised. The delusions of a respondent with mental illness may impair his or her understanding of the need for medical care, appropriate residential choice, and adequate nutrition. The court relies upon the evaluator to test for and relay this type of functional information.

Differences of opinion exist as to whether the evaluation should include an opinion on the ultimate issue of whether the respondent is incompetent. Those who believe that the evaluator should include this opinion in the report argue that the purpose of the report is to advise the court of the evaluator's expert opinion, which results from the evaluator's testing, interviewing, and record review. To provide a report without reaching a conclusion leaves the court without the guidance needed to make a decision.

Those who oppose including such ultimate issue opinions in the report typically raise three objections. First, incompetency is a legal, not psychological or medical conclusion and must be made by the court after considering the report along with other documentary and testamentary evidence at the hearing. If the evaluator were to testify in person at the hearing, a court could sustain an objection to testimony on the ultimate issue and, therefore, the same opinion should not be allowed when put in writing. Second, there is no guarantee that the evaluator understands the legal definition of incompetency or is using that term in the same manner that the court does. Finally, in situations in which a written report is provided without the live testimony of the evaluator, the evaluator will not have had the opportunity to hear testimony at the hearing and, given the live testimony, change his or her opinion based upon information not available at the time the evaluation was performed.

Ultimately, the decision as to whether the evaluation should include this opinion rests with the court. Some courts may not only want, but expect, the evaluator's opinion. Other courts do not want to read a conclusion on the ultimate issue. The authors often review reports that include the evaluator's opinion as to competency and sometimes as to the identity of the most appropriate guardian. We do not oppose these opinions in reports because, regardless of the evaluator's stated opinion on the ultimate issue, we make our own decisions based upon the totality of the evidence presented at the hearing and the relevant statutory standard. Courts should be careful to evaluate the report for what it offers, and not blindly follow any conclusions beyond the purview of the evaluator.

GUARDIANSHIP AND RESTORATION ISSUES

Most states today provide for "limited" or "partial" guardianship (American Association of Retired Persons Policy Institute: Limited guardianship of the person). Some states that do not specifically provide for this type of guardianship have statutory policy statements requiring guardians to encourage the ward's development of maximum self-reliance and independence. The idea of limited guardianship is a recent development, based upon the belief that only those rights that the ward cannot exercise should be removed and placed in the hands of a guardian. The concept of incompetency has evolved from a view that a person is either competent or not (i.e., an all-or-nothing judgment) to a view in which incompetency is a spectrum in which some wards can retain some rights and decisions when they have adequate capacity to exercise those rights and make those decisions. To determine whether a guardianship should be limited, the court must first determine that although the respondent is in fact incompetent, he or she remains competent in some matters and should retain the right to engage in those matters without control of the guardian. The retained rights can be an entire classification of rights, such as the right to make residential or vocational decisions, or it can be a portion of a right, such as the right to handle a certain amount of money or to obtain a residence of the ward's own choosing in a particular city.

To create a limited guardianship, a court must enter a specific order or judgment that states with specificity which rights and decisions the ward retains or which rights and decisions are assigned to the guardian. To do this, the court needs detailed information as to the specific abilities of the ward. These cases often require more detailed information than in evaluations in all-or-nothing cases. The court must determine issues such as the respondent's ability to live alone, count and handle money, understand what is read, and comprehend the nature of his or her impairment as it relates to employment.

Another factor for the court to consider is the effect that the guardianship will have on the ward's physical and emotional health. An elderly ward who has lived an independent life may be emotionally distraught over an adjudication of incompetence and loss of the right to make independent decisions regarding housing, medical, and financial matters. The negative impact of an adjudication of incompetence can be minimized for the ward by a limited guardianship in which the ward retains the right, for example, to manage spending money of a certain amount and control any other matter he or she has the capacity to control.

Once a person is adjudicated incompetent and a guardian is appointed, the court may at some time thereafter restore the person to competency, thus ending the guardianship. Restoration occurs when the ward's condition has improved to the extent that his or her rights can be restored. Restoration of competency most often occurs in cases in which the ward has sustained a brain injury or suffered the effects of mental illness. Restoration can, however, occur in other situations. For example, restoration may be appropriate when an immature young ward with mild mental retardation subsequently matures and begins to make good decisions and manage his or her own affairs independently. When restoration is the issue before the court, a recent evaluation is particularly valuable. The court looks to the evaluator for an opinion, based upon the applicable jurisdictional legal standard, as to whether the ward now has the requisite capacity to handle his or her own affairs. To illustrate, the authors are aware of a case in which the ward petitioning for restoration admitted to having a long history of auditory hallucinations and to experiencing auditory hallucinations at the time of the restoration hearing, but presented evidence of good decision-making ability and adequate functioning notwithstanding the current hallucinations. He met the jurisdictional evidentiary burden and was restored to competency.

A ward may be restored to competency completely or partially. Complete restoration may be accomplished in one court setting or over time with several court settings. In the latter cases, the court fashions a limited guardianship at each setting to accommodate the ward's newly acquired areas of capacity. Following this latter path, the court may eventually restore the ward to complete competency over time. The court may rely upon an evaluator's report for guidance at each step of the way, although it is unlikely that a full evaluation is needed at each step unless rights are restored over a long period of time.

The most problematic competency cases involve respondents with chronic mental illness who cycle between periods of incompetency and competency. These respondents often have a history of multiple hospitalizations for mental illness followed by periods of relative stability. Their cycling sometimes involves periods of medication compliance followed by periods of noncompliance; cycling may also involve periodic instability notwithstanding complete medication and treatment compliance. For other respondents, external factors influence their condition. When wards that fall in this category come before the court seeking restoration, they are usually at their highest level of functioning. The court often finds that the stability of these wards is due to medication and therapy compliance, stable living arrangements, and/or stability within their family unit. Notwithstanding the positive factors presented to the court, the respondent's history of cycling in and out of stability remains problematic for the court. When the ward has a lengthy history of recurring decompensation, a premature restoration may cause the respondent more harm than good. In these situations, it is not uncommon for the ward's family members to appear at the restoration proceeding and testify that they have witnessed the ward's repeated cycling, doubt the ward's ability to remain competent for an extended period of time, and vigorously oppose restoration of rights. In these cases a good solution may be a limited guardianship. The court may restore rights periodically as the ward demonstrates over time that treatment is effective and that he or she has the willingness and ability to maintain treatment compliance. If the ward fails to remain compliant and his or her illness exacerbates, full guardianship can be reinstated. The court may benefit from an evaluation in which the evaluator identifies the ward's mental illness, explains how compliance with treatment affects the ward's ability to function independently, and suggests a specific incremental plan for partial or complete restoration that the court can follow.

Once the court has determined that a person lacks capacity to handle his or her own affairs and, therefore, needs a guardian, the court must decide who the guardian will be. This decision may be as, if not more, difficult than the decision as to the respondent's competence. In some cases the identity of the best available option for appointment is obvious. However, when the best available option is not easily identified, the court may look to the evaluator to evaluate both the respondent's unique needs and the dynamics of the respondent's family. The evaluator can, to the extent allowed by jurisdictional state law and court practice, interview the respondent's family members and other interested persons. In situations in which significant conflict is present within the family, the evaluator can often uncover tension among family members without much prodding. It is not uncommon in those cases for a family member to eagerly tell his or her side of the story and attempt to recruit the evaluator's, and ultimately the court's, support. In cases of family conflict, the court must decide whether any family member can effectively serve as guardian, or if the best option for appointment is a neutral individual or agency. In any case, the court must base the appointment on the best interest of the respondent and make an appropriate appointment without concern for resulting hurt feelings, argument, and tension among family members. However, if it appears to the evaluator that resulting family tension from a particular appointment is likely to negatively impact the respondent over time, the court benefits from the inclusion of that assessment in the evaluation report. It is helpful to the court when the evaluation report includes the identities of the individuals who were interviewed, the recommended guardian, and the basis for the recommendation. The recommendation can be specific, as in "Billy's mother should serve," or more generic, as in "one of Billy's siblings should serve." Some state statutes set forth a specific hierarchy of preference for selection of a guardian. For example, the hierarchy can begin with preference for a close family member, followed by a list of possibilities in decreasing familial closeness to the respondent. The latter category may include a distant family member, a friend, and a disinterested public agency. Where the state statute includes a hierarchy for appointment, the evaluator should be aware of the available options and list recommendations for appointment according to statutory direction.

A final recommendation that is helpful to the court, guardian *ad litem*/visitor/attorney, and possibly the respondent, is whether the respondent should attend the incompetency hearing. Attendance is a legal, not psychological or medical decision. Most state statutes allow the absence of a respondent from court for reasons such as "good cause," "serious risk of harm," or "threat to health" (American Bar Association Commission on Law and Aging: Conduct and findings of guardianship proceedings). The court will not be aware of any reason to excuse attendance unless the issue is raised by some party to the case. Usually this will be the guardian *ad litem*/visitor/attorney. Although it may appear to violate fairness standards for an individual to be absent from a court proceeding in which the court determines retention or deprivation of rights, it is sometimes in the respondent's best interest to be absent. For example, a depressed or frail elderly woman with advanced dementia who does not understand the nature of the proceeding and is conclusively incompetent may have nothing to gain from being brought to court simply to hear her children relate her history of cognitive decline and recite a litany of activities in which she can no longer participate. Similarly, an 18-year-old girl with mental retardation who cannot, in the opinion of her attorney, handle her own affairs and wants to have her parents appointed guardian may not benefit by being present in court to hear her parents outline her cognitive deficiencies. To determine whether a respondent must attend the court proceeding, the court weighs the respondent's legal civil right to be present against a compassionate consideration for the respondent's potential health risks attendant in his or her presence. The evaluator can assist the court in this analysis by providing insight into the benefit of the respondent's presence versus the risk to the respondent's emotional and physical health.

CONCLUSIONS

The statutory recognition of the rights of persons who are alleged to be incompetent has placed increased importance for accurate, understandable, and relevant competency evaluations. As the ultimate consumer of these reports, a court needs a report that is understandable to the trier of fact who is not a trained mental health professional, relevant to the issues of the particular case, customized to the individual being evaluated, and properly supported by testing and background information. This information can assist the court in making the difficult decisions the court often encounters in these cases. Without a thorough evaluation that documents the respondent's cognitive and adaptive functioning and a neutral evaluator's clinical impressions and recommendations, it may be impossible for the court to have a holistic view of the incompetency matter. The evaluator has a unique and privileged role in this important judicial process.

References

American Association of Retired Persons Public Policy Institute: Limited guardianship of the person (as of statutory revisions December 31, 2008). Retrieved from www.abanet.org/aging/legislativeupdates/pdfs/chart_limited.pdf.

American Bar Association Commission on Guardianship and Aging. Capacity definition and initiation of guardianship proceedings (as of statutory provisions December 31, 2009). Retrieved from http://new.abanet.org/aging/PublicDocuments/chart_cap_initiation_08_10.pdf.

American Bar Association Commission on Guardianship and Aging. Conduct and findings of guardianship proceedings (as of statutory provisions December 31, 2009). Retrieved from http://new.abanet.org/aging/PublicDocuments/chart_conduct_08_10.pdf.

American Bar Association Commission on Law and Aging. Representation and investigation in guardianship proceedings (as of statutory revisions December 31, 2009). Retrieved from http://new.abanet.org/aging/PublicDocuments/chart_rep_invest_08_10.pdf.

Kentucky Revised Statutes 387.570.1.

New Hampshire Revised Statutes 464-A: 8.

Wyoming Statutes 3–2-104 (a).

15

Looking Ahead: Directions for Future Research in Civil Capacities

GEORGE J. DEMAKIS

Psychologists' role in capacity evaluations is likely to continue, if not grow, with the aging of our society and our increasing comfort in the legal area. This volume was written to improve our role in the evaluation of civil capacity, and, in my view, the various chapters go a long way toward doing that. Even so, there is still room for improvements in research and practice. The purpose of this final chapter is to provide a broad roadmap for future research in various aspects of civil capacity and competency evaluations.

FUTURE DIRECTIONS IN CIVIL CAPACITY RESEARCH

Practice patterns: In my Introduction (Chapter 1), I detailed what little we know about how neuropsychologists conduct capacity evaluations. These "on-the-ground" data are useful, but are quite limited and are based only on self-report. An exception is work by Moye et al. (2007) in which evaluations written for guardianship in three states were evaluated, but some of these were completed by nonpsychologists and several of the assessed variables were fairly crude and not particularly illustrative (e.g., they assessed only whether functional abilities were included and not the actual measures used). Cleary, more research is needed in this area. For each of the various capacities described in this volume, it would be beneficial to know how psychologists are actually conducting these evaluations. What psychological tests are used, for instance, to evaluate financial decision making? On what sources of evidence do psychologists subsequently form their opinion? Once formed, do these opinions address the ultimate issue in the report? How do psychologists use relevant legal statutes and state competency statutes to guide their report and ultimate opinion? Of course, there are many more unanswered questions; these demonstrate only the paucity of extant information and, without such data, it is difficult to offer recommendations for improving psychological report-writing and consulting. Clearly there exist both practical and conceptual issues to address, but other areas of forensic psychology have done such work. For example, Christy, Douglas, Otto, and Petrila (2004) evaluated the characteristics of mental health professionals' (mostly psychologists) reports of juveniles evaluated for competency to proceed to trial, whereas Borum and Grisso (1995) surveyed forensic psychologists and psychiatrists to determine which tests they used and the perceived importance of various domains of testing (e.g., objective personality testing) in competency to stand trial and criminal responsibility evaluations. This work has been useful to practitioners.

Psychological tests: Although much of the second part of this volume discusses tests used to evaluate various capacities, more empirical work in this area would be of value. In particular, more robust and comprehensive psychometric data (i.e., reliability and validity) would likely enhance practice, as would empirical comparisons of the various capacity tests. One recent study by Baird, Solcz, Gale-Ross, and Blake (2009), for instance, examined the relationships between the Hopemont Capacity Assessment Instrument, Independent Living Scales, and several other measures in a sample of healthy older adults. The two former measures were moderately correlated with one another, but only the Hopemont was correlated with measures of literacy skills (e.g., Wechsler Test of Adult Reading). Another study found that tests of medical decision making (e.g., MacArthur Competency Assessment Tool—Treatment and Capacity to Consent to Treatment Interview) evidenced fair to good agreement for overall treatment decision-making capacity and for treatment understanding in mild to moderate dementia (Gurrera, Karel, Azar, & Moye, 2007). There was poor agreement for treatment appreciation, reasoning, and expression of a choice. These comparative studies can point to inconsistencies between constructs or models of various types of capacity and, ideally, stimulate enhanced empirical and conceptual work. Moving beyond the relationships between the various instruments, future work that assesses which test best predicts the ultimate legal ruling would also be ideal. Of course, this is not to say that other aspects of the evaluation are not useful in understanding a particular capacity—they are—but cognitive testing and functional testing remain a core aspect of many evaluations and are unique tools that neuropsychologists bring to these evaluations.

How the trier of fact uses psychological evaluations: The psychological report or testimony is ultimately designed to assist the trier of fact or legal decision maker about a civil capacity issue. Yet relatively little is known about how these legal professionals regard, use, and integrate psychological data into their decisions. For instance, in deciding a case about testamentary capacity, how do they weigh psychological testing of memory impairment as compared to, for instance, collateral reports or behavioral observations of these same deficits? In what sorts of cases do they believe that testing improves their decision making? Although a somewhat controversial issue in forensic psychology circles, what do they think about psychologists offering opinions about the ultimate issue? Examination of these and other similar questions is certainly not simple, but in my view, would improve psychological practice. In the criminal realm, for instance, Ackerson, Brodsky, and Zapf (2005) identified the functional abilities that judges considered important for making decisions about whether a defendant was competent to be executed and Spar, Hankin, and Stodden (1995) evaluated probate judges' opinions on mental capacity and susceptibility to undue influence. This research has likely improved both legal and psychological practice.

Multicultural considerations: Relatively little attention has been devoted to how ethnic or racial differences might affect capacity issues as well as aspects of guardianship. This is problematic given the increasing diversity of American society—Vincent and Velkoff's (2010) demographic research demonstrates that this is true even for older adults—and the important ways in which culture influences psychological constructs that may be relevant for capacity evaluations. There may be, for instance, differences on cognitive test performance, behavioral presentation during an interview, styles of interacting with healthcare providers, treatment adherence, and even end-of-life decision making and preferences. Although these potential differences are too vast to be considered for this chapter, two issues are particularly relevant for capacity assessments. First, if there are racial differences in capacity test performance these should be, at minimum, considered in data interpretation and, ideally, controlled for. If certain racial or ethnic groups perform below norms that are typically entirely or mostly developed on whites, a classification of an individual's performance as impaired may occur. This inappropriate classification may be used to assert that the individual has experienced a decline from premorbid levels of functioning and thus possibly be used to diagnose dementia erroneously (see Heaton, Taylor, & Manly, 2003). Instead, the individual may be performing at premorbid levels and has not experienced a drop in cognitive or adaptive functioning. Although research has not yet examined whether there are racial differences on capacity instruments, there are some differences on neuropsychological measures frequently used in capacity assessments that are controlled (see, for example, Heaton, Miller, Taylor, & Grant, 2004).

Second, as various capacity evaluations require interviewing and working with families and making determinations about the care a family can provide, accounting for cultural differences is important. African-American families, for instance, as compared to white families, are more likely to be matriarchal, to share or swap resources, and to exist within a network of community, extended family, and friends (see Aulette, 2007, pp. 104–134). A strong spiritual orientation may be present with close ties to a local church that can provide various sources of support for a family. Latino families emphasize the group rather than the individual and stress family unity, welfare, and honor; they are also more likely to be deal with immigration and acculturation-related stressors (Garica-Preto, 2005). Consideration of these factors is a must to best understand these families and the types of resources they may be able to provide. In my own clinical work, I have evaluated several African-Americans for whom the proposed guardian was not an immediate family member, but a distant family member or friend; other family members who were more closely related agreed to these arrangements as they believed that these individuals were best able to serve as guardian. Moreover, in reflecting on the chapters of this volume, it is noteworthy that the importance of attending to and sensitively interpreting such factors is most clearly articulated by the legal decision makers (see Chapter 14). Perhaps this reflects their experience in working with diverse respondents and families, and the general paucity of psychological research on cultural issues and capacity and guardianship. Overall, culture matters, and it affects family structure, nature and types of relationships, social support, as well as an examinee's goals, preferences, and values in decision making.

Testamentary capacity: With the aging of the United States and the increase in various forms of blended families, an increase in will disputes is likely. Chapter 5 details legal rulings in this area, characteristics of examinees referred for this type of evaluation, and information to guide psychological assessment in this area. This information should be helpful to improve practice, but it is notable that a model of testamentary capacity has yet to be developed from either a psychological or neuropsychological perspective. Perhaps as a result of this, we also know very little empirically about the cognitive correlates of will making and will revising. It is also likely that issues of testamentary capacity are less likely to arise than other capacity issues in the course of clinical practice. Complicating the picture is that some of these evaluations may be done retrospectively when, for instance, a decedent's change of his or her will is challenged. When such cases are referred to a psychologist, the capacity opinion is formed based on available medical records, testing before or at the end of a change in will (if available), and perhaps collateral interviews. In general, although research in this area does present unique challenges it also seems to lag behind the considerable conceptual and empirical work done, for instance, on driving and financial and medical decision making.

Family conflict and undue influence: Relatively little research has been done from a psychological perspective on families in conflict surrounding a capacity issue or when undue influence may be present. Peisah, Brodaty, and Quadrio's (2006) article is an exception as they described families in conflict with an older adult with dementia. In their series of 50 cases before a Guardianship Tribunal in Australia, they found that conflict occurred most often between siblings of an older adult with mild to moderate dementia. In the majority of sibling conflicts, several siblings were in alliance against one "black sheep" sibling who had typically assumed primarily caretaking responsibility and who, in about half of the cases, suffered from a mental illness. To my knowledge, this is the only work in this area and more work would be welcome, particularly research that could provide a richer understanding of the dynamics between the older adult and his or her adult children, as well as between the adult children. In terms of undue influence or exploitation, some of the work in this area comes from a nursing/social work perspective and is pragmatic, dealing with recognition and intervention strategies (Quinn, 2002), whereas there has also been some conceptual work from a psychiatric perspective (Shulman, Cohen, Kirsh, Hull, & Champine, 2007). Related conceptual work has detailed indicia for voluntarism (Roberts, 2002), a core concept in informed consent, but one that can be broadly applied to capacity issues that is violated when an individual is unduly coerced or influenced to make decisions against personal values or prior stated wishes (e.g., a will). Empirical psychological work in this area would be a valuable addition. For instance, what is the cognitive and psychological functioning of those who have been exploited? Do certain cognitive deficits make individuals particularly vulnerable? It might be supposed that executive processing deficits would be most problematic, but this remains an empirical question and might be difficult to tease out in an individual with broader dementia-related deficits. In terms of exploitation, a better understand of the mechanisms by which influence is exerted would be beneficial. In addition to obvious financial indicia of exploitation (e.g., money transfers), are their particular behavioral manifestations of it, such as increasing isolation from other family members, a high level of identification with the exploiter, and/or other changes in psychological functioning? Because of the complexity of the dyad and even family dynamics in these cases, input from researchers with expertise in clinical psychology and family systems would likely be of value.

CONCLUSIONS

Civil capacity evaluations, in whatever form, are already likely to be a part of many neuropsychologists' practices and they are likely to increase with the aging of our society. Although there clearly have been societal advances in this work (e.g., many states reformed competency and guardianship statutes through the 1980s and 1990s), there have also been crucial conceptual, empirical, and psychometric developments from psychology. With further developments in the areas described above, psychological practice could be further improved and, ideally, better serve the examinees we evaluate and the legal professionals we consult and to whom we provide feedback.

References

Ackerson, K. S., Brodsky, S. L., & Zapf, P. A. (2005). Judges' and psychologists' assessments of legal and clinical factors in competence for execution. *Psychology, Public Policy, and Law, 11*, 164–193.

Aulette, J. R. (2007). *Changing American families* (2nd ed.). Boston: Pearson.

Baird, A. D., Solcz, S. L., Gale-Ross, R., & Blake, T. M. (2009). Older adults and capacity-related assessment: Promise and caution. *Experimental Aging Research, 35*, 297–316.

Borum, R., & Girsso, T. (1995). Psychological test use in criminal forensic evaluations. *Professional Psychology: Research and Practice, 26*, 465–473.

Christy, A., Douglas, K. S., Otto, R. K., & Petrila, J. (2004). Juveniles evaluated incompetent to proceed: Characteristics and quality of mental health professionals' evaluations. *Professional Psychology: Research and Practice, 35*, 380–388.

Garcia-Preto, N. (2005). Latino families: An overview. In M. McGoldrick, J. Giordano, & N. Garcia-Preto (Eds.), *Ethnicity and family therapy* (3rd ed.) (pp. 153–165). New York: Guilford.

Gurrera, R. J., Karel, M. J., Azar, A. R., & Moye, J. (2007). Agreement between instruments for rating treatment decisional capacity. *American Journal of Geriatric Psychiatry, 15*, 168–173.

Heaton, R. K., Miller, S. W., Taylor, M. J., & Grant, I. (2004). *Revised comprehensive norms for an Expanded Halstead-Reitan battery: Demographically adjusted neuropsychological norms for African American and Caucasian adults*. Lutz, FL. Psychological Assessment Resources.

Heaton, R. K., Taylor, M. J., & Manly, J. (2003). Demographic effects and use of demographically corrected norms with the WAIS-III and WMS-III. In D. S. Tulsky, G. J. Chelune, R. J. Ivnik, A. Prifitera, D. H. Saklofske, R. K. Heaton, R. Bornstein, & M. F. Ledbetter (Eds.), *Clinical interpretation of the WAIS-III and WMS-III* (pp. 181–210). San Diego, CA: Academic Press.

Moye, J., Wood, E., Edelstein, B., Wood, S., Bower, E. H., Harrison, J. A., & Armesto, J. C. (2007). Statutory reform is associated with improved court practice: Results of a tri-state comparison. *Behavioral Sciences and the Law, 25*, 425–426.

Peisah, C., Brodaty, H., & Quadrio, C. (2006). Family conflict in dementia: Prodigal sons and black sheep. *International Journal of Geriatric Psychiatry, 21*, 485–492.

Quinn, M. J. (2002). Undue influence and elder abuse: Recognition and intervention strategies. *Geriatric Nursing, 23*, 11–16.

Roberts, L. W. (2002). Informed consent and the capacity for voluntarism. *American Journal of Psychiatry, 159*, 705–712.

Shulman, D. I., Cohen, C. A., Dirsh, F. C., Hull, I. M., & Champine, P. R. (2007). Assessment of testamentary capacity and vulnerability to undue influence. *American Journal of Psychiatry, 14*, 722–727.

Spar, J. F., Hankin, M., & Stodden, A. B. (1995). Assessing mental capacity and susceptibility to undue influence. *Behavioral Sciences and the Law, 13*, 394–403.

Vincent, G. K., & Velkoff, V. A. (May, 2010). The older population in the United States: 2010 to 2050. Population estimates and projections. *Current Population Reports*. Washington, D.C.: Bureau of the Census.

Index

Note: Page numbers followed by "*f*" and "*t*" denote figures and tables, respectively.

The manufacturer's authorised representative in the EU for product
safety is Oxford University Press España S.A. of El Parque Empresarial
San Fernando de Henares, Avenida de Castilla, 2 - 28830 Madrid
(www.oup.es/en or product.safety@oup.com). OUP España S.A. also acts
as importer into Spain of products made by the manufacturer.
Printed and bound by CPI Group (UK) Ltd, Croydon, CR0 4YY
14/09/2026
02216286-0013